Optical Coherence Tomography

ESASO Course Series

Vol. 4

Series Editor

F. Bandello Milan
B. Corcóstegui Barcelona

Optical Coherence Tomography

Volume Editors

Gabriel Coscas Créteil/Paris
Anat Loewenstein Tel Aviv
Francesco Bandello Milan

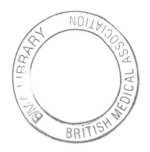

137 figures, 97 in color, and 9 tables, 2014

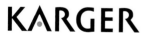

Basel · Freiburg · Paris · London · New York · Chennai · New Delhi ·
Bangkok · Beijing · Shanghai · Tokyo · Kuala Lumpur · Singapore · Sydney

Gabriel Coscas
Department of Ophthalmology
University of Paris Est Créteil
Centre Hospitalier Intercommunal de Créteil
40, avenue de Verdun
FR–94010 Créteil (France)

Anat Loewenstein
Tel Aviv Medical Center
Department of Ophthalmology
6 Weizmann Street
IL–64239 Tel Aviv (Israel)

Francesco Bandello
Department of Ophthalmology
Vita-Salute University
San Raffaele Scientific Institute
IT–20132 Milan (Italy)

Library of Congress Cataloging-in-Publication Data

Optical coherence tomography (Coscas)
  Optical coherence tomography / volume editors Gabriel Coscas, Anat
Loewenstein, Francesco Bandello.
     p. ; cm. -- (ESASO course series, ISSN 1664-882X ; vol. 4)
  Includes bibliographical references and index.
  ISBN 978-3-318-02563-7 (hard cover : alk. paper) -- ISBN 978-3-318-02564-4
(electronic)
  I. Coscas, Gabriel, editor of compilation. II. Loewenstein, Anat, editor
of compilation. III. Bandello, F. (Francesco), editor of compilation. IV.
Title. V. Series: ESASO course series ; v. 4. 1664-882X.
  [DNLM: 1. Tomography, Optical Coherence. WN 206]
  RC78.7.T6
  616.07'57--dc23
                                      2013045766

Bibliographic Indices. This publication is listed in bibliographic services, including Current Contents®.

© Copyright 2014 by S. Karger AG, P.O. Box, CH–4009 Basel (Switzerland)
www.karger.com
Printed in Germany on acid-free and non-aging paper (ISO 9706) by Kraft Druck, Ettlingen
ISSN 1664–882X
e-ISSN 1664–8838
ISBN 978–3–318–02563–7
eISBN 978–3–318–02564–4

Contents

List of Contributors

Francesco Bandello
Department of Ophthalmology
Vita-Salute University
San Raffaele Scientific Institute
Via Olgettina 60
IT–20132 Milan (Italy)
E-Mail Bandello.francesco@hsr.it

Maurizio Battaglia Parodi
Department of Ophthalmology
Vita-Salute University
San Raffaele Scientific Institute
Via Olgettina 60
IT–20132 Milan (Italy)
E-Mail battagliaparodi.maurizio@hsr.it

Gianluigi Bolognesi
Department of Ophthalmology
Vita-Salute University
San Raffaele Scientific Institute
Via Olgettina 60
IT–20132 Milan (Italy)
E-Mail bolognesi.gianluigi@hsr.it

Enrico Borrelli
Department of Ophthalmology
Vita-Salute University
San Raffaele Scientific Institute
Via Olgettina 60
IT–20132 Milan (Italy)
E-Mail e.borrelli@studenti.unisr.it

Ferdinando Bottoni
Eye Clinic, Luigi Sacco Hospital, University of Milan
Via G.B. Grassi 74
IT–20157 Milan (Italy)
E-Mail ferdinando.bottoni@fastwebnet.it

Maria Lucia Cascavilla
Department of Ophthalmology
Vita-Salute University
San Raffaele Scientific Institute
Via Olgettina 60
IT–20132 Milan (Italy)
E-Mail marialuciacascavilla@gmail.com

Matteo Giuseppe Cereda
Eye Clinic, Luigi Sacco Hospital, University of Milan
Via G.B. Grassi 74
IT–20157 Milan (Italy)
E-Mail matteo.cereda@gmail.com

Marco Codenotti
Department of Ophthalmology
Vita-Salute University
San Raffaele Scientific Institute
Via Olgettina 60
IT–20132 Milan (Italy)
E-Mail codenotti.marco@hsr.it

Florence Coscas
Department of Ophthalmology
University of Paris Est Créteil
Centre Hospitalier Intercommunal de Créteil
40, avenue de Verdun
FR–94010 Créteil (France)
E-Mail coscas.f@gmail.com

Gabriel Coscas
Department of Ophthalmology
University of Paris Est Créteil
Centre Hospitalier Intercommunal de Créteil
40, avenue de Verdun
FR–94010 Créteil (France)
E-Mail gabriel.coscas@gmail.com

Maxime Delbarre
Hôpital d'Instruction des Armées du Val de Grâce
Service d'Ophtalmologie
74, boulevard de Port Royal
FR–75005 Paris (France)
E-Mail maximedelbarre@yahoo.fr

Claudia Del Turco
Department of Ophthalmology
Vita-Salute University
San Raffaele Scientific Institute
Via Olgettina 60
IT–20132 Milan (Italy)
E-Mail delturco.claudia@hsr.it

Hussam El Chehab
Hôpital d'Instruction des Armées du Val de Grâce
Service d'Ophtalmologie
74, boulevard de Port Royal
FR–75005 Paris (France)
E-Mail elchehab_hussam@hotmail.fr

Ali Erginay
Service d'Ophtalmologie
Hôpital Lariboisière
AP-HP, Université Paris 7 – Sorbonne Paris Cité
2, rue Ambroise Paré
FR–75475 Paris Cedex 10 (France)
E-Mail ali.erginay@lrb.aphp.fr

Jean Remi Fenolland
Hôpital d'Instruction des Armées du Val de Grâce
Service d'Ophtalmologie
74, boulevard de Port Royal
FR–75005 Paris (France)
E-Mail fenolland@gmail.com

Marlène Francoz
Hôpital d'Instruction des Armées du Val de Grâce
Service d'Ophtalmologie
74, boulevard de Port Royal
FR–75005 Paris (France)
E-Mail francozmarlene@yahoo.fr

Marco Gagliardi
Department of Ophthalmology
Vita-Salute University
San Raffaele Scientific Institute
Via Olgettina 60
IT–20132 Milan (Italy)
E-Mail Gagliardi.marco@hsr.it

Anouk Georges
Department of Ophthalmology
University of Paris Est Créteil
Centre Hospitalier Intercommunal de Créteil
40, avenue de Verdun
FR–94010 Créteil (France)
E-Mail ageorges@student.ulg.ac.be

Jean-Marie Giraud
Hôpital d'Instruction des Armées Sainte Anne
Boulevard Sainte Anne
FR–83000 Toulon (France)
E-Mail jean-marie-giraud@wanadoo.fr

Dafna Goldenberg
Tel Aviv Medical Center, Department of Ophthalmology
6 Weizmann Street
IL–64239 Tel Aviv (Israel)
E-Mail dafnagoldenberg@gmail.com

Pierluigi Iacono
Department of Ophthalmology, Vita-Salute University
San Raffaele Scientific Institute
Via Olgettina 60
IT–20132 Milan (Italy)
E-Mail pierluigi.iacono@libero.it

Francesca Ingegnoli
Gaetano Pini
Piazza Cardinale Andrea Ferrari, 1
IT–20122 Milan (Italy)
E-Mail francesca.ingegnoli@unimi.it

Lorenzo Iuliano
Department of Ophthalmology
Vita-Salute University
San Raffaele Scientific Institute
Via Olgettina 60
IT–20132 Milan (Italy)
E-Mail iuliano.lorenzo@hsr.it

Adrian Koh
Eye & Retina Surgeons
Camden Medical Centre #13-03, 1 Orchard Boulevard
Singapore 248649 (Singapore)
E-Mail dradriankoh@eyeretinasurgeons.com

Jean Francois Le Rouic
Clinique Sourdille
3 place Anatole France
FR–44000 Nantes (France)
E-Mail jflerouic@gmail.com

Anat Loewenstein
Tel Aviv Medical Center
Department of Ophthalmology
6 Weizmann Street
IL–64239 Tel Aviv (Israel)
E-Mail anatlow@netvision.net.il

Bruno Lumbroso
Centro Oftalmologico Mediterraneo
Via Brofferio 7
IT–00195 Rome (Italy)
E-Mail bruno.lumbroso@gmail.com

Pascale Massin
Hôpital Lariboisière
AP-HP, Université Paris 7
Sorbonne
FR–Paris Cité (France)
E-Mail pascale.massin@lrb.aphp.fr

Franck May
Hôpital d'Instruction des Armées du Val de Grâce
Service d'Ophtalmologie
74, boulevard de Port Royal
FR–75005 Paris (France)
E-Mail ophtimum@aol.com

Elisabetta Miserocchi
Department of Ophthalmology
Vita-Salute University
San Raffaele Scientific Institute
Via Olgettina 60
IT–20132 Milan (Italy)
E-Mail miserocchi.elisabetta@hsr.it

Davide Panico
Department of Ophthalmology
Vita-Salute University
San Raffaele Scientific Institute
Via Olgettina 60
IT–20132 Milan (Italy)
E-Mail davidepaniko@libero.it

Marco Pellegrini
Eye Clinic, Luigi Sacco Hospital, University of Milan
Via G.B. Grassi 74
IT–20157 Milan (Italy)
E-Mail mar.pellegrini@gmail.com

Luisa Pierro
Department of Ophthalmology, Vita-Salute University
San Raffaele Scientific Institute
Via Olgettina 60
IT–20132 Milan (Italy)
E-Mail pierro.luisa@hsr.it

Giuseppe Querques
Department of Ophthalmology
University of Paris Est Créteil
Centre Hospitalier Intercommunal de Créteil
40, avenue de Verdun
FR–94010 Créteil (France)
E-Mail giuseppe.querques@hotmail.it

Jean-Paul Renard
Hôpital d'Instruction des Armées du Val de Grâce
Service d'Ophtalmologie
74, boulevard de Port Royal
FR–75005 Paris (France)
E-Mail pr_renard@yahoo.fr

Marco Rispoli
Centro Oftalmologico Mediterraneo
Via Brofferio 7
IT–00195 Rome (Italy)
E-Mail rispolimarco@gmail.com

Maria Cristina Savastano
Department Ophthalmology, Catholic University
Largo Agostino Gemelli 8
IT–00168 Rome (Italy)
E-Mail crisav8@virgilio.it

Roy Schwartz
Tel Aviv Medical Center, Department of Ophthalmology
6 Weizmann Street
IL–64239 Tel Aviv (Israel)
E-Mail royschwartz@gmail.com

Eric H. Souied
Department of Ophthalmology,
University of Paris Est Créteil
Centre Hospitalier Intercommunal de Créteil
40, avenue de Verdun
FR–94010 Créteil (France)
E-Mail eric.souied@chicreteil.fr

Giovanni Staurenghi
Eye Clinic, Luigi Sacco Hospital, University of Milan
Via G.B. Grassi 74
IT–20157 Milan (Italy)
E-Mail giovanni.staurenghi@unimi.it

Foreword

The innovation of no other diagnostic technique in the field of ophthalmology has had a greater impact on the management of patients than optical coherence tomography (OCT). Clinical activities, diagnostic guidelines, and multicenter trial protocols have been substantially modified by the introduction of OCT in the last 20 years.

The reasons for this success lie in the numerous advantages granted by the use of OCT compared with the other older techniques: simplicity, quickness of execution, noninvasiveness, reliability, repeatability and quantification of measures, and results which are easy to read and understand are only a few of these advantages; these explain well the planetary success obtained in only a few years.

More recently, OCT has also been useful to allow a different interpretation of some retinal diseases, and in the future the contribution of OCT images to the knowledge of pathogenic mechanisms involved in many retinal diseases will certainly be useful.

For some time after its introduction, OCT had only been used in highly specialized centers, but after a while it started to be offered in any outpatient service; the only limitation for its wider distribution was the relatively high costs. Recently, thanks to the availability of several machines on the market, the costs have been reduced, and the number of available instruments is continuing to increase.

Another important factor which contributed to the great success of OCT was the introduction of the intravitreous approach to the therapy of many retinal diseases. OCT is in fact able to detect a very small amount of fluid inside or under the retina, and this helps a lot when deciding whether intravitreous injections are needed or not. The combination of a new diagnostic tool with a new therapy is comparable to what happened in the 1970s and 1980s when fluorescein angiography and laser photocoagulation were introduced into the clinical practice. Also, at that time the interpretation and the therapies of many retinal diseases improved a lot, and for many patients the prognosis changed significantly.

This new volume in the *ESASO Course Series* is published thanks to the enthusiasm of Professor Gabriel Coscas and Professor Anat Lowenstein who recently chaired an ESASO Course on new developments in the use of OCT and who were able to collect the contributions from all the speakers in a very short period of time.

I hope that you will enjoy reading these contributions as much as they enjoyed working on the project.

Francesco Bandello, Milan

Preface

Optical coherence tomography (OCT) is a noninvasive, patient-friendly imaging modality for eye structures. Thanks to recent advances in the technology with its ensuing increasing specificity and sensitivity, OCT has become the modality of choice in visualizing retinal pathologies as well as response to treatment.

The role of OCT has been dramatically enlarging in the last decade, suffice would be to say that it has revolutionized the way we screen, manage and monitor the treatment of retinal disease.

The ESASO intensive course in OCT is a must for any ophthalmologist as well as ophthalmologist in training. After a swift tour of the equipment available and basic techniques, the participants will learn the imaging features of pathological findings in retinal diseases starting with the outer layers including new modalities for choroid imaging, out-layer disease such as various types of macular degeneration, retinal disease such as diabetic retinopathy and vascular occlusion, and retina-vitreous interface pathologies.

Special lectures are dedicated to teaching the practicality of using OCT in pre- and postsurgical evaluation of the posterior segment, in the differential diagnosis of vitreoretinal diseases and in the management of patients with retinal and neuro-ophthalmological diseases.

Pre- and post-treatment cases are presented in a didactical manner. This is followed by a special case presentation elaborating on diagnosis and management.

Gabriel Coscas, Créteil/Paris
Anat Loewenstein, Tel Aviv

Coscas G, Loewenstein A, Bandello F (eds): Optical Coherence Tomography.
ESASO Course Series. Basel, Karger, 2014, vol 4, pp 1–8 (DOI: 10.1159/000355854)

Evolution of Optical Coherence Tomography Technology Comparison of Commercially Available Instruments

Luisa Pierro · Marco Gagliardi

Department of Ophthalmology, Vita-Salute University, San Raffaele Scientific Institute, Milan, Italy

Abstract

The present investigation was designed to appraise the agreement among the commercially available optical coherence tomography (OCT) devices, and to evaluate intra- and interoperator reproducibility in macular thickness, retinal nerve fiber layer (average thickness and four-quadrant values) and cornea thickness in healthy subjects without ocular pathologies. Owing to the increasing number of commercially available spectral domain OCTs, some patients examined with one OCT instrument may indeed receive subsequent examinations with other OCT devices during the follow-up. Therefore, it is of the utmost importance to evaluate the agreement in thickness measurements among the different OCT instruments. In conclusion, the same results were obtained for the macula, retinal nerve fiber layer and cornea measurement thickness reproducibility. A great variability in thickness and reproducibility was registered among the different OCT instruments in all the subjects. The anterior segment spectral domain-OCT technology instruments are not interchangeable for thickness measurements.

A new generation of optical coherence tomography (OCT) devices [1] was recently introduced and currently is in clinical use for the detection and monitoring of a variety of macular, retinal nerve fiber layer (RNFL) and cornea diseases. Indeed, high-speed and high-resolution imaging of central corneal thickness has become feasible with the recent introduction of anterior segment spectral domain-OCT technology.

These devices, called spectral domain (SD) use a spectrometer that can sample more than 20,000 A-scans per second and, therefore, collect far more data than is possible using the time-domain system, which functions at approximately 500 A-scans per second. SD OCT is able to gather in-depth data from the spectra of the OCT signal.

The SD OCT technique offers better axial resolution (5 μm) and increases the speed of data collection by a factor of more than 40 times. The increased speed of SD OCT means there is less eye movement during scans, thus resulting in more stable images. The image stack across the macula can be processed to produce 3-dimensional structural representations.

Segmentation of three-dimensional images permits better visualization of the retinal layers than visualization with time domain-OCT and also allows three-dimensional eye mapping [2].

Due to the increasing number of commercially available SD-OCTs, the patients examined with one OCT instrument may receive subsequent examinations with other OCT devices during the follow-up. Therefore, it is of the utmost importance to evaluate the agreement in macular, RNFL and cornea thickness measurements among the different OCT instruments.

Moreover, measurement reproducibility is an essential parameter when determining the clinical usefulness of a device. Many studies have offered variable and contrasting results regarding macula, RNFL and cornea reproducibility with different OCTs [3–17].

Our goal was to determine the intra- and interoperator reproducibility of macula, RNFL and cornea thickness measurement in normal eyes using commercially available SD OCT devices.

Methods

Macula
Macular thickness was assessed in 18 randomly chosen consecutive eyes of 18 healthy volunteers from the staff of our department by 2 masked operators, L.P. (A) and E.M. (B), with similar practical OCT experience.

Six SD OCT devices were used: Spectral OCT/SLO (Opko/OTI; software version November 2007); 3D OCT-1000 (version 2.12); RTVue-100, (software version 3.0); Cirrus HD-OCT (software version 3.0); SOCT Copernicus (software version 3.03); Heidelberg Spectralis HRA_OCT (software version 3.1.5), and 1 time-domain OCT device was used: Stratus OCT (software version 4.0.1; Carl Zeiss Meditec, Inc.).

Only subjects with no history or evidence of intraocular surgery, retinal disease, or glaucoma, and with refractive error less than 2 dptr were qualified as normal. Both observers repeated 2 consecutive measurements on 1 eye of each subject during the same day at the same time for each instrument used. All subjects underwent OCT imaging using each of the 7 devices at various times from 2007 through 2008.

Central foveal thickness was determined automatically and was analyzed by OCT software. The pupil was not dilated. In all OCT maps, automated macular thickness detection was performed without manual operator. If a scan showed a segmentation error, the information was not included in the statistical analysis. Only good quality images were included in the study.

Retinal Nerve Fiber Layer
Thirty-eight healthy volunteers from the staff of our department were used as control. The inclusion criteria for all participants consisted of a best-corrected visual acuity of 20/20 or better, spherical refraction between +2.0 and –2.0 dptr, axial length <24 mm, normal optic nerve without abnormality of the neuroretinal rim, cup-to-disc ratio greater than 0.2, and normal anterior chamber with open angle.

Exclusion criteria were as follows: any ocular disease, history of ocular hypertension or glaucoma, refractive error greater than 2 dptr, history of ocular surgery, and axial length >24 mm.

The right eye of each subject was scanned using all of the OCT instruments. The peripapillary RNFL thickness (average) was analyzed, comparing six SD-OCTs and one time-domain OCT, by two experienced, masked operators in an observational prospective study. Both operators repeated two consecutive measurements on the same day at the same time. For each OCT, results from two separate scan sets were then averaged to generate the final data for each eye.

Measurements of the peripapillary RNFL (average and four-quadrant values) were obtained by using Spectral OCT/SLO (OPKO Health Instrumentation, Miami, Fla., USA), 3D-OCT 2000 (Topcon, GB Ltd., Newbury, Berkshire, UK), Cirrus HD 100 (Carl Zeiss Meditec, Dublin, Calif., USA), OCT RS-3000 (NIDEK, Gamagori, Japan), RTVue-100 (Optovue Inc., Fremont, Calif., USA), Spectralis (Heidelberg Engineering, Heidelberg, Germany), and Stratus OCT (Car Zeiss Meditec).

All subjects underwent a complete ophthalmologic examination, including assessment of LogMAR visual acuity, refractive error, slit-lamp biomicroscopy, intraocular pressure measurement, and fundus examination. If a scan showed a segmentation error, the information was not included in the statistical analysis. Only good quality images were included in the study.

Table 1. Macular thicknesses mean values and SDs of seven different OCT instruments

Instrument	Operator 1	Operator 2
Stratus OCT[1]	202.88±13.56	206.27±18
Spectral OCT/SLO[2]	213.02±10.03	215.02±10.39
3D OCT-1000[3]	224.41±18.19	225.30±25.66
RTVue-100[4]	233.22±10.32	236.91±9.76
Cirrus HD OCT[5]	253.94±9.73	253.72±9.75
SOCT Copernicus[5]	172.66±7.92	172.88±8.51
Spectralis HRA+OCT[5]	273.19±8.29	272.55±8.88

Mean values ± SD. Analysis of variance: instrument factor, $p < 0.001$; operator factor, $p = 0.042$; instrument × operator, $p = 0.32$. Post hoc test for differences among instruments: [1] $p < 0.005$ against all except Spectral OCT/SLO; [2] $p < 0.005$ against all except Stratus OCT and 3D OCT-1000; [3] $p < 0.005$ against all except Spectral OCT/SLO and RTVue-100; [4] $p < 0.005$ against all except 3D OCT-1000; [5] $p < 0.005$ against all.

Cornea

Central corneal thickness (CCT) was measured in the right eye of 34 randomly chosen healthy subject (18 women, 16 men, mean age 44 ± 10,6 years) by 2 masked operators using 1 ultrasound device (Pachmate DGH55, DGH Instruments, Inc.), 6 SD-OCT (Spectral OCT/SLO, Opko; Cirrus HD-OCT, Zeiss; 3D OCT-2000, Topcon; RS-3000, Nidek; RtvUe-100, Optovue; SS-1000 CASIA, Tomey), 1 TD-OCT (Visante, Zeiss) and 1 Scheimpflug Camera (Sirius, C.T.O.).

To avoid subjective bias, the operators determined all first measurements of each subject, and then all the second measurements, so that they would not remember the CCT value from the previous corneal image for each patient.

Exclusion criteria were history of corneal and anterior segment surgery, corneal diseases, and use of contact lens. Both operators repeated two consecutive measurements of each subject during the same day. If a scan showed a segmentation error, the information was not included in the statistical analysis. Only good quality images were included in the study.

For all the three types of measurements in these three studies, informed consent was obtained from the subjects after explanation of the nature and possible consequences of the study. Our research was approved by the institutional review board of the Scientific Institute San Raffaele. Our research adhered to the tenets of the Declaration of Helsinki.

Statistical Analysis

For all the studies, inter- and intraoperator reproducibility was evaluated by intraclass correlation coefficient (ICC), coefficient of variation (CV) and Bland-Altman plot. Instruments-to-instruments reproducibility was determined by ANOVA for repeated measures.

Results

Macula

With regard to the macular thickness, mean macular thickness for observers A and B are reported in table 1. The ICC (95% CI) for observer A ranged from 0.75 (RTVue-100) to 0.96 (Spectralis HRA+OCT and Cirrus HD OCT). The ICC for observer B was slightly higher, but showed the same trend. The CV for operator A ranged from 2.75 (Stratus OCT) to 0.44 (Spectralis HRA+OCT), and the CV for operator B ranged from 2.66 (Stratus OCT) to 0.43 (Spectralis HRA+OCT).

Bland-Altman analysis evaluated the mean interoperator differences. The best interoperator agreement was observed with Spectralis HRA-OCT. However, the worst agreement was seen

Table 2. RNFL thicknesses mean values and SDs of seven different OCT instruments

	OPKO OTI OCT/SLO	Zeiss Cirrus	Topcon 3D-OCT 2000	NIDEK RS-3000	Zeiss Stratus	Optovue RTVue-100	Heidelberg Spectralis
Average	103.58±7.26	90.08±6.28	106.51±8.35	102.43±6.54	99.63±8.62	103.90±6.16	93.30±5.18
Nasal	88.76±13.50	69.77±7.52	95.77±15.48	86.32±11.27	80.08±12.87	83.2±13.53	70.73±8.12
Temporal	71.98±14.53	63.31±12.35	81.82±15.19	71.76±12.49	70.14±14.38	79±11.84	70±15.46
Inferior	128.77±9.90	116.96±11.39	127.83±14.25	128.41±7.71	126.16±12.64	129.73±13.14	120.44±8.78
Superior	124.25±13.49	109.72±10.97	120.11±15.91	122.72±14.90	121.27±16.35	123.65±16.39	111.74±11.15

Mean ± SD. ANOVA: instrument factor, p < 0.001. Post hoc for differences among instruments. p < 0.005 against all in all sectors.

with the 3D OCT-1000. The analysis of variance, which was also evaluated in a post hoc manner, showed that the interinstrument factor was statistically significant (p < 0.001); the mean interoperator results were not very different, but were still statistically significant (p = 0.042); instrument-operator interaction was not statistically significant (p = 0.32).

Similar differences in the mean thickness were found when the 2 observers used different instruments.

Retinal Nerve Fiber Layer
Cirrus HD-OCT and Spectralis HRA+OCT showed thinner RNFL thickness (average RNFL thickness was 90.08 and 93.30 μm, respectively), whereas Topcon 3D-OCT 2000 showed the highest value (average RNFL thickness was 106.51 μm) (table 2).

As expected, RNFL thickness was higher in superior and inferior quadrants than in nasal and temporal quadrants, using all the instruments (instrument factor, p < 0.001; post hoc test for differences among instruments, p < 0.005 against all in all sectors) (table 2). Heidelberg Spectralis, Zeiss Stratus, NIDEK RS-3000, and Topcon 3D-OCT 2000 gave the best results for the superior sector. Zeiss Cirrus and Optovue RTVue-100, on the contrary, gave the best results for the inferior sector, while OPKO OTI OCT/SLO and Heidelberg

Spectralis, once again, and gave the best results for the temporal sector. On the contrary, the lowest reproducibility was observed with Heidelberg Spectralis, Zeiss Cirrus, Optovue RTVue-100, and OPKO OTI OCT/SLO in the nasal sector, with Topcon 3D-OCT 2000 and Zeiss Cirrus in the temporal sector, and with NIDEK RS-3000 in the inferior sector.

As expected, intraoperator reproducibility was better than interoperator average reproducibility showed that the best correlation was found with Heidelberg Spectralis (ICC 0.92; CV 1.65%), Zeiss Cirrus HD-OCT (ICC 0.90; CV 2.20%), and Zeiss Stratus (ICC 0.91; CV 2.01%), according to the ICC and the CV tests and the Bland-Altman test. As expected, intraoperator reproducibility was better than interoperator reproducibility for all instruments.

Cornea
Mean CCT ranged from 536.38 μm (SD 42.13) to 576.92 μm (SD 39.72). Visante and Sirius showed the lowest value in all measurements, while 3D OCT 2000 and Spectral OCT/SLO showed the highest (fig. 1).

While ICC and CV showed excellent inter- and intraoperator reproducibility for all optic-based devices (best results obtained by CASIA with CV <0.06% and ICC = 1 for both inter- and intraoperator reproducibility), inter- and intra-

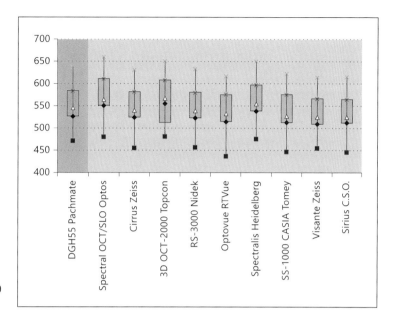

Fig. 1. Box-plot representation of 10 devices CCT measurements.

operator reproducibility for Pachmate DGH55 was just good (CV <1.01% and ICC >0.87 for both inter- and intraoperator reproducibility).

Discussion

Macula

In our study, we noted differing mean macular thickness measurements from instrument to instrument. Our mean macular thickness values ranged from 172 µm with SOCT Copernicus to 272 µm with Spectralis HRA+OCT. Unlike the previous reports, the lowest macular thickness value was recorded with SOCT Copernicus and not with Stratus OCT. On the contrary, the highest value was recorded with Spectralis, followed by Cirrus, as in previous studies [3–7].

Based on differences in the reflectance pattern, all OCT software locates the inner retina on the vitreoretinal interface. The segmentation of the outer retinal border differs significantly from instrument to instrument. The Stratus OCT system shows the outer retinal layers (retinal pigment ep-

ithelium-photoreceptor complex) as 2 hyper-reflective bands. The segmentation software of Stratus OCT uses the inner hyper-reflective band for segmentation.

The new SD OCT system typically shows the outer retinal layers as 3 hyper-reflective bands. The bands may correspond to the external limiting membrane, the junction of the inner segment and the outer segment of the photoreceptors, and the retinal pigment epithelium. The SOCT Copernicus, Spectral OCT/SLO, RTVue-100, and 3D OCT-1000 use the second inner hyper-reflective band as the outer border of the retina. Cirrus HD-OCT and Spectralis HRA+OCT identify the external reflective band as the outer border. These positions are regulated by the software of each instrument and have been chosen arbitrarily by the manufacturers. This is the reason why measurements tend to differ.

Many factors may influence differing instrument-to-instrument reproducibility. Each device uses its own scan parameters, such as the number of A-scans for each B-scan raster and the frame acquisition per second. The number of A-scan lines for each B-scan line is identical for certain devices, such as Cirrus HD OCT, 3D OCT-1000, and Spectral OCT/SLO, and is different for others, such as RTVue-100, SOCT Copernicus, and Spectralis HRA+OCT.

The number of B-scan lines also varies from instrument to instrument, and this means that the grid density is different for each device. A greater number of B-scan lines should mean superior reproducibility. However, the longer time it takes to carry out this procedure does not favor this result. Each device, in fact, has a different acquisition time because the sampling time is also different. The Spectralis HRA+OCT, for example, takes longer to carry out the scan because every B-scan line is the result of the average of 6 lines based on the average carried out while creating the map.

The main result of our study is that macular thickness absolute value differs for each device. For this reason, the devices are not interchangeable. This problem has to be solved, perhaps by using a conversion factor or maybe looking for common measurement parameters, including the boundary line detection of the retinal thickness to compare mean retinal values.

Retinal Nerve Fiber Layer

Our study about optic nerve showed that average RNFL thickness measurement carried out by several different instruments generates significantly different average and sector values, as already reported. It is plausible that segmentation differences in the definition of the outer border of RNFL and optical interaction with tissue due to different light sources and laser camera system sensor may determine this variability. We obtained a greater variability among instruments either for thickness or reproducibility. In particular, we analyzed the potential influence of different conditions related to RNFL thickness.

First of all, we considered different standard diameters. It is well known that RNFL thickness increases with increasing proximity to the optic disc. We hypothesize that measurement closer

than 3.4-mm diameter around the disc, as with Stratus and Topcon 3D-OCT 2000, may explain the greater thickness of the nerve [26, 29]. Spectral OCT/SLO, Cirrus, RTVue, Spectralis, and NIDEK work with a 3.46-mm diameter. Nevertheless, Topcon's RNFL assessment had a higher value (106.51 mm) than that of Stratus (99.63 mm), even if both devices have the same scanning diameter (3.40 mm).

We also analyzed the influence of image quality on RNFL variability. Even if we acquired only images with the same quality level value (>6), the signal strengths differ among the instruments and may determine the variability that we found among RNFL thickness measurements. The effect of blood vessels was also studied. The presence of blood vessels around the optic disc can modify the optic nerve profile and may interfere with thickness. Specifically, comparing Topcon, Heidelberg, and OPKO OCTs, the vascular patterns around the optic disc were obtained by the test-retest function of the instrument and automatically identified in successive scans. It is noteworthy that even though Topcon, Heidelberg, and OPKO have the same options, the results greatly differed.

In an attempt to investigate the effects on reproducibility, other aspects should be considered. First of all, the differences among the instrument scan circle placement may greatly influence the RNFL thickness measurement. In clinical practice, accurate centering of the measurement circle can be difficult. Imprecise measurement caused by an off-center scan circle may be a source of measurement variability. Cirrus has completely automatic scan circle placement obtained by a raster cube scan, whereas all the other OCTs require manual placement of the circular scan set down of the optic disc edge by the operator. RTVue uses a combination of radial and circular scans that require more software interpolation. However, reproducibility results are good also in devices with manual placement of the circle scan.

Another condition refers to the incidence angle of the illuminating beam that may produce different responses. Although some authors have demonstrated that the angle of incidence of the illuminating beam makes the RNFL image on the nasal side dimmer, and therefore less identifiable by the measurement algorithm and also less reproducible, we noticed a wide reproducibility variability involving all the sectors, and not only in the nasal sector, as we have previously reported.

Moreover, we tried to evaluate the effect of eye tracking. Eye tracking can improve reproducibility, as happens with Spectralis and OCT/SLO, but it does not seem fundamental if we consider that Stratus, which is the least updated of the available instruments and does not have this function, shows excellent reproducibility. Eventually, the scanning time may also theoretically affect reproducibility. The instrument scanning time is also very different among OCTs. Spectral OCT/SLO and NIDEK have similar scanning time (1.5 s for three circle scans), whereas that of Stratus and Spectralis is 1.92 s, and that of Cirrus is 2.4 s. On the other hand, Topcon has 0.05. Calibration curves for Optovue RTVue-100 (right) and NIDEK OCT RS-3000 (left) are using OPKO OTI OCT/SLO as reference. OPKO OTI OCT/SLO values are plotted on the y-axis. Black spots describe the true corresponding measurement among coupled devices.

RNFL Thickness Assessment by OCT Instrument Model 5917 s for each circle scan and RTVue has 0.39 s, suggesting that fast scanning times do not necessarily mean good reproducibility. Therefore, scanning time should not be considered as an influencing factor for reproducibility.

In conclusion, great variability in thickness and reproducibility can be registered among different OCT instruments, for both average and sector values [8–13].

In the absence of a clear gold standard demonstrating the real RNFL thickness, it is difficult to establish the most accurate assessment of each instrument. In light of our error analysis results, we found that a scale bias among instruments could interfere with a thorough RNFL monitoring, suggesting that best monitoring is obtained with the same operator and the same device.

Cornea

Considering cornea thickness in terms of repeatability, this study showed that two SD-OCT (SS-1000 CASIA Tomey and RS-3000 Nidek) had the best inter- and intra-operator repeatability, whereas DGH55 Pachmate the worst.

The higher axial resolution of SD-OCT provides enhanced images because of higher reflectivity that improves edge detection. Moreover, rapid acquisition scanning minimizes ocular movement artefacts and might make ocular movement negligible during measurement, which also accounts for lower variability. Therefore, SD-OCT devices might become the gold standard for measuring CCT because clinicians and patients demand non-invasive reliable procedures.

Several authors have reported discrepancies between SD-OCT and ultrasonic pachymetry, resulting in under or overestimation of measurements. These discrepancies are likely to arise because ultrasonic is highly examiner dependent for the difficult to maintain the probe perpendicular to the cornea, to center the probe on the corneal vertex and to avoid compression of the cornea by the probe. Moreover, the accuracy of ultrasound measurement might be influenced by changes in corneal hydration. In fact, the speed of the sound increases in less-hydrated tissue [14–17].

Once again we believe that the most important factor in CCT measurement is the algorithm and type of software used, as we found in our macular thickness and RNFL thickness reproducibility studies. Despite the outstanding repeatability value obtained, devices considered in our study are not totally interchangeable for the measurement of central corneal thickness. In conclusion, also for the cornea measurements the devices considered are not inter-changeable.

References

1 Hee MR, Izatt JA, Swanson EA, Huang D, Schuman JS, Lin CP, Puliafito CA, Fujimoto JG: Optical coherence tomography of the human retina. Arch Ophthalmol 1995;113:325–332.

2 Drexler W, Fujimoto JG: State-of-the-art retinal optical coherence tomography. Prog Retin Eye Res 2008;27:45–88.

3 Pierro L, Giatsidis SM, Mantovani E, Gagliardi M: Macular thickness inter operator and intra operator reproducibility in healthy eyes using 7 optical coherence tomography instruments. Am J Ophthalmol 2010;150:199–204.

4 Legarreta JE, Gregori G, Punjabi OS, Knighton RW, Lalwani GA, Puliafito CA: Macular thickness measurements in normal eyes using spectral domain optical coherence tomography. Ophthalmic Surg Lasers Imaging 2008;39(4 suppl):S43–S49.

5 Leung CK, Cheung CY, Weinreb RN, Lee G, Lin D, Pang CP, Lam DSC: Comparison of macular thickness measurements between time domain and spectral domain optical coherence tomography. Invest Ophthalmol Vis Sci 2008;49:4893–4897.

6 Chen TC, Cense B, Pierce MC, et al: Spectral domain optical coherence tomography: ultra-high speed, ultra-high resolution ophthalmic imaging. Arch Ophthalmol 2005;123:1715–1720.

7 Forte R, Cennamo GL, Finelli ML, Crecchio GD: Comparison of time domain Stratus OCT and spectral domain SLO/OCT for assessment of macular thickness and volume. Eye (Lond) 2009;23:2071–2078.

8 Pierro L, Gagliardi M, Iuliano L, Ambrosi A, Bandello F: Retinal nerve fiber layer thickness reproducibility using seven different OCT instruments. Invest Ophthalmol Vis Sci 2012;53:5912–5920.

9 Menke MN, Knecht P, Sturm V, Dabov S, Funk J: Reproducibility of nerve fiber layer thickness measurements using 3D fourier-domain OCT. Invest Ophthalmol Vis Sci 2008;49:5386–5391.

10 Buchser NM, Wollstein G, Ishikawa H, Bilonick RA, Ling Y, Folio LS, Kagemann L, Noecker RJ, Albeiruti E, Schuman JS: Comparison of retinal nerve fiber layer thickness measurement bias and imprecision across three spectral-domain optical coherence tomography devices. Invest Ophthalmol Vis Sci 2012;53:3742–3747.

11 Savini G, Carbonelli M, Barboni P: Retinal nerve fiber layer thickness measurement by Fourier-domain optical coherence tomography: a comparison between cirrus-HD OCT and RTVue in healthy eyes. J Glaucoma 2010;19:369–372.

12 Bendschneider D, Tornow RP, Horn FK, Laemmer R, Roessler CW, Juenemann AG, Kruse FE, Mardin CY: Retinal nerve fiber layer thickness in normals measured by spectral domain OCT. J Glaucoma 2010;19:475–482.

13 Rao HL, Kumar AU, Kumar A, Chary S, Senthil S, Vaddavalli PK, Garudadri CS: Evaluation of central corneal thickness measurement with RTVue spectral domain optical coherence tomography in normal subjects. Cornea 2011;30:121–126.

14 Amano S, Honda N, Amano Y, Yamagami S, Miyai T, Samejima T, Ogata M, Miyata K: Comparison of central corneal thickness measurements by rotating Scheimpflug camera, ultrasonic pachymetry, and scanning-slit corneal topography. Ophthalmology 2006;113:937–941.

15 Zhao PS, Wong TY, Wong WL, Saw SM, Aung T: Comparison of central corneal thickness measurements by visante anterior segment optical coherence tomography with ultrasound pachymetry. Am J Ophthalmol 2007;143:1047–1049.

16 Jonuscheit S, Doughty MJ: Evidence for a relative thinning of the peripheral cornea with age in white European subjects. Invest Ophthalmol Vis Sci 2009;50:4121–4128.

17 Pierro L, Gagliardi M, Parrinello G, Rama P, Bandello F: Healthy Eyes Central Corneal Thickness Reproducibility Using 8 Optical Instruments and 1 Ultrasonic Instrument. ARVO Meeting Abstracts March 26, 2012, vol 53, p 132.

Dr. Luisa Pierro, MD
Department of Ophthalmology, Vita-Salute University
San Raffaele Scientific Institute
Via Olgettina 60, IT–20132 Milan (Italy)
E-Mail pierro.luisa@hsr.it

Coscas G, Loewenstein A, Bandello F (eds): Optical Coherence Tomography.
ESASO Course Series. Basel, Karger, 2014, vol 4, pp 9–16 (DOI: 10.1159/000355863)

Optical Coherence Tomography Pathologic Findings in the Vitreoretinal and Macular Interface

Dafna Goldenberg · Roy Schwartz · Anat Loewenstein

Tel Aviv Medical Center, Department of Ophthalmology, Sackler Faculty of Medicine, Tel Aviv University, Tel Aviv, Israel

Abstract

The vitreous body is bounded posteriorly by the retina and is adherent to it. Abnormalities in the adhesion between the vitreous and the macula, or vitreoretinal interface, are involved in the pathogenesis of several macular conditions. Optical coherence tomography is a noninvasive in vivo ophthalmic imaging technique, which allows for a better understanding and improved diagnosis of disease processes that involve the vitreoretinal interface. The aim of this paper is to describe optical coherence tomography findings in vitreomacular disorders, namely epiretinal membrane, idiopathic macular hole, lamellar macular hole, and vitreomacular traction syndrome, in order to assist in the diagnosis and proper treatment of these syndromes.   © 2014 S. Karger AG, Basel

The vitreous body is bounded posteriorly by the retina and is adherent to it. It is formed by collagen fibrils that insert superficially into the internal limiting membrane (ILM) of the retina [1]. Attachment to the ILM is facilitated by macromolecules such as laminin, fibronectin, chondroitin and heparan sulfate proteoglycans [2]. The vitreous is firmly attached to the lens capsule, retinal vessels, optic nerve, and to the macula. Abnormalities in the adhesion between the vitreous and the macula, or vitreoretinal interface, are involved in the pathogenesis of several macular conditions.

Optical coherence tomography (OCT) is a noninvasive in vivo ophthalmic imaging technique. Technological advancements, including the introduction of high-resolution spectral-domain OCT (SD-OCT) in 2004, have allowed for a better understanding and improved diagnosis of disease processes that involve the vitreoretinal interface. Nowadays, OCT has become a valuable tool for assessment of the vitreoretinal interface.

The aim of this chapter is to describe OCT findings in vitreomacular disorders, namely epiretinal membrane (ERM), idiopathic macular hole (MH), lamellar MH, and vitreomacular traction syndrome, in order to assist in the diagnosis and proper treatment of these syndromes.

Epiretinal Membrane

An ERM is a fibrocellular membrane on the inner retinal surface that is adherent to the ILM of the retina. It is believed to arise as a result of proliferation of glial cells, retinal pigment epithelium, or hyalocytes at the vitreoretinal interface.

ERMs are classified as idiopathic or secondary to a plethora of conditions, including retinal vascular occlusive disease, diabetes mellitus, ocular inflammatory diseases, ocular trauma, ocular surgery and others.

Clinically, ERMs may have various appearances on biomicroscopy. Mild ERMs may appear as a glistening layer on the retinal surface, as an irregular light reflex – the so-called cellophane maculopathy, or as retinal striae, resulting from wrinkling of the ILM. Denser ERMs appear as a gray sheet overlying the retina. When the pathology is more advanced, contraction of the ERM may lead to retinal distortion, vascular traction, macular edema due to increased permeability of contracted vessels, and formation of a pseudo-hole. Moderate-to-severe cases of ERM contracture are also termed macular pucker.

On OCT, ERMs appear as a highly reflective layer on the inner retinal surface. They may appear adherent to the retina (fig. 1Aa) or separated from the inner retina (fig. 1Ab), partially or completely.

Since epiretinal membranes may appear completely detached from the retinal surface, they may be confused with a detached posterior hyaloid on OCT images. One distinction is the reflection caused by the two entities. The posterior hyaloid usually has a thin reflection compared to the denser reflection of an ERM. Another way to differentiate between the two is the degree of separation from the inner retina, which is usually greater for the posterior hyaloid (fig. 1B). When still not certain, one can examine an OCT slice containing the optic nerve head. The posterior hyaloid tends to adhere to it while an ERM does not.

An ERM may distort the foveal contour or lead to its flattening (fig. 1Aa). It may lead to superficial retinal folds, or a saw-tooth pattern (fig. 1Ab, C). Retinal folds should not be mistaken for choroidal folds. The latter will also include folds in the outer retinal layers. Other helpful modalities in this distinction are the infra-red image accompanying an OCT image and the B-mode ultrasound of the eye. The latter may also shed light on the etiology behind the choroidal folds.

As mentioned above, contraction of the membrane may lead to the creation of a pseudo-hole. A pseudo-hole (fig. 1C), as opposed to a MH (see p. 12), which is a retinal break or defect, appears due to thickening of the retinal layers on both sides of the foveola, may lead to the false appearance of a true partial MH. A number of features assist in recognizing pseudo holes and differentiating them from true holes. The first is the existence of a distinct ERM alongside the pseudo-hole. Second, the foveal contour tends to appear punched out, well delineated, and steepened. Another important characteristic of a pseudo-hole, which is almost pathognomonic for the condition, is verticalization of the foveal pit – its edges on both sides tend to be straight and vertical, as opposed to the rounded edges of a MH or lateral splits of a lamellar hole (see p. 14). As the pathology arises from thickening of the perifoveal retina, a moderately increased thickness of the surrounding macula will be seen, usually with a normal central foveal thickness.

Another result of contraction of an ERM is the creation of traction on the inner retinal layers, leading to the formation of macular edema. In most cases, edema in ERM is diffuse and not cystic (fig. 1Da). In the rare occasions of a cystic edema caused by an ERM, it tends to appear central and symmetric (fig. 1Db).

A final subject of significance in the interpretation of ERM images on OCT is the photoreceptor-retinal pigment epithelial (PR-RPE) layers. When looking at the outer retinal layer in an OCT image, one should note the integrity of the PR layer. PR disruption was found to be a predictor of poor visual outcome in eyes with idiopathic

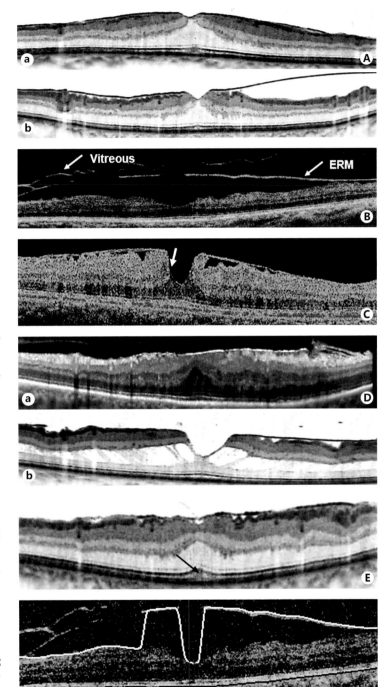

Fig. 1. A Epiretinal membrane as seen on spectral-domain OCT (SD-OCT). ERMs may appear as a highly reflective layer adherent to the retinal inner surface (**a**), or partially separated from the ILM (**b**). The membrane is creating a saw-tooth pattern in this image, seen to the left of the fovea. **B** Posterior hyaloid face versus ERM on SD-OCT. Notice the thinner reflection of the vitreous in comparison to the ERM and the degree of separation from the inner retina, which is greater for the posterior hyaloid. **C** Pseudo-hole created by an epiretinal membrane. Notice the steepening of the foveal contour, the verticalization of the foveal pit (arrow), and the increased thickness of the surrounding macula. **D a** Diffuse edema caused by an ERM on SD-OCT. **b** The rarer form of cystic edema along with an ERM, characterized by a symmetrical pattern. **E** SD-OCT image showing an ERM. Notice the complete integrity of the PR layer. Also note the subfoveal sediment between the PR and RPE layers (arrow). **F** Segmentation inner line breakdown results in inaccurate quantitative analysis.

ERMs. Moreover, early ERM removal may prevent further progression of PR damage in those patients [3]. Another feature in these layers is the existence of reflective sediment between the PR and RPE layers which may be found in eyes with an ERM. The clinical significance of such sediments has not been proven (fig. 1E).

Finally, when interpreting a thickness map of patients with an ERM, one should not rely solely on the measurements made by the OCT software, as they can lead to erroneous treatment decisions. OCT segmentation lines are automatically drawn on the ILM as the inner line. However, segmentation inner line breakdown frequently occurs secondary to ERMs and vitreomacular traction (VMT), resulting in irregular topographic mapping and inaccurate quantitative analysis. The segmentation made by the OCT software may confuse an ERM for an ILM, leading to the false detection of macular edema (fig. 1F). SD-OCT devices allow for segmentation line correction, so the inner lines can be manually manipulated and moved to the correct location.

Macular Hole

A MH results from a vertical split in the foveal neurosensory retina. MHs are more common in females, and tend to occur in the sixth to eighth decades of life. They may be idiopathic, or may be secondary to a variety of conditions, including trauma (physical, electrical, laser), cystoid macular edema, retinal vascular diseases, macular pucker, rhegmatogenous retinal detachment, and hypertensive retinopathy. This chapter focuses on idiopathic MHs.

Investigations using OCT and ultrasonography suggest that idiopathic MHs are caused by vitreoretinal abnormalities and vitreoretinal traction [4].

Patients with MHs may complain of metamorphopsia and diminished central visual acuity.

On biomicroscopy a MH appears as a small yellow spot in the fovea. It may be differentiated from a pseudohole (see p. 12) or a lamellar hole (see p. 14) by the Watzke-Allen test, in which a thin beam of light is shined over the area of the spot. A positive test, indicating a true MH, requires that the patient perceive a 'break' in the slit beam.

In 1988, long before the introduction of OCT, Gass defined 4 stages in the development of MHs, based solely on clinical observation. He believed that idiopathic MHs development was attributed to tangential traction rather than anteroposterior forces [5]. The introduction of OCT provided better understanding of the disease pathogenesis and allowed clinicians to follow the sequence of events which lead to the development of full thickness MHs. It has led to the understanding that oblique traction, rather than tangential traction, results in MH. OCT imaging re-defined Gass' stages and is composed of 3 MH stages rater than 4.

Stage I (or impending MH) – This stage is divided into two stages. Stage Ia MH: (fig. 2Aa) foveal 'pseudocyst', or horizontal splitting (schisis), associated with a vitreous detachment from the perifoveal retina.

If the tractional forces persist, the pseudocyst might extend through the entire foveal thickness resulting in stage Ib MH (fig. 2Ab) where there is a break in the outer foveal layer of the pseudocyst.

A stage I MH may resolve spontaneously following separation of perifoveal vitreous adhesion in as many as 50% of cases. In other cases it may become a lamellar hole (see p. 14) or a full thickness MH (stage II).

When a tractional break develops in the 'roof' of the stage Ib pseudocyst a stage II full-thickness MH forms.

Stage II (fig. 2Ac) is defined as a full-thickness MH (FTMH) with posterior hyaloid (operculum) which remains attached to either side of the MH.

Stage III (fig. 2B) is defined as a FTMH along with foveal posterior hyaloid detachment. The posterior hyaloid may be seen with an operculum suspended over the hole.

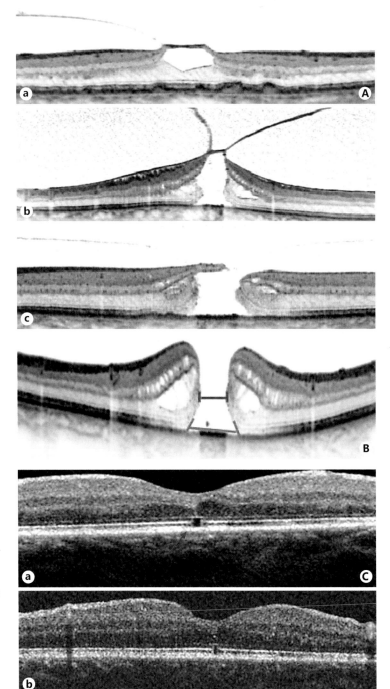

Fig. 2. A Stages of a MH, as seen on OCT. a Stage Ia – a pseudocyst appears. b Stage Ib – the 'floor' of the cyst (or its outer layer) is broken. c Stage II – the 'roof' (or inner layer) of the cyst is broken, resulting in a FTMH. The posterior vitreous (the operculum) is still attached to the foveal center. B Stage III – differentiated from stage 2 by the detachment of the hyaloid from the fovea. A stage III MH with cystic changes in the surrounding neurosensory retina. Calipers are placed for maximal (blue) and minimal (red) width. C a A gap in the PR layer 2 months after FTMH closure operation. b The gap closed spontaneously after 4 months.

Fig. 2. D Fellow eyes of a FTMH eye with stage 0 MH. **a** Attachment of the posterior hyaloid to only one side of the fovea. **b** Attachment of the posterior hyaloid to both sides of the fovea puts this patient at 50% risk of developing a FTMH in the fellow eye.

When describing an OCT image of a FTMH, a few variables need to be addressed. First, the stage of the MH, as described previously. Second, the size of the hole. There are a few available methods for measuring MH sizes. The most common method entails measuring the maximum FTMH width at the level of the RPE or minimum FTMH width between the closest edges of the hole (fig. 2B). A third consideration is the existence of edge elevation, which signifies a more advanced state of a FTMH. Lastly, one should note whether cystic changes appear in the neurosensory retina engulfing the hole. It is believed that the defect of the inner retinal layers allows infiltration of vitreal fluid to within the retina, leading to intraretinal cysts and MH enlargement.

SD-OCT serves as an excellent prognostic tool before surgical intervention. The photoreceptor layer most commonly has to have continuity in order to function properly after surgical closure of a hole. Recent studies have shown that in certain cases a gap in the photoreceptor layer may close with time, leading to an improvement in visual acuity (fig. 2C).

Another prognostic consideration is the completeness of the external limiting membrane. It was shown that damage to this layer affects post-surgical prognosis.

When examining a MH, it is important to address the fellow eye. Chan et al. [6] coined the idea of a 'stage 0' MH, in which a perifoveal vitreous detachment develops. In their study, fibers of the posterior hyaloid seemed to insert into the fovea obliquely, flattening to the periphery and reinserting outside of the foveal area. Based on their study, they proposed that the presence of a stage 0 MH in the fellow eye signified an almost 6-fold increase in the risk for developing a MH in the fellow eye. They have stratified the risks of developing a MH in a fellow eye of an eye with a FTMH. The lowest risk (0%) belongs to eyes with a complete vitreous detachment. A perifoveal insertion on one side of the fovea increases the risk to 25%, while bilateral foveal attachment raises it to 50% (fig. 2D).

Lamellar Macular Hole

Lamellar holes represent a break in the inner fovea with intact foveal photoreceptors.

They may result from an abortive process of MH formation (de roofing of pseudocyst of stage Ia with preservation of foveal base) (fig. 3) (see p. 12) or may be a complication of chronic CME, when a cyst or number of cysts in the complex open.

Some unique features in the presentation of a lamellar hole on OCT may aid in distinguishing it from similar entities, such as a pseudo-hole (see p. 10). First, there will be thinning of the foveal

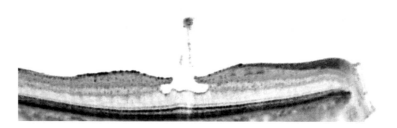

Fig. 3. Lamellar MH resulting from 'de-roofing' of a pseudocyst.

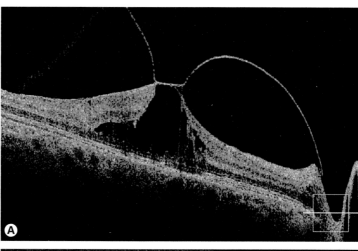

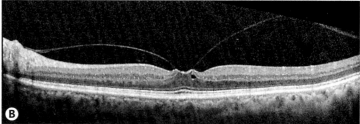

Fig. 4. A Vitreomacular traction syndrome. Notice the cystoid macular edema resulting from the tractional forces. **B** A mild form of VMT syndrome resulting in a small cystic foveal change. Biomicroscopic examination of this patient seemed normal, but the patient was complaining of visual deterioration.

floor, as opposed to a pseudo-hole, in which foveal thickness does not change. Another unique feature is intraretinal splitting laterally on either side of the hole, resulting from a split between the inner and outer retinal layers (fig. 3). When a retinal splitting is not seen but a lamellar hole is suspected, different sections of the OCT image may reveal this configuration, specifically a star-shaped section. As opposed to a pseudo-hole, no thickening of the surrounding macula is seen in a lamellar hole.

Vitreomacular Traction Syndrome

A VMT syndrome results from tangential tractional forces on the foveal and parafoveal regions applied by the vitreous, as a result of partial PVD. Patients may complain of decreased visual acuity as a result of distortion of the normal macular architecture or secondarily to the development of macular edema as a result of the tractional forces (fig. 4A).

As opposed to MHs and epiretinal membranes, diagnosis of a VMT syndrome may be missed by biomicroscopy alone. First generations of OCT allowed the discovery of the syndrome in maculas that seemed normal clinically. The increase in axial resolution introduced in SD-OCT has improved dramatically our ability to visualize the vitreomacular interface and posterior hyaloid membrane [7], allowing for even mild cases of VMT syndrome to be detected (fig. 4B).

References

1 Johnson MW: Perifoveal vitreous detachment and its macular complications. Trans Am Ophthalmol Soc 2005; 103:537–567.
2 Ponsioen TL, Hooymans JMM, Los LI: Remodelling of the human vitreous and vitreoretinal interface – a dynamic process. Prog Retinal Eye Res 2010;29:580–595.
3 Suh MH, Seo JM, Park KH, et al: Associations between macular findings by optical coherence tomography and visual outcomes after epiretinal membrane removal. Am J Ophthalmol 2009; 147:473–480.
4 Michalewska Z, Michalewski J, Sikorski BL, et al: A study of macular hole formation by serial spectral coherence tomography. Clin Exp Ophthalmol 2009;37: 373–383.
5 Gass JD: Idiopathic senile macular hole. Its early stages and pathogenesis. Arch Ophthalmol 1988;106:629–639.
6 Chan A, Duker JS, Schuman JS, Fujimoto JG: Stage 0 macular holes. Observations by optical coherence tomography. Ophthalmology 2004;111:2027–2032.
7 Wolf S, Wolf-Schnurrbusch U: Spectral-domain optical coherence tomography use in macular diseases: a review. Ophthalmologica 2010;224:333–340.

Dafna Goldenberg
Tel Aviv Medical Center
Department of Ophthalmology
6 Weizmann Street, Tel Aviv 64239 (Israel)
E-Mail dafnagoldenberg@gmail.com

Coscas G, Loewenstein A, Bandello F (eds): Optical Coherence Tomography.
ESASO Course Series. Basel, Karger, 2014, vol 4, pp 17–25 (DOI: 10.1159/000356337)

Optical Coherence Tomography in the Inner Retinal Layers

J.M. Giraud[a] · H. El Chehab[b] · M. Francoz[b] · J.R. Fenolland[b] ·
M. Delbarre[b] · F. May[b] · J.P. Renard[b]

[a]A Hôpital d'Instruction des Armées Sainte Anne, Toulon, [b]Hôpital Instruction des Armées du Val de Grâce,
Service Ophtalmologie, Paris, France

Abstract

Optical coherence tomography (OCT) in the inner retinal layers is a new and very interesting tool for glaucoma diagnosis and follow-up. New spectral domain-OCT with layer segmentation analysis is able to measure thickness from the 3 layers containing parts of the retinal ganglion cells. Dendrites from the retinal ganglion cells form the inner plexiform layer, cellular bodies form the ganglion cell layer and axons form the nerve fiber layer. Glaucomatous apoptosis of ganglion cells causes thinning of the inner layers. Numerous OCT devices produce macular maps of thickness for theses layers, with a reference to a normative database. Nevertheless, the thickness difference between normal and glaucomatous patients is small and OCT must be realized and analyzed very carefully to avoid false results due to artifacts or poor quality scanning. Macular inner layers mapping is a very promising tool for glaucoma, complementary with peripapillary retinal nerve fiber layer and optic nerve head analysis.

© 2014 S. Karger AG, Basel

Glaucoma diagnosis at the beginning of treatment, and during follow-up, to determine disease progression is often a difficult challenge.

Clinical optic disc examination proves the existence of physiological excavations in normal patients as well as in glaucoma patients with small discs without excavation. Even experienced clinicians find it difficult to affirm progression on successive disc examinations.

Defects on the visual field are delayed compared with structural changes. At long-term follow-up, fluctuations are found that could be confused with disease progression.

Glaucomatous neuropathy causes insidious apoptosis of the retinal ganglion cells (RGC). This is followed by progressive thinning of the inner retinal layers. Different parts of the RGC create 3 different inner retinal layers: dendrites from the RGC form the inner plexiform layer (IPL), cellular bodies form the ganglion cell layer (GCL) and axons form the nerve fiber layer (NFL).

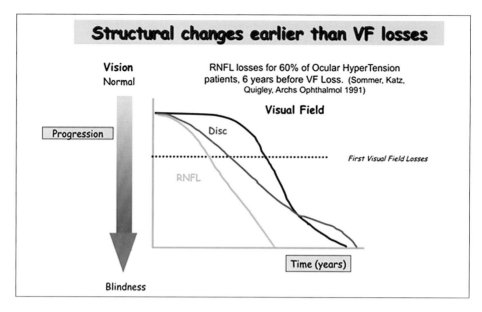

Fig. 1. Structural loss is earlier than functional loss. RNFL losses for 60% of ocular hytension patients 6 years before loss of visual field. From Sommer et al. [1].

In the macular area, precise and reproducible measurements from tissular structural changes on the RGC could bring substantive input for the diagnosis and follow-up of glaucoma.

We here describe the new possibilities offered by spectral domain-optical coherence tomography (OCT) for this macular analysis (OCT also provides a very contributive analysis of the peripapillary retinal nerve fiber layer (RNFL) and direct optic disc excavation measurements, but this is not described here).

Structural Changes Are Earlier than Visual Field Losses

Histopathologic studies showed long ago that structural damage occurs earlier than functional loss. Visual field peripheral defect occurs after 30–35% RGC losses and visual field central defect occurs in 50% of RGC losses. RNFL losses occur in 60% of patients with ocular hypertension, i.e. 6 years' visual field loss [1] (fig. 1).

OCT Macular Analysis and Glaucoma

In 2004, a study compared full macular thickness and peripapillary RNFL measurements with time domain-OCT, for glaucoma diagnosis [2]. It found macular thinning in glaucomatous patients, but full macular thickness appears less sensitive than RNFL for glaucoma detection.

With spectral domain-OCT, higher resolution and powerful software, segmentation of the retinal layers and separate thickness analysis of each layer throughout the macular area has become possible. Results are compared with a normative database with healthy subjects of the same ages.

The macular ganglion cell complex (GCC) is defined as the three innermost retinal layers: it represents 30% of the full retinal thickness. The NFL is composed of RGC axons, the bodies form the GCL, and RGC dendrites form the IPL (fig. 2).

The GCC only is damaged in glaucoma (photoreceptors do not seem to be lost in glaucoma).

Giraud · El Chehab · Francoz · Fenolland · Delbarre · May · Renard

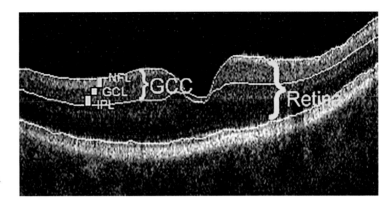

Fig. 2. The three retinal inner layers. Courtesy of Optovue®.

With thickness measurements, the machine's software built macular maps of the GCC, as reported to a normative database. Normative databases are segmented according to age categories.

Optical Coherence Tomography Devices

Many companies have built and sell more and more advanced OCT devices. Here are the characteristics of some models.

Optovue® RT Vue
This was the first OCT device used to measure the GCC. The acquisition protocol was named the MM7 protocol. It acquired 7-mm long scans, 1 horizontal scan and 15 vertical scans spaced 0.5 mm apart (fig. 3). The acquisition area is shifted by 1 mm on the temporal side of the fovea.

After scan acquisition, the RT Vue computes 3 GCC macular maps: a thickness map where blue-colored areas indicate a 20–30% GCC loss and black areas indicate a 50% loss, a deviation map where percentage of thickness loss is reported to the normative database, and a significance map with three colors: red for statistically significant deviation p < 1%, yellow for p < 5% and green for normal values for age category (fig. 4).

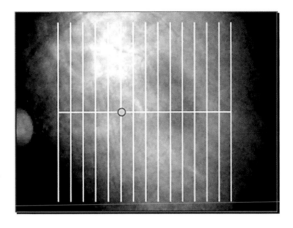

Fig. 3. MM7 scan acquisition protocol on RtVue®.

Analysis software also calculates two very interesting indexes: FLV (focal loss volume in %) is significant volume losses reported to the macular area, and GLV (global loss volume in %) is total volume of significant GCC loss.

Nidek® OCT
The Nidek OCT has the largest macular acquisition area. Scan acquisitions take a macular cube 9 × 9 mm.

Then, scan analysis is done on 6 or 9 mm with128 B scans (512 A scans) and delivers 3 maps: a thickness map, a deviation map, and a thickness compared to normative database map.

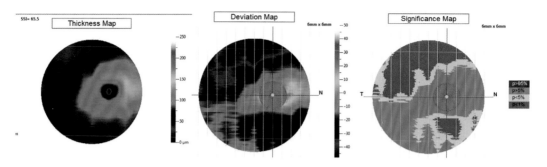

Fig. 4. RtVue macular maps for GCC.

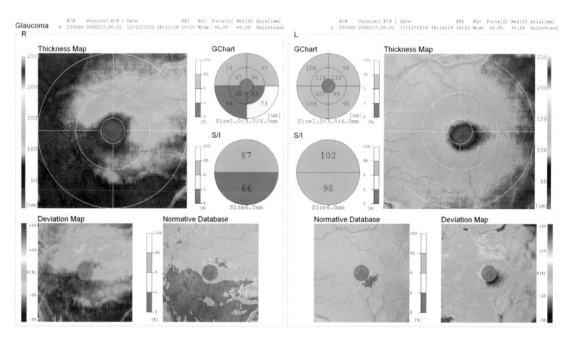

Fig. 5. Nidek macular maps for GCC.

The G Chart grid cuts the macular area into 8 regions. One grid shows the mean thickness values in the 8 regions and the other shows the hemisuperior and hemiinferior thicknesses [3] (fig. 5).

Topcon® 3D OCT 2000
Scan acquisition takes a macular cube 7 × 7 mm in size (512 × 128 scans).

Data analyses produce a report with a thickness map, a significance map and an asymmetry superior-inferior map. It is possible to choose to analyze the thickness of one or of contiguous retinal layers. The report also gives the values of the average, superior and inferior thicknesses. The Topcon is the only device to acquire a color fundus photograph at the same time [4] (fig. 6).

Giraud · El Chehab · Francoz · Fenolland · Delbarre · May · Renard

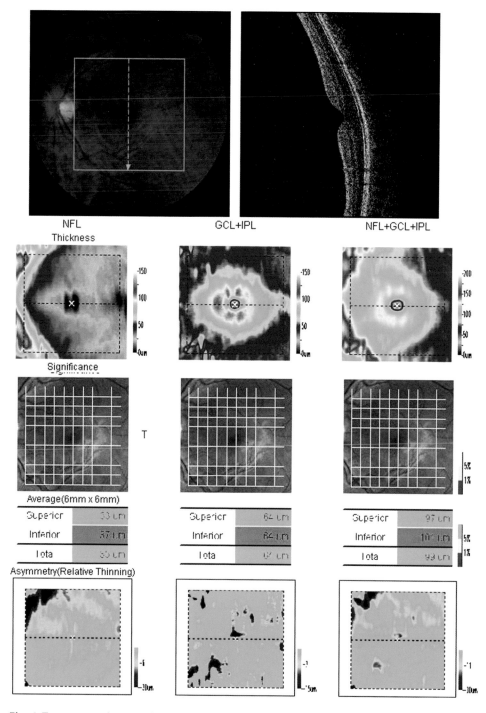

Fig. 6. Topcon macular maps for GCC.

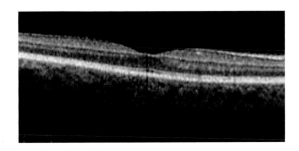

Fig. 7. Cirrus GCA = GCL + IPL (without RNFL).

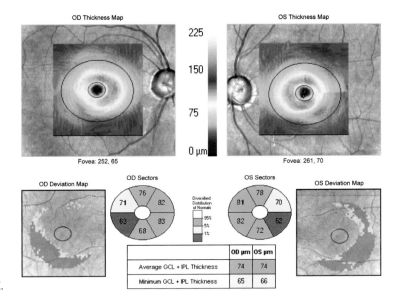

Fig. 8. Cirrus macular maps for GCC.

Zeiss® Cirrus HD OCT

Acquisition takes a photograph of a macular cube with 6 × 6 sides (200 × 200 or 512 × 128 scans). The latest versions are fitted with an eye tracker. Analysis uses ganglion cell analysis (GCA). GCA is different from GCC because it does not include the RNFL. Zeiss consider that the RNFL have too many variations. The RNFL are axons that extend from the ganglion cells to converge on the optic disc. On one defined area, the RNFL layer is a mix of axons of local ganglion cells and fibers coming from other areas (fig. 7).

Cirrus GCA = GCL + IPL (without RNFL)
The Zeiss Cirrus® provides both a thickness map and a deviation map. It shows the thickness values in 6 sectors. The global average thickness and minimum thickness could be a signal of a beginning defect (fig. 8).

Canon® HS 100
This device offers a double eye tracking system (on pupil and fundus vessels) to correct micromovement artifacts. It acquires 70,000 A-scans/s with a resolution of 3 μm. It is able to realize a full retinal segmentation (fig. 9).

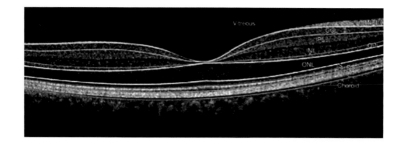

Fig. 9. Canon HS 100® full segmentation.

Acquisition of Data and Analysis of Spectral Domain-OCT Reports

Many factors could influence the acquisition of images. It is important to consider the patient-related and the machine-related factors.

Patient-Related Factors
First, the axial length: when the axial length increases, the RNFL thickness decreases [5]. The size, shape and variations of the optic disc influence the peripapillary RNFL but not the MGC complex. So, macular GCC or GCA measurements could be better than peripapillary measurements. GCC could be interesting in 3 instances: with small discs, the RNFL thickness decreases, with large discs, the RNFL thickness increases, and with diversion discs, the peripapillary measurements are very irregular.

OCT-Related Factors
The index of quality (sometimes called 'signal strength' or by other names) exists on all OCT devices. Operators and ophthalmologists must take good notice of this index. If the index is low, segmentation and analysis could not be accurate. Images must be acquired again.

The color codes: red zones on maps or red overlining of bad values could be a help …or a trap … Ophthalmologists should not reduce the patient's evaluation to flashy color codes: green = normal patient, red = abnormal patient! Color codes are relevant for good normative databases

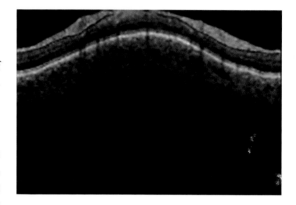

Fig. 10. Signal outside the acquisition window: false result.

(and many databases are built with a too small number of patients in each age class). It is important to remember that many patients could be 'border line'. If there is a successive report, it is useful to always compare the reports and each value very carefully to evaluate if any disease progression has occurred.

Numerous traps could exist in OCT reports. These reports must always be read with a critical eye. Some classic examples of the traps are:
– All macular pathologies: high myopia with macular atrophy, epiretinal membranes, and age-related macular degeneration will modify the thickness of the macular layers.
– If the signal is outside of the acquisition window, the device will make a false analysis (fig. 10).

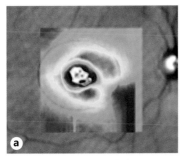

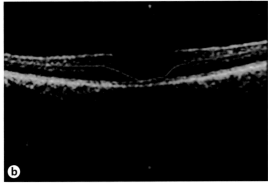

Fig. 11. a, b Lens opacity causing a defect in acquisition.

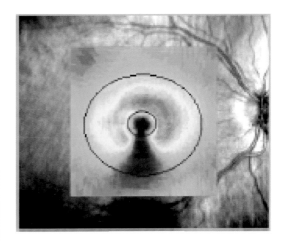

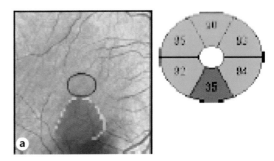

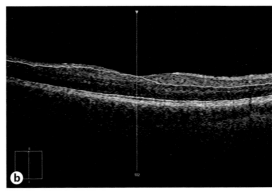

Fig. 12. a, b Bad quality scan, low signal: errors in segmentation.

– A dense crystal lens opacity in the visual axis will induce segmentation errors and produce a false GCC map (fig. 11a, b).
– A bad quality scan (low index of quality) will induce errors of segmentation and a false defect on the report (fig. 12a, b).
– Multifocal intraocular lenses couls cause wavy horizontal artifacts on the OCT images [6].

To get a reliable report, it is most important to make a good image acquisition to avoid artifacts and misinterpretations. Guidelines for optimal acquisition are:

– To analyze images only if they have a good index of quality.
– If there is a narrow pupil or weak acquisition signal, it is possible to enhance the quality under mydriasis. The operator has to administer mydriatic drops and realize a new scan acquisition under mydriasis.

– If abnormalities appear on the report, it is crucial to control the segmentation. The operator must read each scan and do manual corrections if the segmentation is false.

Giraud · El Chehab · Francoz · Fenolland · Delbarre · May · Renard

– It is very important to always associate RNFL and GCC measurements to get a richer structural analysis.

Main Indications

The main indications for inner retinal layers OCT are patients suspected of having glaucoma, and follow-up of ocular hypertension. With glaucomatous patients, follow-up of all stages of glaucoma as well as peripapillary RNFL and ONH analysis is important. Analysis is also very interesting with 'difficult' or special-shaped optic discs. A complete OCT analysis is very useful with low reliability visual fields examinations. In advanced glaucoma, analysis of the inner layers could be interesting and show a progression when peripapillary RNFL and sometimes the visual field do no longer show any progression [7].

Conclusions

GCC is a good new structural parameter but it is far better to consider all the different structural and functional parameters together. OCT does not replace clinical or visual field examination, all are complementary methods and bring light to the clinical strategy. GCC seems of great interest for early ganglion cells loss (pre-perimetric) and in advanced glaucoma, and could be the last index to show progression. In moderate glaucoma, the diagnostic power of GCC and RNFL are equal. Deviation maps, significance maps, and indexes like FLV or GLV are of great interest for diagnosis and progression follow-up.

GCC analysis has particular interest in high myopia and papillary diversion (when peripapillary RNFL and ONH analysis are inoperative).

Analysis of the inner retinal layers is a promising additional good structural analysis tool, complementary with RNFL and TNO analysis.

References

1 Sommer A, Katz J, Quigley HA, Miller NR, Robin AL, Richter RC, Witt KA: Clinically detectable nerve fiber atrophy precedes the onset of glaucomatous field loss. Arch Ophthalmol 1991;109:77–83.
2 Wollstein G, Schuman JS, Price LL, Aydin A, Beaton SA, Stark PC, Fujimoto JG, Ishikawa H: Optical coherence tomography (OCT) macular and peripapillary retinal nerve fiber layer measurements and automated visual fields. Am J Ophthalmol 2004;138:218–225.
3 Morooka S, Hangai M, Nukada M, et al: Wide 3D Macumar GCC imaging with SDOCT in glaucoma. Invest Ophthalmol Vis Sci 2012;53:4805–4812.
4 Nakatani Y, Higashide T, Ohkubo S, et al: Evaluation of macular thickness and pRNFL for detection of early glaucoma using OCT. J Glaucoma 2011;20:252–259.
5 Öner V, Aykut V, Tas M, et al: Effect of refractive status on peripapillary RNFL thickness a study by RTVue SD OCT. Br J Ophthalmol 2013;97:75–79.
6 Inoue M, Bissen-Miyajima H, Yoshino M, Suzuki T: Wavy horizontal artifacts on optical coherence tomography line-scanning images caused by diffractive multifocal intraocular lenses. J Cataract Refract Surg 2009;35:1239–1243.
7 Renard JP, Fénolland JR, El Chehab H, Francoz M, Marill AM, Messaoudi R, Delbarre M, Maréchal M, Michel S, Giraud JM: Analysis of macular ganglion cell complex (GCC) with spectral-domain optical coherence tomography (SD-OCT) in glaucoma (in French). J Fr Ophtalmol 2013;36:299–309.

Jean-Marie Giraud
Chef du Service d'Ophtalmologie
Hôpital d'Instruction des Armées Sainte Anne
Boulevard Sainte Anne, FR–83000 Toulon (France)
E-Mail jean-marie-giraud@wanadoo.fr

Coscas G, Loewenstein A, Bandello F (eds): Optical Coherence Tomography.
ESASO Course Series. Basel, Karger, 2014, vol 4, pp 26–33 (DOI: 10.1159/000355870)

Optical Coherence Tomography of the Outer Retinal Layers

Adrian Koh

Eye and Retina Surgeons, ESASO Asia, Singapore National Eye Centre, Singapore Eye Research Institute,
National University Hospital, Singapore, Singapore

Abstract

Spectral domain optical coherence tomography (OCT) provides high-resolution images of the different layers of the macula approximating histological sections. It plays a significant role in the management of outer retinal diseases such as exudative age-related macular degeneration, central serous chorioretinopathy, and polypoidal choroidal vasculopathy. The OCT is an important complementary tool in detecting activity of diseases such as choroidal neovascularization and polypoidal choroidal vasculopathy, and is indispensable in monitoring the response to treatment and decision-making regarding retreatment. The use of OCT, together with anti-vascular endothelial growth factor therapy, has greatly improved visual outcomes of many outer retinal diseases.

© 2014 S. Karger AG, Basel

An understanding of the normal outer retinal structure, as represented on the spectral domain optical coherence tomography (OCT) (fig. 1), is crucial in the evaluation of the morphological changes which result from retinal diseases. Using the time-domain OCT, the detailed imaging of the individual layers and structures of the outer retina was not possible. This has changed with excellent spatial resolution afforded by spectral domain OCT technology, which delivers sections of the macula closely approximating histological specimens viewed microscopically.

The outer retinal layers of the normal eye show three distinct bands on the spectral domain OCT: (1) retinal pigment epithelium (RPE) band – consisting of the RPE, Bruch's membrane and choriocapillaris; (2) anterior to the RPE – comprising external limiting membrane, inner segment-outer segment (IS-OS) line, and Verhoeff's membrane; (3) posterior to the RPE – middle and outer layers of the choroid.

Further, Pircher et al. [1] described four distinct bands as follows:
– Band 1: external limiting membrane.
– Band 2: interface of the inner and outer segments of the photoreceptor layer (IS-OS junction).
– Band 3: outer segment RPE interdigitation (Verhoeff's membrane).
– Band 4: RPE/Bruch's membrane complex (fig. 2).

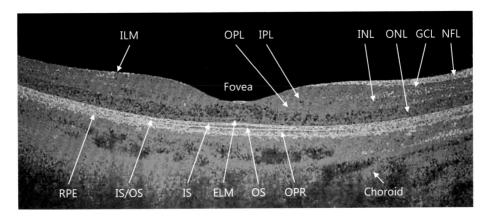

Fig. 1. Spectral domain OCT of the normal macula. NFL = Nerve fiber; OPL = outer plexiform layer; ILM = internal limiting membrane; ONL = outer nuclear layer; GCL = ganglion cell layer; ELM = external limiting membrane; IPL = inner plexiform layer; IS = photoreceptor inner segment; INL = inner nuclear layer; OS = photoreceptor outer segment; RPE = retinal pigment epithelium; IS/OS = interface between IS and OS.

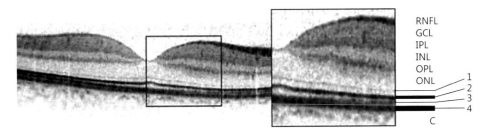

Fig. 2. Four distinct bands of the outer retina on spectral domain OCT according to Pircher et al. [1]. Band 1: ELM. Band 2: interface of the inner and outer segments of the photoreceptor layer (IS-OS junction). Band 3: outer segment-RPE interdigitation (Verhoeff's membrane). Band 4: RPE/ Bruch's membrane complex. RNFL = Retinal nerve fiber layer; GCL = ganglion cell layer; IPL = inner plexiform layer; INL = inner nuclear layer; OPL = outer plexiform layer; ONL = outer nuclear layer; C = choriocapillaris and choroidea.

How to Evaluate the Macular OCT

(1) Study carefully the distinct most prominent hyper-reflective RPE band: look for irregularities, thickening, fragmentation, breaks, disruption, shadowing and separation of RPE from Bruch's membrane.

(2) Turn your attention to the zone anterior to the RPE band, taking note of the following features: retinal thickness, presence of cavities, deposits and hyper-reflective dots.

(3) Analyze the neurosensory retinal layers, membranes and vitreoretinal interface.

(4) Examine the zone posterior to the RPE band to determine if there is hyper-reflectivity (choroidal atrophy) or hyporeflectivity (shadowing).

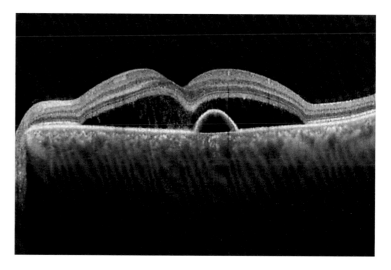

Fig. 3. Neurosensory detachment in CSC, with a small pigment epithelial detachment just temporal to the fovea. Elongated outer segments of photoreceptors are clearly visible on the underside of the neural retina. The 'septae' traversing the subretinal space on the nasal aspect of the detachment represent retinoschisis, indicative of the long-standing nature of the detachment.

OCT Features of Central Serous Chorioretinopathy

The classic OCT finding in active central serous chorioretinopathy (CSC) is localized neurosensory detachment. In addition, elongated outer segments and pigment epithelial detachment may accompany the neurosensory fluid. Long-standing cases may show a 'split' in the neural retina (retinoschisis), or RPE thinning and atrophy (fig. 3).

Some cases may be caused by an optic disc pit, which shows a deep defect in the optic nerve margin, associated with a schisis-like separation between the inner and outer retina. Enhanced depth imaging (EDI)-OCT is a new imaging modality to enable high-resolution OCT imaging of external retinal layers, the choroid and lamina cribrosa [2].

In a study of 19 patients with CSC, Imamura et al. [3] found a mean subfoveal choroidal thickness of 505 μm (SD 124 μm, range 439–573 μm), significantly higher than normative data reported previously. Among those who had unilateral CSC, choroidal thickness was also increased in the disease-free fellow eye [4]. Increased choroidal thickness is thought to be due to increased circulation and vascular dilatation, consistent with indocyanine green (ICG) angiography studies which show diffuse ICG leakage in the choroid in both eyes, even if only one eye has clinically demonstrable CSC. Furthermore, Maruko et al. [5] have shown that choroidal thickness is reduced after successful treatment with photodynamic therapy compared to laser photocoagulation. Photodynamic therapy is thought to reduce choroidal vascular hyperpermeability, leading to reduction in choroidal thickness as measured on EDI-OCT (fig. 4).

OCT in Age-Related Macular Degeneration (AMD)

The OCT shows different features depending on the type of age-related macular degeneration (AMD). In dry AMD, OCT shows drusen and geographic atrophy. In wet AMD, the OCT findings include choroidal neovascularization (CNV type I, II), pigment epithelial detachment, RPE tear/rip, retinal angiomatous proliferation (RAP) and polypoidal choroidal vasculopathy (PCV).

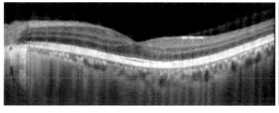
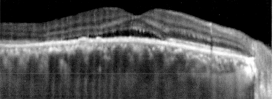

Fig. 4. Normal choroidal thickness on EDI-OCT (right); marked increased choroidal thickness on EDI-OCT (left) in a patient with acute CSC. The diffuse choroidal vascular hyperpermeability results in significant thickening of the choroid as measurable on EDI-OCT. With verterporfin photodynamic therapy, the choroidal thickness normalizes, unlike focal laser photocoagulation, in which the choroidal thickness remains unchanged.

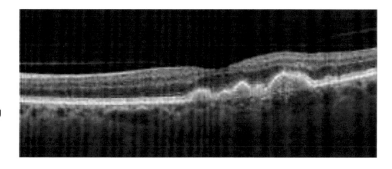

Fig. 5. The OCT in dry AMD showing nodular deposits between the RPE and Bruch's membrane, causing focal elevation of the RPE.

OCT in Dry Age-Related Macular Degeneration

Soft drusen may be visualized as focal, shallow elevations of well-defined RPE band depositions between the RPE basal lamina and the inner collagenous layer of Bruch's membrane (fig. 5). Geographic atrophy manifests as reduced macular thickness, loss of RPE cells, shown as thinning or absence of the RPE band, increased deep reflectivity stemming from the unimpeded penetration of light allowed when RPE melanin is absent and collapse of the outer retinal layers immediately adjacent to the zone of atrophy.

Choroidal Neovascularization

Typical features of wet AMD include macular thickening from neurosensory, intraretinal and sub-RPE fluid; RPE fragmentation, fusiform

thickening, splitting or disruption; and high reflectivity of the choriocapillaris (fig. 6).

Two main types of CNV based on the location of the lesion in relation to the RPE layer have been described. The clinical observations were correlated to histopathology sections and predated OCT examination. Type 1 CNV was described as sub-RPE CNV, where the lesion was limited to the area between the RPE and Bruch's membrane. This is clearly illustrated in OCT imaging of type 1 CNV. Type 2 CNV is described as neovascularization which occurs in the subretinal space above the level of the RPE. Since this early classification system, other authors have added a type 3 CNV, which refers to retinal angiomatous proliferation within the deep neural retina [6].

The OCT is indispensable in detecting exudative activity of the CNV in AMD. Figure 7 shows a case which illustrates the difficulty in determining the cause of reduced vision and metamorphopsia in a patient with confluent soft drusen at the macula. The fluorescein angiogram is equivocal for presence of leakage. The OCT, however, clearly demonstrates the presence of a small neurosensory detachment, confirming activity of CNV, and confirming the need for anti-VEGF therapy.

Retinal Angiomatous Proliferation

RAP is an uncommon but important cause of exudative maculopathy in AMD. The main OCT features include intraretinal edema in association with a serous pigment epithelial detachment, presence of a deep retinal hyper reflective mass, intraretinal hemorrhage, supported by ICG evidence of retinochoroidal anastomosis, most visible using SLO video angiography. RAP is associated with a poorer visual outcome and usually requires more frequent and longer anti-VEGF treatment compared to choroidal neovascularization [7].

Comparison between Fluorescein Angiography and OCT in Age-Related Macular Degeneration

Fluorescein angiography has been the gold standard of evaluation of AMD in the era before OCT was available. Indeed, the OCT has not replaced the FA in the diagnosis of exudative AMD. Both investigations are complementary and FA should not be omitted in the initial evaluation of every patient presenting with exudative AMD. The FA shows the vascular component of the fibrovascular CNV membrane, topography and area covered by CNV, and presence of leakage, pooling or RPE transmission window defects from atrophy. However, its main disadvantages are: it is an invasive procedure with rare potentially serious adverse events, it does not show whether CNV are located beyond or upon the RPE nor reveal extent of retinal damage caused, and it cannot provide quantitative measurement of macular thickness.

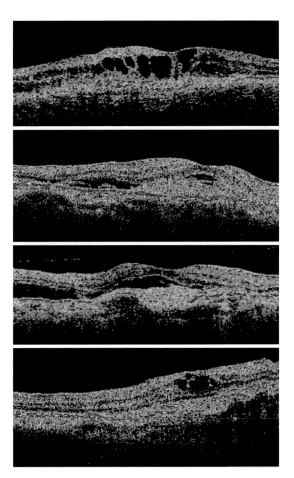

Fig. 6. OCT signs of wet AMD are demonstrated in these examples (from top to bottom): RPE fragmentation; fusiform thickening of the RPE-Bruch's line; splitting and disruption of the RPE with increased reflectivity of the underlying choriocapillaris; and macular edema, consisting of intra- and subretinal fluid.

Role of OCT in Wet Age-Related Macular Degeneration

There are two major roles of the OCT in the management of wet AMD. Firstly, the quantitative OCT ('fast' scanning protocols) allows accurate and repeatable measurements of the macula, especially the center-point thickness, also known as central subfield thickness. Comparison of central subfield thickness before and after treatment al-

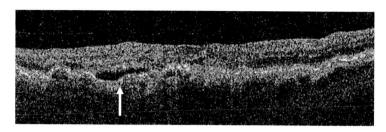

Fig. 7. This patient presented with large soft confluent drusen and recent metamorphopsia, although visual acuity remained unchanged. The clinical examination did not show any signs of choroidal neovascularization, but the OCT clearly demonstrated new neurosensory fluid (arrow) at the macula, indicating disease activity and necessitating anti-VEGF therapy.

lows objective assessment of the effectiveness of treatment and helps determine if further treatment is necessary. All major treatment trials for AMD have employed the evaluation of central subfield thickness as an outcome measure of treatment.

Besides quantitative changes on the OCT, qualitative OCT ('regular' scanning protocols) changes are as, if not more, important because these protocols define specific structural changes caused by CNV leak, such as the presence of diffuse retinal edema, intraretinal cysts, subretinal fluid and sub-RPE fluid.

Because the aim of the new treatments of AMD is not to destroy CNV but to limit their extension and stop exudation, qualitative criteria of efficacy have become more important. Some of these criteria include the flattening of serous retinal detachment; elimination of any fluid; normalization of macular thickness; and restoration of outer retinal bands, e.g. IS-OS line.

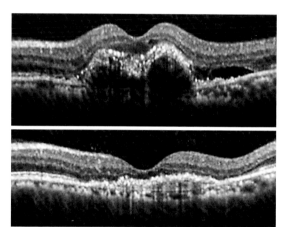

Fig. 8. This patient was treated successfully with anti-VEGF therapy for occult choroidal neo vascularization (top), but visual acuity did not improve significantly because the IS-OS junction was already disrupted before treatment and remained so despite flattening of the macula (bottom).

Inner Segment-Outer Segment Line

The IS-OS line represents the junction between the inner and outer segments of the macular photoreceptor cells. In the normal state, it should appear smooth, linear and complete without disruption. The IS-OS line may be broken or disrupted, deformed by folds or RPE detachments, thickened or even absent from pathological processes.

Shin et al. [8] found that foveal photoreceptor integrity was closely associated with final visual acuity in neovascular AMD after treatment. Ini-

tial visual acuity, IS/OS and external limiting membrane integrity, central macular thickness, and choroidal neovascularization height were correlated with final photoreceptor integrity, and they would be visual prognostic factors after resolution of exudation (fig. 8).

Outer Retinal Hyper-Reflective Dots

These foci are discrete areas of hyper-reflectivity within the inner and outer retinal layers as seen on the spectral domain OCT. The lower resolu-

OCT of the Outer Retinal Layers

31

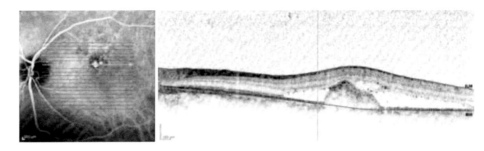

Fig. 9. Characteristic features of polypoidal choroidal vasculopathy on SD-OCT include a sharply inverted V-shaped elevation of the RPE, polypoidal lesions between the RPE and Bruch's membrane, irregular undulation of the RPE representing the branching vascular network, and adjacent neurosensory detachment.

Table 1. Typical pathological findings of outer retinal diseases on the OCT

Outer neural retina
    Diabetic macular edema
    Macular telangiectasia
    Acute macular neuroretinopathy
Subretinal space
    Central serous chorioretinopathy
    Type II (classic) CNV
    Photoreceptor layer
    Cone rod dystrophy
    Macular hole
RPE/Bruch's membrane
    Dry AMD: drusen, geographic atrophy
    Wet AMD: pigment epithelial detachment, type I
        (occult) CNV, RAP, RPE tear/rip
    Polypoidal choroidal vasculopathy
    Pseudo-AMD: vitelliform macular degeneration
    Best disease
    Angioid streaks

---

tion and pixilation in time-domain OCTs do not allow adequate visualization of these lesions. These lesions have been described for the first time by Coscas et al. [9], in AMD and a variety of retinal vascular diseases, such as diabetic macular edema [10], retinal vein occlusions [11] and parafoveal telangectasia [12].

These lesions are thought to represent activated microglial cells, reflective of an underlying inflammatory mechanism of retinal vascular diseases [9]. These foci correlate with visual prognosis, integrity of the external limiting membrane and IS/OS line. With successful treatment, these lesions resolved and their resolution was associated with better final visual acuity.

Polypoidal Choroidal Vasculopathy

While the gold standard for the diagnosis of PCV is indocyanine green angiography, there are characteristic features of PCV on spectral domain OCT [13] which help support the diagnosis (fig. 9).

The most reliable of these signs is a sharp inverted V-shaped elevation of RPE, usually lying between the RPE and Bruch's membrane. This sign may correspond to an orange-red subretinal nodule, which is a clinical hallmark of the disease. In addition to the visualization of polypoidal structures, the OCT sometimes reveals irregular undulation of RPE representing the branching vascular network.

When active, the lesion is exudative; hence an adjacent neurosensory detachment and pigment epithelial detachment are common accompanying signs on the OCT. As in wet AMD, OCT signs of activity help guide retreatment decisions.

Outer Retinal Tubulations

This lesion was first described in 2009 [14]. Degenerating photoreceptors may become arranged in a circular or ovoid fashion. They are best visualized with en face C-scan, which show single straight or branching tubules to complex cavitary networks, usually overlying areas of pigment epithelial alteration or subretinal fibrosis. These lesions remain stable over time. About 25% of any disease affecting the outer retina and retinal pigment epithelium may show this finding, which are often misinterpreted as intraretinal or subretinal fluid, prompting unnecessary anti VEGF therapy.

Conclusions

The spectral domain OCT is an invaluable tool in analysis of the outer retinal layers: RPE-Bruch's complex, anterior to the RPE, posterior to the RPE.

Different macular conditions have characteristic OCT features which aid diagnosis and monitoring of natural history or response to treatment.

Analysis of the IS-OS line is useful for evaluation of integrity of photoreceptors, and hence visual prognosis.

Today, the OCT has become indispensable in the management of outer retinal diseases such as wet AMD.

References

1 Pircher M, et al: Human macula investigated in vivo with polarization-sensitive optical coherence tomography. Invest Ophthalmol Vis Sci 2006;47:5487–5494.
2 Spaide RF, Koizumi H, Pozzoni MC: Enhanced depth imaging spectral-domain optical coherence tomography. Am J Ophthalmol 2008;146:496–500.
3 Imamura Y, et al: Enhanced depth imaging optical coherence tomography of the choroid in central serous chorioretinopathy. Retina 2009;29.10:1469–1473.
4 Iida T, et al: Persistent and bilateral choroidal vascular abnormalities in central serous chorioretinopathy. Retina 1999; 19:508–512.
5 Maruko I, et al: Subfoveal choroidal thickness after treatment of central serous chorioretinopathy. Ophthalmology 2010;117:1792–1799.
6 Freund KB, et al: Type 3 neovascularization: the expanded spectrum of retinal angiomatous proliferation. Retina 2008; 28:201–211.
7 Viola F, et al: Retinal angiomatous proliferation: natural history and progression of visual loss. Retina 2009;29:732–739.
8 Shin HJ, Chung H, Kim HC: Association between foveal microstructure and visual outcome in age-related macular degeneration. Retina 2011;31:1627–1636.
9 Coscas G, et al: Hyper-reflective dots: a new spectral-domain optical coherence tomography entity for follow-up and prognosis in exudative age-related macular degeneration. Ophthalmologica 2013;229.1:32–37.
10 Uji A, et al: Association between hyper-reflective foci in the outer retina, status of photoreceptor layer, and visual acuity in diabetic macular edema. Am J Ophthalmol 2012;153:710–717.
11 Ogino K, et al: Characteristics of optical coherence tomographic hyperreflective foci in retinal vein occlusion. Retina 2012;32.1:77–85.
12 Baumuller S, et al: Outer retinal hyperreflective spots on spectral-domain optical coherence tomography in macular telangiectasia type 2. Ophthalmology 2010;117:2162–2168.
13 Ojima Y, et al: Improved visualization of polypoidal choroidal vasculopathy lesions using spectral-domain optical coherence tomography. Retina 2009;29.1: 52–59.
14 Zweifel SA, et al: Outer retinal tubulation: a novel optical coherence tomography finding. Arch Ophthalmol 2009; 127.12:1596–1602.

Dr. Adrian Koh, MD, FRCS, MMed (Ophth), FRCOphth, FAMS
Eye & Retina Surgeons, Camden Medical Centre #13-03
1 Orchard Boulevard
Singapore 248649 (Singapore)
E-Mail dradriankoh@eyeretinasurgeons.com

Coscas G, Loewenstein A, Bandello F (eds): Optical Coherence Tomography.
ESASO Course Series. Basel, Karger, 2014, vol 4, pp 34–45 (DOI: 10.1159/000355893)

Optical Coherence Tomography Findings in the Choroid

Gabriel Coscas[a, b] · Florence Coscas[a, b]

[a]Department of Ophthalmology, University Paris Est Créteil, Centre Hospitalier Intercommunal de Créteil, Créteil, and [b]Centre d'Ophtalmologie de l'Odéon, Paris, France

Abstract

We discuss the role of optical coherence tomography (OCT) in the evaluation of the changes in the choroid from normal to different diseases, according to age and refractive status. Advances in spectral domain (SD)-OCT have enabled clinicians to visualize in detail the various structures of the choroid using the enhanced depth imaging technique, and, more recently, with the new generation of prototypes swept source (SS)-OCT (1,050 nm and higher scan rate). The software update version (5.4) automatically produced inverted capturing images and the eye tracking technology improves image quality, with a high inter- and intraobserver reproducibility but without automatic measuring software. Choroidal thickness (CT) is defined as the distance between the outer borders of the RPE to the hyper-reflective line of the choroid/sclera boundary at predefined intervals of the inner surface of the sclera. The boundaries of the choroid are difficult to define: not so much for the anterior limit (posterior limit of RPE band), but mainly because of the posterior limit that varies in appearance. Normal choroidal thickness has been described with the Spectralis® as 287 ± 76 μm and with the Cirrus® as 272 ± 81 μm, with a statistically significant reproducibility (Bland and Altman). CT is thickest subfoveally and thins nasally more than temporally. There is a negative correlation between CT and age (decrease of 1.56 per year). Subfoveal CT in subjects aged more than 70 years is 224.8 ± 52.9 μm. These results are statistically different from CT in wet age-related macular disease (171.2 ± 38.5 μm) and from CT in dry early age-related macular disease (177.4 ± 49.7 μm), as well as from CT in vascular polypoidal choroidopathy (438.3 ± 87.8 μm) and CT in central serous choroidopathy (367.81 ± 105.56 μm).
© 2014 S. Karger AG, Basel

Optical Coherence Tomography Findings in the Choroid

The choroid plays an important role in ocular physiology by providing metabolic support to the retinal pigment epithelium (RPE) and outer retina. Understanding the anatomic structures of the choroid may provide insight to the pathophysiology of diseases of the choroid and the retina.

Visualization of the choroid was difficult by indirect ophthalmoscopy and fluorescein angiography, easier and more efficient with SLO-ICG-A, but without 3D evaluation. With the advancement of spectral domain-optical coherence tomography (SD-OCT), in vivo images of the choroid are now available.

In typical SD-OCT, the signal strength, posterior to the RPE, is decreased due to the use of near-infrared wavelengths (850 nm) that penetrate well into the retina, whereas deeper penetration is limited because of the high back-scattering induced by the RPE.

This is compensated by new and enhanced software which enables visualization of the choroid and its boundaries and will allow choroidal thickness measurements.

Advances in SD-OCT have enabled clinicians to visualize in detail the various structures of the choroid using the enhanced depth imaging (EDI) technique, and, more recently, with the new generation of prototypes of swept source-OCT (SS-OCT) (1,050 nm and higher scan rate).

EDI-OCT Protocol

The method of obtaining EDI-OCT images (Spectralis®, Heidelberg) has been reported with published data [1, 2] and that enabled the cross-sectional thickness to be evaluated.

The software update version (5.4), automatically produced inverted capturing images and the eye tracking technology improves image quality, with a high inter- and intraobserver reproducibility (but without automatic measuring software).

Choroidal Thickness

Choroidal thickness (CT) is defined as the distance between the outer borders of the RPE to the hyper-reflective line of the choroid/sclera boundary, measured at predefined intervals of the inner surface of the sclera subfoveally and at 1,500-, 1,000- and 500-μm intervals from center to nasal to temporal and from superior to inferior.

Boundaries of the Choroid

The boundaries of the choroid are difficult to define: not so much for the anterior limit (posterior limit of RPE band), but mainly for the posterior limit that varies in appearance. It is usually called the 'choroidal-scleral junction', but is frequently difficult to define.

This needs to consider either (fig. 1):
– the 'lamina fusca' (LF), natural anatomical boundary, not always visible, or
– the 'suprachoroidal space' (SCS), thin OCT dark layer, sometimes virtual, or
– the 'outer vascular limit' (OVL), frequently the only landmark available.

Choroid Thickness Measurements

Choroid thickness measurements are affected by boundary criteria:

In our study of 96 eyes, the *OVL* is only visible in 50% (48 eyes). In which no SCS or LF were detectable. Including 28 eyes (60%) that were high myopic with choroid thinning.

The *LF* was detectable in 35% (34 eyes) without the SCS being visible. In these cases, the measurements are easier but LF is too rarely visible.

Presence of the *SCS* must be remembered as visible in 15% (14 eyes). It may be more frequently associated with myopia or retinal pathology.

A common posterior boundary definition is necessary to avoid significant measurements bias. In future studies, it could become compulsory to define precisely which posterior limit (OVL or LF or SCS) has been selected.

Normal Choroidal Thickness

Since the development of the EDI technique, many investigations have been published, related to bi-dimensional detailed thickness analysis.

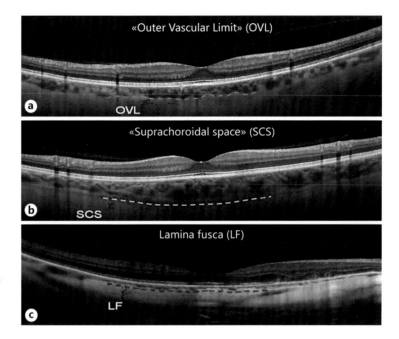

Fig. 1. The posterior boundaries of the choroid. **a** OVL. Frequently the only landmark available. **b** SCS: thin OCT dark layer, sometimes virtual. **c** LF. Natural anatomical boundary but not always visible.

Normal choroidal thickness has been described by Margolis et al. [3] with Spectralis, as 287 ± 76 μm, and by Manjunath et al. [4] with Cirrus®, as 272 ± 81 μm, with a statistically significant reproducibility (Bland and Altman). CT has been shown to be thickest subfoveally and thinner nasally more than temporally.

A negative correlation has been evidenced between CT and age, with a decrease of 1.56 per year and the mean subfoveal CT in subjects aged more than 70 years is 224.8 ± 52.9 μm.

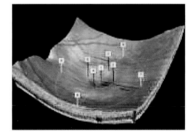

Fig. 2. Measurements at predefined intervals, subfoveally and at 1,500-, 1,000- and 500-μm intervals from center to nasal and to temporal and from superior to inferior.

Values in Different Diseases

These values in normal subjects are statistically different in different diseases:

The mean CT in wet age-related macular degeneration (AMD) is 171.2 ± 38.5 μm and, similarly, the mean CT in dry AMD is 177.4 ± 49.7 μm. These values are clearly different from the mean CT in vascular polypoidal choroidopathy (438.3 ± 87.8 μm). They are also different from the mean CT values in central serous choroidopathy (367.81 ± 105.56 μm).

Method of Measurement of Choroidal Thickness

All measurements are made at predefined intervals of the inner surface of the retina, subfoveally and at 1,500-, 1,000- and 500-μm intervals from center to nasal to temporal and from superior to inferior (fig. 2–4).

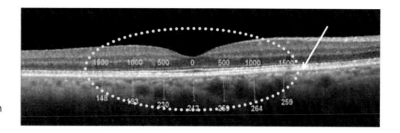

Fig. 3. Measurements: at the fovea center, ±500, ±1,000 and ±1,500 μm away from the fovea center.

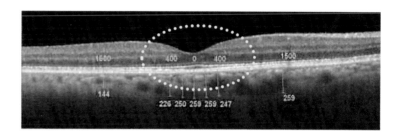

Fig. 4. Measurements: at the fovea center, ±200, ±400 and ±1,500 μm.

Results

The mean CT in SD-OCT has been evaluated in three different groups of patients: group 1 – normal and myopic, group 2 – high pathologic myopia, group 3 – myopia + choroidal new vessels (CNV) (fig. 5).

In group 1, CT was thicker subfoveally than nasally or temporally.

In group 2, CT was similar in different localizations (out of staphyloma).

In group 3, CT was irregular but thinner with severe myopia.

Mean Choroidal Thickness Variations According to Age

In healthy subjects, there was a significant decrease in CT according to age in all localizations.

Other studies have shown no change according to gender, or to moderate refractive errors (fig. 6).

Reproducibility and Repeatability

Reproducibility and repeatability have been studied by many investigators and are highly correlated across different SD-OCT systems (Spectralis, Optovue, Cirrus, Topcon) with good reproducibility and no significant CT changes [5–8].

There were no changes according to gender or to moderate refractive errors. A significant but moderate diurnal variation in CT was observed (29 + 6/−16 μm) [9, 10].

Many recent studies are oriented to choroidal volume analysis that could be a better tool to evaluate chorioretinal diseases [11, 12].

In many cases of healthy, normal eyes, measurements showed an accentuated asymmetry (fig. 7).

Choroidal Imaging, Choroidal Thickness and Disease

Recently, the choroid has been reported to be involved in the pathogenesis of various ocular diseases:

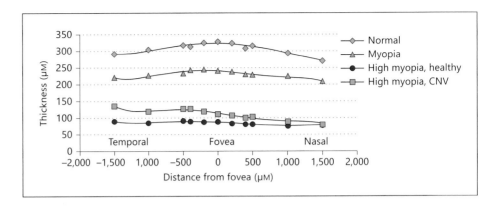

Fig. 5. Mean CT. Evaluation in SD-OCT in the three different groups: normal and myopic; high pathologic myopia; myopia + CNV.

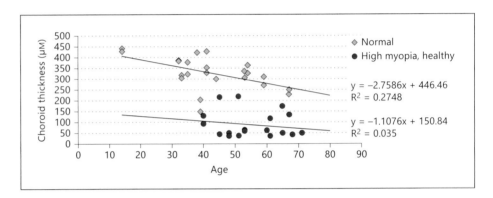

Fig. 6. Significant CT decrease according to age in the fovea and in all localizations.

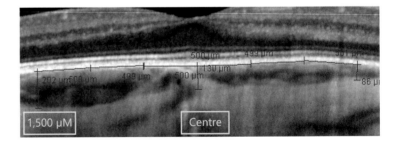

Fig. 7. Healthy, normal eye but accentuated asymmetry.

– Either diseases with *thinner choroid*, including pathologic myopia, exudative AMD and dry AMD, proliferative diabetic retinopathy, diabetic macular edema, multifocal choroiditis, retinitis pigmentosa, and glaucoma.

– Or, diseases with *thicker choroid*, including central serous chorioretinopathy (CSC), polypoidal choroidal vasculopathy (PCV), adult-onset foveomacular vitelliform dystrophy (AOFVD), and Vogt-Koyanagi-Harada syndrome.

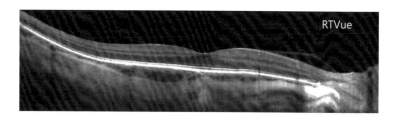

Fig. 8. Moderate myopia. Irregular thickness, nasal and temporal thinning and relatively good visual acuity (myopic eye, –8.00 dptr, 20/32, 44 years, female, horizontal scan).

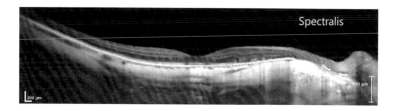

Fig. 9. Degenerative high myopia. Accentuated thinning (less than 50 µm), including nasal and temporal areas: relative conservation of VA (20/63), highly myopic eye, –16.00, 67 years old, female, RE, horizontal scan.

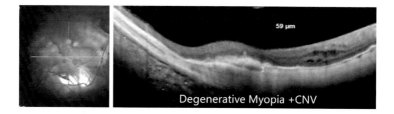

Fig. 10. Severe degenerative myopia, with CNV. Extreme thinning (less than 50 µm), but irregular with still some large vessels.

Diseases with Thinner Choroid: Pathologic Myopia

Excessive elongation affects also choroid and BM. In histology, choroidal thinning seems to be due initially to thinning of chorio-capillaris and focal lack of vessels.

The mean choroidal thickness has been measured: 93.2 ± 62.5 at a mean age of 59.15 ± 17.6 and a refractive error of 11.9 ± 3.7 [13].

The CT is negatively correlated with age, refractive error and presence of CNV.

CT may be a predictive factor for visual acuity but here are many unexpected differences and not always a positive correlation between CT and visual acuity.

Thinning of the choroid may be moderate in refractive myopic error, with irregular thickness, nasal and temporal thinning and relatively good visual acuity. Usually, only one layer of vessels is visible, with diminution of caliber (fig. 8).

In a highly myopic eye, there is an accentuated thinning (less than 50 µm), including nasal and temporal areas, sometimes with unexpected relative conservation of visual acuity (fig. 9).

In severe degenerative myopia, with CNV, there is usually extreme thinning (less than 50 µm), but irregular with some large vessels remaining (fig. 10).

Diseases with Thinner Choroid: Exudative AMD and Dry AMD

Abnormalities in choroidal circulation have been suggested to contribute to the development of AMD.

Fig. 11. Dry AMD eye, 71 years old, female, OS, horizontal scan. Note the severe thinning of the choroid, 50 µm, comparable to high myopia.

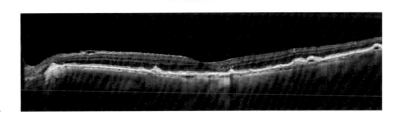

Fig. 12. Exudative AMD. Accentuated thinning 111–123 µm (only one layer of choroidal vessels).

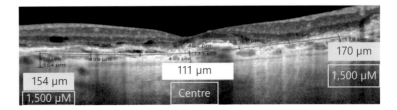

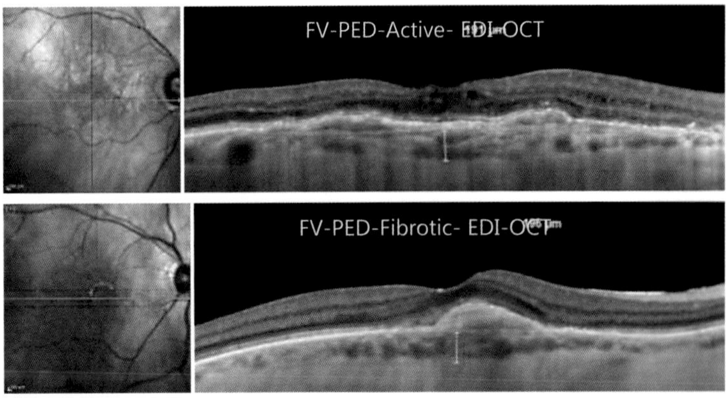

Fig. 13. FV-PED. Moderate thinning (191–196 µm) – quite similar in the active and late stages (only one layer of the choroidal vessels is distinctly visible).

Variations in choroid thickness may indicate the presence or progression of a disease, or provide insights into its prognosis.

Choroidal thinning has been observed, not only in dry AMD (177.4 ± 49.7 µm), but also in wet AMD (171.2 ± 38.5 µm) (fig. 11–13) [14].

The choroid thinning is usually moderate and quite similar in the active and late stages, but only one layer (the most peripheral) of choroidal vessels is distinctly visible.

The choroidal thinning is more accentuated in severe late fibrosis after CNV with atrophy of the sensory retina than in the less severe late stages of dry AMD.

These data have to be compared to healthy aged (75 years; 224.8 ± 52.9 µm) and to CT in PCV (438.3 ± 87.8 µm), or to CT in CSC (367.8 ± 105.56 µm) and also in early AMD, with a mean CT of 179 ± 27 vs. control (202 ± 18), p = 0.008 [15].

Diseases with Thinner Choroid: Diabetic Macular Edema

Choroidal thinning has been reported in diabetic macular edema (mean 63.3 µm), and in proliferative DR (mean 69.6 µm) [16].

Other studies reported less accentuated thinning, suggesting more or less reduction of choroi-

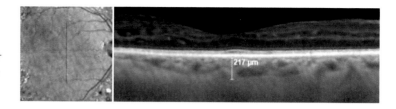

Fig. 14. Diabetic retinopathy. Choroidal thinning has been reported, macular edema (mean 63.3 µm), and in proliferative DR (mean 69.6 µm).

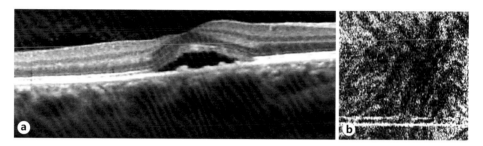

Fig. 15. CSC. **a** OCT B-scan: note the thick choroid, mainly at the level of the Haller vessels' layer; hyper-reflective stroma in the Sattler layer. **b** 'En face' OCT: thick large choroidal vessels.

dal blood flow and associated choroidal vasculopathy (obstruction of the choriocapillaris, microaneurysms, and neovascularization shown in histology) (fig. 14).

Diseases with Thicker Choroid

Recently, the choroid has also been reported to be involved with an increase of its thickness in the pathogenesis of various ocular diseases, including CSC, PCV, AOFVD, and Vogt-Koyanagi-Harada syndrome.

Diseases with Thicker Choroid: Central Serous Chorioretinopathy

Significant choroidal thickening has been shown in many publications, in CSC, with a range of 439–573 µm [16].

This thickening is usually bilateral and regressive posttreatment, particularly after treatment with PDT (fig. 15, 16).

The increase of thickness is commonly associated with diffuse hyperpermeability, clearly detectable in SLO-ICG.

These clinical changes, easy to evaluate with OCT examination may be used as useful parameter for diagnosis.

It was also found in other diseases with accumulation of subretinal fluid as in PVC and more recently in AOFVD.

In active chronic CSC, there is an Increase of CT in the whole area of the macula, with hyperpermeability and hyper-reflective dots visible in the retina and in the choroid (fig. 17).

Diseases with Thicker Choroid: Polypoidal Choroidal Vasculopathy

In PCV, there is an increase of CT in the whole posterior pole, contrasting with all the other forms of AMD.

This is also observed in the fellow eye, with dilatation of middle and large veins. In PCV, an increase in CT is associated to hyperpermeability and dilatation of the choroidal vessels [17] (fig. 18).

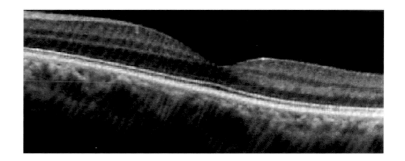

Fig. 16. CSC. Retina flattening, but only limited changes in CT after treatment with PDT.

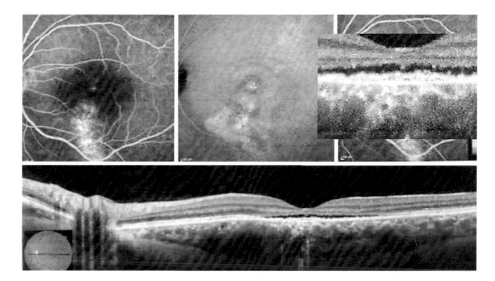

Fig. 17. Active chronic CSC. Increase of CT in the whole area of the macula. Note the hyperpermeability and the hyper-reflective dots; also note the retinal *and* choroidal increased thickness. From Jirarattanasopa et al. [18].

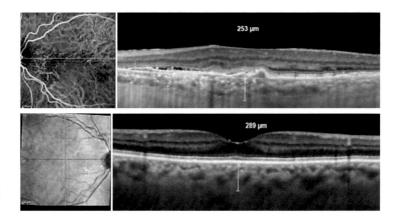

Fig. 18. PCV. Increase of CT in the whole posterior pole, also observed in the fellow eye.

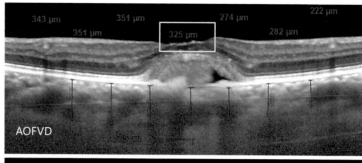

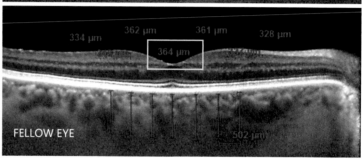

Fig. 19. Typical vitelliform lesion. Choroidal thickness (325 μm) thicker than in a normal person of the same age than in subjects with wet and dry AMD. In the fellow eye of same patient, choroidal thickness (364 μm) was thicker than in a normal person of the same age than in subjects with wet and dry AMD.

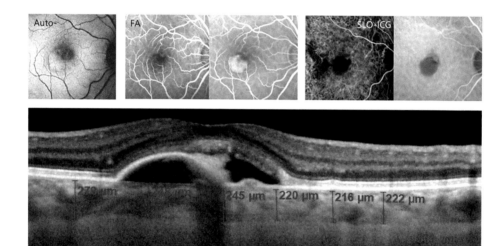

Fig. 20. Advanced stage of AOFVD with fluid accumulation (vitelliruptive stage). Increase of choroidal thickness could bring additional information to help the decision for treatment, and should be confirmed during follow-up [14].

Increase of CT Could Help in Differentiating AMD and PCV (Particularly Asiatic Forms)
In PCV, an increase of CT is associated with hyperpermeability, and dilatation of choroidal vessels.

Choroidal thickness has been evaluated in adult-onset foveomacular dystrophy versus dry and exudative AMD. In a recent study [14], we found that the differences between
- subfoveal CT in AOFVD with subretinal fluid (325.66 ± 86 μm),
- versus CT in exudative AMD (168.21 ± 57.7 μm), and

– versus CT in dry AMD (158.77 ± 68 μm) were statistically significant, with both p < 0.001 and p < 0.001,
– and, versus CT in elderly normal subjects (238.33 ± 83 μm), also statistically significant with p = 0.002.

The increase of CT was similar in the affected and the fellow eyes (325.66 ± 86 versus 317.52 ± 92.7 μm; difference not significant at p = 0.64).

Diseases with Thicker Choroid: Adult-Onset Foveomacular Vitelliform Dystrophy

In the typical vitelliform lesion, the choroid was thicker in normal subjects of the same age than in subjects with wet and dry AMD. In the fellow eye of the same patient, choroidal thickness was also thicker in normal subjects of the same age than in subjects with wet and dry AMD (fig. 19).

In the advanced stage of AOFVD with fluid accumulation (vitelliruptive stage), sometimes masquerading the presence of CNV, the increase in choroidal thickness could bring additional information to help in the decision for treatment (fig. 20).

The increase of thickness could be explained by the presence of dilated choroid vessels. This increase is not as much as in CSC or polyps.

But there is some continuum in these three diseases (CSC, PCV and AOFVD). CT measurement could become the criteria in case of a challenging diagnosis between exudative AMD and advanced stage of AOFVD with fluid accumulation and for decision of the treatment, with an eventual delay or contraindication for anti-VEGF intravitreous injection.

Conclusion

Analysis and evaluation of the choroid is already a normal part of the OCT examination. New developments will include swept source, Doppler color OCT, identifying the different vascular layers, arteries and veins, 'en face' OCT with specific segmentation, and probably many other new findings.

References

1 Spaide RF, Koizumi H, Pozzoni MC: Enhanced depth imaging spectral-domain optical coherence tomography. Am J Ophthalmol 2008;146:496–500.
2 Spaide RF: Enhanced depth imaging optical coherence tomography of retinal pigment epithelial detachment in age-related macular degeneration. Am J Ophthalmol 2009;147:644–652.
3 Margolis R, Spaide RF: A pilot study of enhanced depth imaging optical coherence tomography of the choroid in normal eyes. Am J Ophthalmol 2009;147: 811–815.
4 Manjunath V, Taha M, Fujimoto JG, Duker JS: Choroidal thickness in normal eyes measured using Cirrus HD optical coherence tomography. Am J Ophthalmol 2010;150:325–329.

5 Rahman W, Chen FK, Yeoh J, Patel P, Tufail A, Da Cruz L: Repeatability of manual subfoveal choroidal thickness measurements in healthy subjects using the technique of enhanced depth imaging optical coherence tomography. Invest Ophthalmol Vis Sci 2011;52:2267–2271.
6 Branchini L, Regatieri CV, Flores-Moreno I, Baumann B, Fujimoto JG, Duker JS: Reproducibility of choroidal thickness measurements across three spectral domain optical coherence tomography systems. Ophthalmology 2012;119:119–123.
7 Yamashita T, Yamashita T, Shirasawa M, Arimura N, Terasaki H, Sakamoto T: Repeatability and reproducibility of subfoveal choroidal thickness in normal eyes of Japanese using different SD-OCT devices. Invest Ophthalmol Vis Sci 2012;53:1102–1107.

8 Coscas G, Zhou Q, Coscas F, Zucchiatti I, Rispoli M, Uzzan J, De Benedetto U, Savastano MC, Soules K, Goldenberg D, Loewenstein A, Lumbroso B: Choroid thickness measurement with RTVue optical coherence tomography in emmetropic eyes, mildly myopic eyes, and highly myopic eyes. Eur J Ophthalmol 2012;22:992–1000.
9 Chakraborty R, Read SA, Collins MJ: Diurnal variations in axial length, choroidal thickness, intraocular pressure, and ocular biometrics. Invest Ophthalmol Vis Sci 2011;52:5121–5129.
10 Tan CS, Ouyang Y, Ruiz H, Sadda SR: Diurnal variation of choroidal thickness in normal, healthy subjects measured by spectral domain optical coherence tomography. Invest Ophthalmol Vis Sci 2012;53:261–266.

11 Hirata M, Tsujikawa A, Matsumoto A, Hanga M, Ooto S, Yamashiro K, Akiba M, Yoshimura N: Macular choroidal thickness and volume in normal subjects measured by swept-source optical coherence tomography. Invest Ophthalmol Vis Sci 2011;52:4971–4978.

12 Chahablani J, Barteselli G, Wang H, El-Emam S, Kozak I, Doede AL, Bartsch DU, Cheng L, Freeman WR: Repeatability and reproducibility of manual choroidal volume measurements using enhanced depth imaging optical coherence tomography. Invest Ophthalmol Vis Sci 2012;53:2274–2280.

13 Fujiwara T, Imamura Y, Margolis R, Slakter JS, Spaide RF: Enhanced depth imaging optical coherence tomography of the choroid in highly myopic eyes. Am J Ophthalmol 2009;148:445–450.

14 Coscas F, Puche N, Coscas G, Srour M, Français C, Clacet-Bernard A, Querques G, Souied EH: Comparison of macular choroidal thickness in adult onset foveomacular vitelliform dystrophy and age-related macular degeneration. Invest Ophthalmol Vis Sci 2014;55:64–69.

15 Wood A, Binns A, Margrain T, Drexler W, Považay B, Esmaeelpour M: Retinal and choroidal thickness in early age-related macular degeneration. Am J Ophthalmol 2011;152:1030–1038.

16 Regatieri CV, Branchini L, Carmody J, Fujimoto JG, Duker JS: Choroidal thickness in patients with diabetic retinopathy analyzed by spectral-domain optical coherence tomography. Retina 2012;32:563–568.

17 Chung SE, Kang SW, Lee JH, Kim YT: Choroidal thickness in polypoidal choroidal vasculopathy and exudative age-related macular degeneration. Ophthalmology 2011;118:840–845.

18 Jirarattanasopa P, Ooto S, Tsujikawa A, Yamashiro K, Hangai M, Hirata M, Matsumoto A, Yoshimura N: Assessment of macular choroidal thickness by optical coherence tomography and angiographic changes in central serous chorioretinopathy. Ophthalmology 2012;119:1666–1678.

Prof. Gabriel Coscas, MD
Department of Ophthalmology, University of Paris Est Créteil
Centre Hospitalier Intercommunal de Créteil
40, avenue de Verdun, FR–94010 Créteil (France)
E-Mail gabriel.coscas@gmail.com

Coscas G, Loewenstein A, Bandello F (eds): Optical Coherence Tomography.
ESASO Course Series. Basel, Karger, 2014, vol 4, pp 46–53 (DOI: 10.1159/000356055)

Pre- and Postsurgical Evaluation of the Retina by Optical Coherence Tomography

Marco Pellegrini · Ferdinando Bottoni · Matteo Giuseppe Cereda · Giovanni Staurenghi

Eye Clinic, Department of Biomedical and Clinical Science 'Luigi Sacco', Luigi Sacco Hospital, University of Milan, Milan, Italy

Abstract

Optical coherence tomography (OCT) is a noninvasive imaging technique providing high-resolution cross-sectional images of the retina, optic nerve and the anterior segment. OCT examination reveals to be instrumental in the diagnostic process and management of several medical and surgical conditions. A detailed study of sequential OCT images, moreover, allows a better understanding of the physiopathology of these affections and accurately depicts the dynamic healing processes after surgery is performed. An overview of some surgical entities with representative images and review of the literature is offered in this chapter.   © 2014 S. Karger AG, Basel

Since its introduction in 1991, optical coherence tomography (OCT) has become an essential tool for a noninvasive assessment of the retina providing high-resolution cross-sectional images [1]. Moreover, this technique allows a detailed analysis of the optic nerve and a comprehensive study of the anterior segment. As a consequence, the use of OCT in addition to other imaging studies (autofluorescence, fluorescein and indocyanine green angiography), has better clarified the pathophysiology of several affections. Enhanced depth imaging OCT, in particular, has later allowed a better view of the outer retina, choroid and retrobulbar structures [2].

For these reasons, OCT nowadays represents an instrumental imaging technique for the management of both medical and surgical affections including age-related macular degeneration, diabetic macular edema, vascular occlusions, uveitis, cellophane maculopathy, idiopathic macular holes, retinal detachments, and retinal and choroidal tumors. One of the most useful applications of OCT is its accuracy and reproducibility in monitoring retinal thickness as previously demonstrated by several studies. This allows a reliable follow-up and a better management of these affections [3].

The purpose of this chapter is to show some applications of this tool with particular attention to its utility in the diagnosis and follow-up of surgical cases.

Optic Pit

Optic disc pit is a congenital anomaly of the optic nerve firstly described by Wiethe in 1882. The prevalence of this condition accounts to 1:11,000 with no apparent predilection for race or gender. This condition is usually sporadic but mutations of PAX2 gene have been described. Optic pit is often asymptomatic and it can sometimes be discovered in adult patients during a routine eye visit. About 65% of cases are complicated by a macular neurosensory detachment [4, 5].

Due to a noncomplete understanding of its pathogenesis, the treatment of optic disk pit maculopathy is still controversial. Several strategies have been attempted in the last decades to manage this complication including argon laser photocoagulation, posterior scleral buckling, and pneumatic retinopexy as well as via pars plana vitrectomy. The rate of success of these strategies has been quantified in a review by Postel et al. [6] as 37% for argon laser photocoagulation on the temporal margin of the optic nerve, 63% for pneumatic retinopexy, 100% for macular buckling, and 97% for via pars plana vitrectomy.

Vitrectomy with induction of a posterior vitreous detachment at the optic disc without gas tamponade or laser photocoagulation seems to be an effective method of managing macular detachment resulting from this affection [7]. Nevertheless, induction of posterior vitreous detachment may be challenging in such a young population.

OCT imaging in eyes affected by optic pit typically displays a multilayer schisis-like configuration affecting both the inner and outer retina, a hole in the outer retina and a pocket of subretinal fluid (fig. 1a, b, 2a, c). A defect in the subarachnoid space with communication with the subretinal space can be noticed. More recently, a swept source OCT report has clearly evidenced a direct communication between the retro-bulbar subarachnoid space and the vitreous cavity [8].

As described by Hirakata and Bottoni, after surgery spectral domain-optical coherence tomography (SD-OCT) images display a gradual improvement with progressive reabsorption of the intraretinal fluid and disappearance of the inner/outer retinoschisis (fig. 1, 2) [8, 9]. The reestablishment of the macular structural integrity typically precedes the progressive reabsorption of subretinal fluid. All these changes usually correspond to an improvement in patients' best-corrected visual acuity (BCVA). A thickening of the photoreceptor outer segments is displayed by OCT as soon as the outer nuclear layer recovers (fig. 1f, 2f–h).

After complete reattachment, a pseudovitelliform lesion can be sometimes discovered as confirmed by fundus autofluorescence (FAF) due to an accumulation of lipofuscin bisretinoids in the outer segments of photoreceptors. The elongation of these structures corresponds to an increase signal at FAF. This hyperautofluorescence can manifest either with a granular or a more homogeneous and diffuse pattern. As hypothesized by Sparrow et al. [10], this FAF pattern likely reflects the increase of lipofuscin bisretinoids.

Diabetic Macular Edema

Diabetic retinopathy represents the first cause of legal blindness in the occidental world. In particular, in the USA its incidence approximately accounts for 75,000 new cases per year [11]. One of the main reasons of decreased BCVA in diabetic retinopathy is represented by macular edema, a condition considered multifactorial in its origin. The etiopathogenesis of this manifestation includes anomalies of the inner blood-retinal barrier, an increase of vascular endothelial growth factor (VEGF) and other vasoactive factors and alterations in the vitreoretinal barrier.

The diagnosis and management of diabetic retinopathy firmly relies on periodical clinical examinations of the fundus and imaging investigations including fluorescein angiography and OCT. In particular, OCT represents the most accurate tool

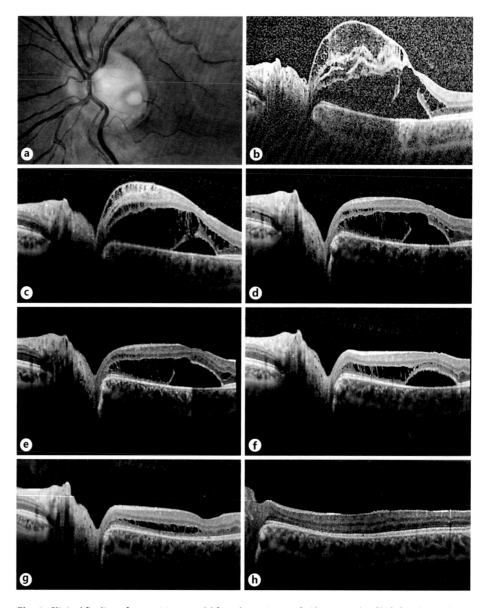

Fig. 1. Clinical findings from a 20-year-old female patient. **a, b** Photograph of left fundus and SD-OCT image before surgery showing a temporal optic disc pit, a multilayered inner and outer retinoschisis, a hole in the outer retina and a macular detachment. **c–h** SD-OCT 2 weeks (**c**), 1 (**d**), 3 (**e**), 6 (**f**), 12 (**g**), and 22 (**h**) months of follow-up after surgery. A progressive reduction of intraretinal and subretinal fluid occurs as long with the elongation of the photoreceptor outer segment (**f**). Images at 22 months after vitrectomy show complete disappearance of both the schisis and the macular detachment with final BCVA rising from 0.1 (baseline) to 1.0 (22-month visit).

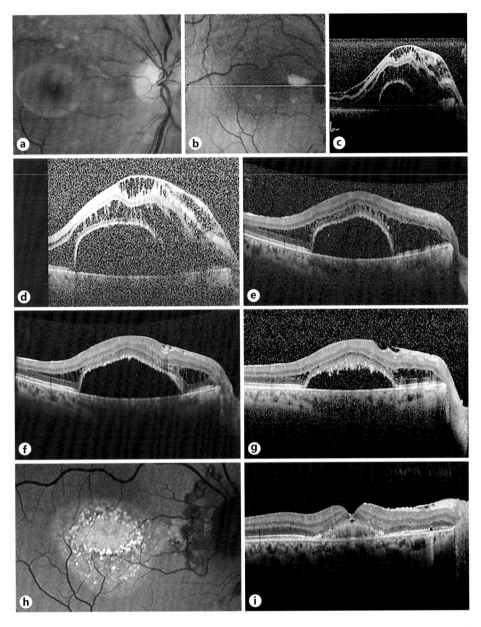

Fig. 2. 35-year-old male patient affected by optic pit in his right eye. **a–c** Clinical picture, FAF and SD-OCT images at baseline. **d–g**, **i** SD-OCT images at 4, 10, 13, 18 and 30 months of follow-up after vitrectomy showing gradual disappearance of intra and subretinal fluid progressively leading to a pseudovitelliform-like lesion. **h** FAF image showing increase autofluorescence corresponding to the thickened outer segments visible at 30 months' follow-up (**i**).

Fig. 3. a, **b** Patient affected by diabetic macular edema with no response to anti-VEGF therapies. **a** Examination before surgery shows a diffuse cystoid macular edema with residual vitreo-retinal adhesion and apparently intact outer retinal structures. **b** Four months after via pars plana vitrectomy and peeling of internal limiting membrane OCT displays reabsorption of intraretinal fluid. **c**, **d** Patient with full-thickness macular hole developing as a complication a few weeks after the surgery in a patient with diffuse macular edema. OCT allows a detailed assessment of inner and outer retina confirming a useful tool for early detection of complications. **e**, **f** Patient developing a lamellar macular hole as a complication of vitrectomy. OCT shows a foveal defect with partial conservation of outer retina and only minor disruption of photoreceptor layers.

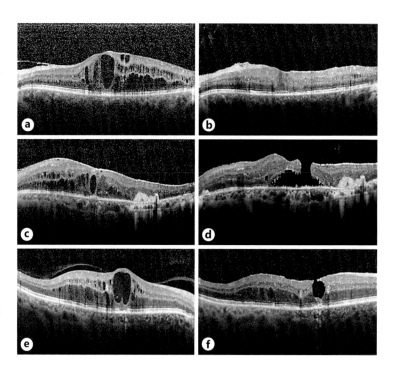

for detecting macular edema, which typically appears as constituted by hyporeflective intraretinal spaces, heterogeneous in size, leading to either focal or diffuse areas of retinal thickening.

Treatment of diabetic macular edema includes several options. Argon laser photocoagulation has represented the gold standard until the advent of the intravitreal therapies era (mainly represented by corticosteroids and anti-VEGF drugs). Nevertheless, via pars plana vitrectomy is another important therapeutic option, confirming the role of the vitreous in the pathogenesis of this affection.

In the preoperative evaluation of a patient undergoing a vitrectomy, OCT offers information regarding the pattern of edema, the distribution of the fluid, a quantification of the central retinal thickness as well as an overview regarding the integrity of the photoreceptors. Evaluation of the external limiting membrane (ELM) and the interface between inner and outer segments of the photoreceptors represents a useful tool, helping

the clinician to predict the prognosis after the treatment [12]. Similarly, after surgery, OCT allows a detailed analysis of the healing processes, displaying progressive changes in retinal thickness, showing the recovery of the physiological retinal morphology and the status of the outer retina. Additionally, OCT assists the surgeon in detecting possible complications, including the onset of macular holes, preretinal membranes, persistence of intra- and subretinal fluid or the appearance of a retinal detachment (fig. 3).

Macular Holes

There is general consensus that OCT plays an instrumental role in the diagnosis, classification and management of macular holes thanks to its ability to visualize the retinal anatomy with near microscopic resolution. Several OCT studies have added valuable information regarding the pathogenesis and course of these conditions; nevertheless, a multi-imaging approach including FAF, especially in the study of lamellar and macular pseudoholes, is recommended.

Lamellar macular holes at SD-OCT examination consist in partial thickness defects of the macula with an irregular foveal contour and a schisis between the inner and outer retinal layers in absence of any defect of the photoreceptors. A contribution to the understanding of the prognosis of this entity has been recently offered by a prospective OCT study. Periodical OCT examinations of 34 consecutive eyes followed over a mean period of 18 months showed a stable size in 79% of the cases with only 5.8% of the cases developing a full-thickness macular hole and requiring surgery [13].

Similarly, in the evaluation of full-thickness macular holes, OCT provides information regarding the entity of the defect, the status of the vitreous (presence of complete, incomplete vitreous detachment and, possibly, a vitreoretinal traction), the concomitant presence of epiretinal membranes, information regarding the integrity or an eventual damage of the outer retinal structures and, indirectly, an estimation of the largest basal diameter. In the last few years, in particular, significant attention has been given to the processes leading to the closure of the retinal defect. Michalewska et al. [14] were the first to examine by SD-OCT a large series of patients showing a gradual restoration of macular morphology that correlated with improved visual acuity. Bottoni et al. [15] prospectively evaluated 19 eyes affected by full-thickness macular holes undergoing vitrectomy with peeling of the internal limiting membrane.

The ELM, in particular, restored more rapidly than the other anatomic structures appearing normal in 53% of the eyes at the 1-month follow-up. In particular, this portion of the outer retina was continuous in 79% of the eyes despite persistent outer foveal alterations. Interestingly, no eyes displayed a continuous ellipsoid portion of the photoreceptors and an interrupted ELM anytime during follow-up. Besides foveal cysts could de-

velop during follow-up, in 45% of cases they gradually filled with a complete recovery of the ellipsoid segment of photoreceptors (fig. 4). An intact outer nuclear layer was described as necessary endpoint to achieve a complete restoration of the photoreceptor microstructure.

Miscellaneous

OCT represents a useful tool for evaluating eyes affected by either anterior segment or vitreoretinal affections. In particular, OCT examination facilitates the diagnostic process, addresses the clinician to the choice of the best treatment and, finally, allows predicting visual acuity prognosis (fig. 5a–e) [16].

In eyes affected by myopic macular schisis, OCT allows a definite diagnosis that was nearly impossible when based just on fundus examination. Additionally, it allows an evaluation in detail of the location of the disease, showing which layers result affected (split of the inner or outer retina). Despite being usually considered a stable condition, complications may occur. In such circumstance, OCT allows a prompt detection of macular holes, retinal detachments as well as recovery after surgery (fig. 5a, b).

The vitreomacular traction syndrome represents a complication of a noncomplete posterior vitreous detachment where the vitreous shows a persistent adherence to the retina in the macular area and optic nerve. Epiretinal membranes may be associated to this condition, appearing at OCT imaging with higher reflectivity and thicker compared to posterior hyaloid. In both vitreomacular traction syndrome and epiretinal membranes; moreover, a hyper-reflective deposit can be detected subfoveally [17]. This finding may correspond to accumulation of bisretinoids of lipofuscin below the retina following the loss of apposition between cone outer segment and retinal pigment epithelium (fig. 5c) [18]. After surgery, OCT examination allows quantifying the reduc-

Fig. 4. Closure of full-thickness macular hole following via pars plana vitrectomy. **a** Before surgery OCT displays a full-thickness macular defect with no chance to visualize the ELM nor the ellipsoid portion of photoreceptors. Some cysts can be detected adjacent to the hole margins. **b** Within 1 month from surgery, OCT allows an accurate assessment of the healing processes showing a progressive reestablishment of the inner retina. ONL appear to be preserved and ELM reveals to be the first structure to recover. At month 3 (**c**), OCT shows a gradual repair of the outer retina with progressive restoration of the ellipsoid portion of photoreceptors by month 6 (**d**) and, at a later stage, normal cone outer segments (**e**, month 9).

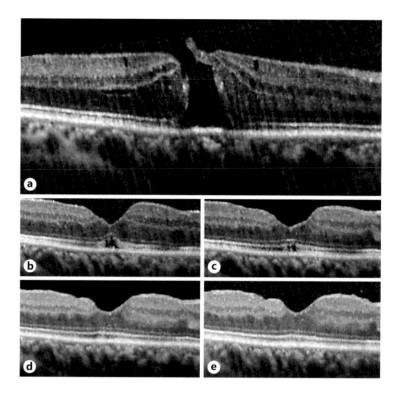

Fig. 5. a, **b** Myopic macular schisis showing a splitting of both the inner and outer retinal layers with thickening at the level of the vitreoretinal interface. After surgery, a normalization of the retinal profile occurs with apparently intact photoreceptors. **c** Macular pucker with evidence of subfoveal hyperreflective deposit (white arrow) likely corresponding to liposfuscin bisretinoids. **d**, **e** Case of cellophane maculopathy associated to an incomplete posterior vitreous detachment. At baseline a loss of physiological foveal depression can be visualized. After 4 months, a spontaneous peeling of the epiretinal membrane occurs concomitant to a posterior vitreous detachment with restoration of the normal foveal profile and minor residual irregularities in the inner layers.

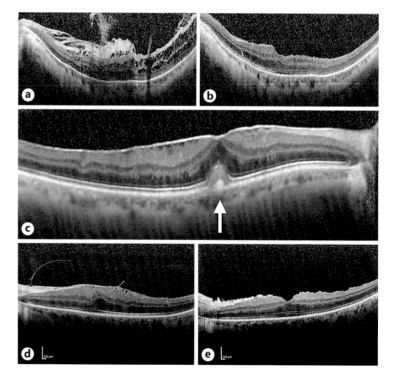

Pellegrini · Bottoni · Cereda · Staurenghi

tion in macular thickness and imaging the healing processes in the outer retina and the integrity of these structures during follow-up visits.

Finally, OCT allows also management of eyes affected by retinal detachment. This topic might be discussed in a dedicate chapter in order to be exposed in detail. Nevertheless, OCT allows an assessment of the macular region with distinction of macula on/macula off retinal detachments, retinal detachment/schisis, a quantification of the subretinal fluid and illustrates the behavior of the retina after treatment. Preoperative OCT, moreover, can display outer retinal corrugations in macula, already described as a predictive landmark of poor visual outcome. This finding, together with evidence of fluid below the fovea, may have implications for the urgency for these eyes to undergo surgical repair [19].

References

1 Huang D, Swanson EA, Lin CP, Schuman JS, Stinson WG, et al: Optical coherence tomography. Science 1991; 254:1178–1181.

2 Spaide RF, Koizumi H, Pozzoni MC: Enhanced depth imaging spectral-domain optical coherence tomography. Am J Ophthalmol 2008;146:496–500.

3 Giani A, Cigada M, Choudhry N, Peroglio Deiro A, et al: Reproducibility of retinal thickness measurements on normal and pathologic eyes by different optical coherence tomography instruments. Am J Ophthalmol 2010;150:815–824.

4 Wiethe T: Ein Fall von angeborener Difformität der Sehnervenpapille. Arch Augenheilk 1882;11:14–19.

5 Kranenburg EW: Crater-like holes in the optic disc and central serous retinopathy. Arch Ophthalmol 1960;64:912–924.

6 Postel EA, Pulido JS, Arch McNamara J, Johnson MW: The etiology and treatment of macular detachment associated with optic nerve pits and related anomalies. Trans Am Ophthalmol Soc 1998;96: 73–88.

7 Hirakata A, Inoue M, Hiraoka T, McCuen BW 2nd: Vitrectomy without laser treatment or gas tamponade for macular detachment associated with an optic disc pit. Ophthalmology 2012;119:810–818.

8 Katome T, Mitamura Y, Hotta F, Mino A, Naito T: Swept-source optical coherence tomography identifies connection between vitreous cavity and retrobulbar subarachnoid space in patient with optic disc pit. Eye (Lond) 2013 doi: 10.1038/eye.2013.175.

9 Bottoni F, Secondi R, Giani A, Cereda M, Staurenghi G: Maculopathy resolution after surgery for an optic disc pit. Ophthalmology 2013;120:877–878.

10 Sparrow JR, Yoon KD, Wu Y, Yamamoto K: Interpretations of fundus autofluorescence from studies of the bisretinoids of the retina. Invest Ophthalmol Vis Sci 2010;51:4351–4357.

11 Bresnik GH: Diabetic macular edema: a review. Ophthalmology 1986;97:989–997.

12 Otani T, Yamaguchi Y, Kishi S: Correlation between visual acuity and foveal microstructural changes in diabetic macular edema. Retina 2010;30:774–780.

13 Bottoni F, Deiro AP, Giani A, Orini C, Cigada M, Staurenghi G: The natural history of lamellar macular holes: a spectral domain optical coherence tomography study. Graefes Arch Clin Exp Ophthalmol 2013;251:467–475.

14 Michalewska Z, Michalewski J, Nawrocki J: Continuous changes in macular morphology after macular hole closure visualized with spectral optical coherence tomography. Graefes Arch Clin Exp Ophthalmol 2010;248:1249–1255.

15 Bottoni F, De Angelis S, Luccarelli S, Cigada M, Staurenghi G: The dynamic healing process of idiopathic macular holes after surgical repair: a spectral-domain optical coherence tomography study. Invest Ophthalmol Vis Sci 2011; 22;52:4439–4446.

16 Mirza RG, Johnson MW, Jampol LM: Optical coherence tomography use in evaluation of the vitreoretinal interface: a review. Surv Ophthalmol 2007;52: 397–421.

17 Tsunoda K, Watanabe K, Akiyama K, Usui T, Noda T: Highly reflective foveal region in optical coherence tomography in eyes with vitreomacular traction or epiretinal membrane. Ophthalmology 2012;119:581–587.

18 Cereda M, Caimi A, Bottoni F, Staurenghi G: Optical coherence tomography in eyes with vitreomacular traction. Ophthalmology 2013;120:e46–e47.

19 Cho M, Witmer MT, Favarone G, Chan RP, D'Amico DJ, Kiss S: Optical coherence tomography predicts visual outcome in macula-involving rhegmatogenous retinal detachment. Clin Ophthalmol 2012;6:91–96.

Prof. Giovanni Staurenghi
Eye Clinic, Luigi Sacco Hospital, University of Milan
Via G.B. Grassi 74, IT–20157 Milan (Italy)
E-Mail giovanni.staurenghi@unimi.it

Coscas G, Loewenstein A, Bandello F (eds): Optical Coherence Tomography.
ESASO Course Series. Basel, Karger, 2014, vol 4, pp 54–61 (DOI: 10.1159/000355917)

Optical Coherence Tomography in the Diagnosis of Challenging Macular Disorders

Giuseppe Querques[a, b] · Enrico Borrelli[b] · Anouk Georges[a] · Eric H. Souied[a]

[a]Department of Ophthalmology, University Paris Est Créteil, Centre Hospitalier Intercommunal de Créteil, Créteil, France; [b]Department of Ophthalmology, University Scientific Institute San Raffaele, Milan, Italy

Abstract

We discuss the role of the optical coherence tomography (OCT) in the diagnosis of challenging macular disorders through the presentation of four clinical cases. The first example describes a case of photic maculopathy secondary to uncomplicated cataract surgery. The OCT revealed a hyporeflective space (a 'partial-thickness hole') and was particularly useful to make the correct diagnosis and follow the spontaneous disease progression. The second example describes a case of posttraumatic photoreceptor disruption. The OCT showed a focal disruption of the inner segment/outer segment junction in the foveal region and was a very useful tool in the diagnosis. The third example describes a case of spontaneous retinal pigmented epithelium rip in nonexudative age-related macular degeneration in which OCT was very useful to exclude choroidal neovascularization and visualize the retinal pigmented epithelium rip. The fourth example shows the usefulness of OCT for diagnosis and follow-up of the vitelliform macular dystrophy preclinical stage: in this phase there is initially a thicker and more reflective appearance of the Verhoeff's membrane.

© 2014 S. Karger AG, Basel

This chapter discusses the importance of optical coherence tomography (OCT) in the diagnosis of challenging macular disorders through the presentation of four clinical cases and typical examples.

Clinical Case No. 01 – Photic Maculopathy Secondary to Uncomplicated Cataract Surgery

Introduction

Photic maculopathy may develop in patients exposed for a long time to an intense light source; moreover, this maculopathy has been well documented after ocular surgery, particularly in the setting of anterior segment procedures [1].

Pathogenesis

Photic maculopathy is the result of photochemical and thermal mechanisms either from sunlight or a microscope. Ultrastructural examination shows that the retinal pigment epithelium (RPE) and outer segments of the photoreceptors are the most susceptible to light insult [2].

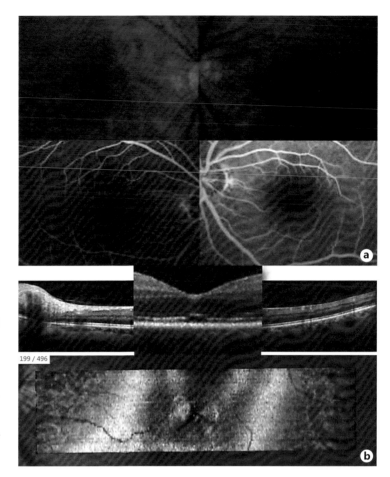

Fig. 1. Clinical case No. 1. **a** Baseline evaluation: fundus color photography and FA showing overall normal findings in both eyes. **b** Baseline evaluation: SD-OCT scan of the left eye shows a hyporeflective space in the outer retina (a 'partial-thickness hole') at the fovea. 'En face' SD-OCT shows a large 'star-shaped' discontinuity in the outer retinal layers centered on the fovea (bottom panel).

199 / 496

Clinical Presentation

Clinically, it is characterized by a yellowish lesion at the fovea, and by a central or para-central scotoma, which diminishes with time.

Case Report

A 36-year-old man presented with blurred vision in his left eye (LE) 1 week after uncomplicated cataract surgery. His best-corrected visual acuity (BCVA) was 20/20 in the right eye (RE) and 20/125 in the LE. Fundus biomicroscopy and fluorescein angiography (FA) showed overall normal findings in both eyes (fig. 1a). Spectral domain (SD)-OCT (Spectralis SD-OCT, Heidelberg Engineering, Heidelberg, Germany) showed normal findings in the RE, and revealed a hyporeflective space (a 'partial-thickness hole') in the outer retina of the LE at the fovea (fig. 1b). Microperimetry (MP1 Nidek Technology, Padova, Italy) revealed a reduction of the central retinal sensitivity in the LE. Multifocal-ERG (mfERG) showed reduced responses within the central 10° in the LE. Based on these findings, the patient was diagnosed with photic maculopathy secondary to uncomplicated cataract surgery. No treatment was undertaken, and the patient was then observed every 2 weeks.

The 1-month follow-up visit showed a BCVA improving to 20/40 in the LE. SD-OCT scans of the LE revealed a reduction of the 'partial-thickness hole' compared with the baseline evaluation

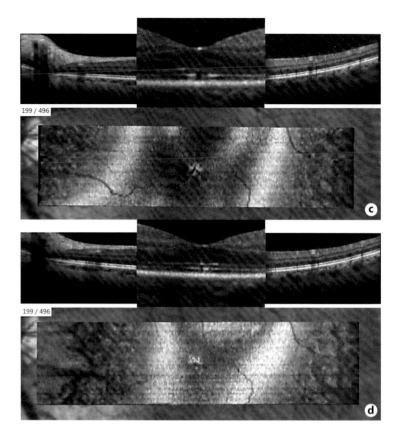

Fig. 1. Clinical case No. 1. **c** One-month follow-up visit: SD-OCT scan of the left fovea after 1 month shows a reduced hyporeflective space in the outer retina (a 'partial-thickness hole') compared with baseline evaluation (top panel, enlarged view). 'En face' SD-OCT centered on the fovea shows a 'star-shaped' discontinuity in the outer retinal layers, which appears reduced compared with baseline evaluation (bottom panel).
d Three-month follow-up visit: SD-OCT scan of the left eye shows an almost normal outer retina (only a slight disruption of the inner segment/outer segment junction) within the fovea (top panel). 'En face' SD-OCT shows a normal outer retinal layers within the fovea (bottom panel). From Querques et al. [1].

(fig. 1c). Microperimetry showed an improved retinal sensitivity and mfERG showed enhanced responses within the central 10° in the LE compared with the baseline examination.

Two months later, BCVA improved to 20/20 in the LE without metamorphopsia and SD-OCT showed an almost complete resolution of the 'partial-thickness hole' (fig. 1d). Both microperimetry and mfERG revealed a return to normal values, compared with the baseline.

Conclusion
SD-OCT is a useful tool in the diagnosis and follow-up of photic maculopathy secondary to uncomplicated cataract surgery. Differently from chronic solar maculopathy, it seems that in photic maculopathy secondary to uncomplicated cataract surgery there is an almost complete resolu-

tion of both morphological and functional changes as soon as 2 months after surgery. Differences in natural history and morphological outcomes in photic lesions are probably the result of varying intensity and length of the light exposure.

Clinical Case No. 02 – Posttraumatic Photoreceptor Disruption

Introduction
Macular injuries after head or eye contusion can consist in a variety of visible lesions, including not only a photoreceptor disruption, but also abnormalities such as retinal or vitreous hemorrhages, macular edema, RPE rip, choroidal neovascularization, macular atrophy and commotion retinae [3, 4].

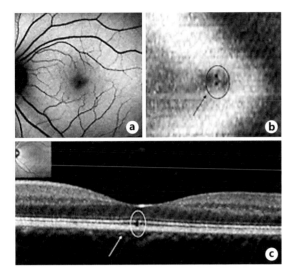

Fig. 2. Clinical case No. 2. **a** Overall normal macular morphology on autofluorescence and infrared images. **b** 'En face' OCT showing a small area of photoreceptor loss. **c** Spectral-domain optical coherence tomographic revealing a focal disruption in the inner segment/outer segment junction of the photoreceptor within the fovea. From Zucchiatti et al. [3].

Pathogenesis

Macular lesions after head contusion may frequently occur because the highest shearing forces in the retina are situated along the posterior vitreous basis [5].

Clinical Presentation

Histological studies have shown changes in the outer retinal structure after a blunt trauma [6], which may correspond to the increased reflectivity in the inner segment/outer segment (IS/OS) junction recently described in vivo using OCT [7]. These changes are generally associated with a typical transient retinal whitening appearance (commotion retinae) on fundus examination [7]. OCT suggests that macular lesions may be reversible as soon as one week after head contusion, probably due to a partial regeneration of the outer segments [8]. Sometimes, the presence and extension of subtle retinal lesions after head or

eye contusion might not be evident on fundus examination, FA, and even conventional OCT scans [9].

Case Report

A 48-year-old woman presented with blurred vision in her LE after head contusion. The patient had already undergone several ophthalmological examinations elsewhere, including FA and OCT reportedly unremarkable in both eyes. Retinal and macular morphology appeared normal on our fundus examination (fig. 2a).

SD-OCT examination, with very close scans centered onto the fovea and 'en face' enhanced depth imaging scan modality, revealed a focal disruption of the IS/OS junction in the foveal region (fig. 2b, c).

Four months later, symptoms of metamorphopsia were still present and visual acuity was unchanged. SD-OCT with follow-up examination showed the persistence of the focal IS/OS disruption.

Conclusion

The presence of a focal disruption of the photoreceptor layer in the foveal area, rather than a hyper-reflectivity in the IS/OS junction, was probably due to a later postacute examination in this patient (which did not allow to detect the hyper-reflectivity in the IS/OS junction, typically seen in the early posttraumatic phases). SD-OCT is a useful tool in the diagnosis and follow-up of maculopathy after head contusion.

Clinical Case No. 3 – Spontaneous Retinal Pigmented Epithelium Rip in Nonexudative Age-Related Macular Degeneration

Introduction

Subretinal drusenoid deposits represent a common phenotypic characteristic in eyes with pigment epithelium detachment (PED) due to non-

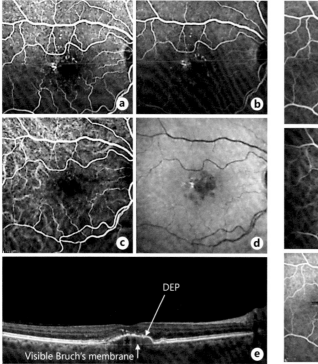

Fig. 3. Clinical case No. 3. **a, b** FA shows in early (**a**) and late (**b**) phases a hyperfluorescence associated to pigment epithelium detachment (DEP). **c, d** Indocyanine green angiography shows in early (**c**) and late (**d**) phases no sign of CNV. **e** SD-OCT of the right eye showed a juxtafoveal DEP, with no sign of exudation. From Mascali et al. [10].

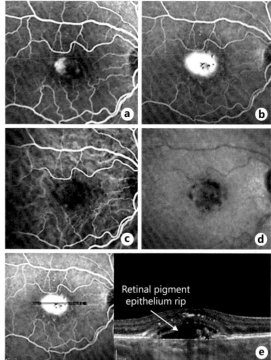

Fig. 4. Clinical case No. 3. **a, b** FA shows in early (**a**) and late (**b**) phases a hyperfluorescence that intensified with time due to 'pooling' effect of the spontaneous RPE tear. **c, d** Indocyanine green angiography showed in early (**c**) and late (**d**) phases no sign of CNV. **e** SD-OCT scan of the right eye showed a RPE rip with a nasal retraction of the RPE (marked by a star). From Mascali et al. [10].

exudative age-related macular degeneration (AMD). Rarely, a PED can spontaneously progress to a RPE tear [10, 11].

Pathogenesis
The pathogenesis of RPE tears is still unknown. Probably, the accumulation of material responsible for the PED results in a mechanical tension that leads over time to a tear.

Clinical Presentation
Clinically, it is characterized by a RPE tear not associated with any signs of neovascularization.

Case Report
A 74-year-old woman presented with sudden loss of vision in the RE. At presentation, BCVA was 20/200 in both eyes. The patient was regularly followed for drusenoid PED in the RE and for atrophic AMD in the LE. On previous ophthalmic examination (1 year before), BCVA was 20/40 in the RE and 20/200 in the LE; both FA and indocyanine green angiography showed the absence of choroidal neovascularization (CNV) in both eyes (fig. 3). As a consequence of this deterioration of BCVA in the RE, we repeated SD-OCT, which showed a RPE tear, not associated with CNV, as confirmed by FA and indocyanine green angiography (fig. 4).

Conclusion

Spontaneous RPE rip may develop in nonexudative AMD and OCT is a very useful tool to exclude CNV and visualize RPE rip.

Clinical Case No. 4 – Preclinical Stage of Best Disease

Introduction

Vitelliform macular dystrophy (VMD), also called Best disease, has an autosomal-dominant inheritance with very variable penetrance and expressivity. VMD is clinically heterogeneous, having a bimodal onset distribution with one maximum peak before puberty and a second following puberty and extending through the fifth decade of life [12, 13].

Clinical Presentation and Preclinical Stage

The onset of Best VMD is characterized by symptoms of metamorphopsia, blurred vision and decrease of central vision. At the fundus, a well-circumscribed 0.5- to 2-disc-diameter 'egg-yolk' lesion within the macula may be observed [14]. This represents the vitelliform stage of the disease, the 2nd of 5 progressive stages defined on the basis of fundus examination. The preclinical stage is characterized by a normal fundus examination of the macula and absence of increased autofluorescence.

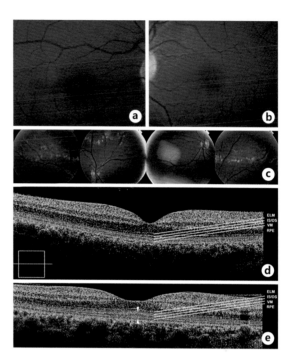

Fig. 5. Clinical case No. 4. Color fundus photography of the macula of the RE and LE showing no major alterations except for foveal granularity (**a**, **b**). Color fundus photography of the RE and LE showing several vitelliform lesions outside the macular area and in mid-periphery (**c**). SD-OCT scan of normal macula (**d**), and SD-OCT scan from the patient's LE (**e**), showing a thicker and more reflective appearance of the layer between the RPE and the interface of IS and OS of the photoreceptor (the Verhoeff's membrane) (arrowheads) in the central region compared with normal human macula. ELM = External limiting membrane; IS = inner segment; OS = outer segment; VM = Verhoeff's membrane. From Querques et al. [12].

Case Report

A 40-year-old woman presented for clinical evaluation because of a family history of VMD. Blood samples from the patient were collected and linkage analysis on genomic DNA revealed that a mutation was present in one allele of *BEST1* (T791C), resulting in the heterozygous change. An electro-oculogram showed an abnormal light peak to dark trough ratio of 0.94 in the RE and 1.17 in the LE. Her BCVA was 20/32 and 20/125 in the RE and LE, respectively.

On fundus biomicroscopy, the macula of both eyes showed no major alterations except for a mild foveal granularity (fig. 5a, b). Several vitelliform lesions were seen outside the macular area and in the mid-retinal periphery (fig. 5c). The presence of lipofuscin within the lesions outside the macular area as well as the apparent absence of vitelliform lesions within the macular area were confirmed by fundus autofluorescence.

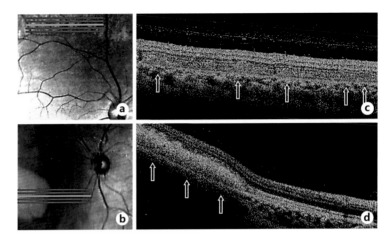

Fig. 6. Clinical case No. 4. SD-OCT scans passing through the vitelliform lesions outside the macular area show small focal hyper-reflective lesions at the level of the RPE/photoreceptor complex (**a**, **b**) (open arrows), as well as a more pronounced thickening of the RPE/photoreceptor complex (**c**, **d**) (open arrows), associated with a focal disruption of the layer corresponding to the inner segment/outer segment (IS/OS) interface (**b**, **d**). From Querques et al. [12].

On SD-OCT macular scans, in both eyes, the layer between the RPE and the IS/OS junction, corresponding to Verhoeff's membrane, had a thicker and more reflective appearance in the central area compared with the normal macula (fig. 5d, e). The vitelliform lesions outside the macular area appeared on SD-OCT scans either as small focal hyper-reflective lesions at the level of the RPE/photoreceptor complex, either as a more pronounced thickening of the RPE/photoreceptor complex, associated with a focal disruption of the layer corresponding to the IS/OS interface (fig. 6).

Conclusion

SD-OCT is useful for the diagnosis and follow-up of the Best VMD preclinical stage. In this phase there is initially a thicker and more reflective appearance of the Verhoeff's membrane [15]. On the other hand, late changes involve the RPE, first undergoing hypertrophy and then disruption and attenuation, as seen in the advanced vitelliform lesions located, in the case here reported, outside the macular area.

References

1 Querques L, Querques G, Cascavilla ML, Triolo G, Lattanzio R, Introini U, et al: Natural course of photic maculopathy secondary to uncomplicated cataract surgery. Clin Exp Optom 2013, E-pub ahead of print.

2 Hope-Ross MW, Mahon GJ, Gardiner TA, Archer DB: Ultrastructural findings in solar retinopathy. Eye (Lond) 1993;7: 29–33.

3 Zucchiatti I, Querques G, Querques L, Cascavilla ML, Introini U, Parodi MB, et al: En face optical coherence tomography visualization of post-traumatic photoreceptor disruption. J Fr Ophthalmol 2013, E-pub ahead of print.

4 Yu W, Zheng L, Zhang Z, Dai R, Dong F: Spectral-domain optical coherence tomography characteristics of macular contusion trauma. Ophthalmic Res 2012;47:220–224.

5 Delori F, Pomerantzeff O, Cox MS: Deformation of the globe under high-speed impact: it relation to contusion injuries. Invest Ophthalmol 1969;8:290–301.

6 Mansour AM, Green WR, Hogge C: Histopathology of commotio retinae. Retina 1992;12:24–28.

7 Oh J, Jung J-H, Moon SW, Song SJ, Yu HG, Cho HY: Commotio retinae with spectral-domain optical coherence tomography. Retina 2011;31:2044–2049.

8 Saleh M, Letsch J, Bourcier T, Munsch C, Speeg-Schatz C, Gaucher D: Long-term outcomes of acute traumatic maculopathy. Retina 2011;31:2037–2043.

9   Stepien KE, Martinez WM, Dubis AM, Cooper RF, Dubra A, Carroll J: Subclinical photoreceptor disruption in response to severe head trauma. Arch Ophthalmol 2012;130:400–402.

10 Mascali R, Querques G, Georges A, Souied E: Spontaneous rupture of a drusenoid pigment epithelium detachment. J Fr Ophtalmol 2013, E-pub ahead of print.

11 Alten F, Clemens CR, Milojcic C, Eter N: Subretinal drusenoid deposits associated with pigment epithelium detachment in age-related macular degeneration. Retina 2012;32:1727–1732.

12 Querques G, Regenbogen M, Soubrane G, Souied EH: High-resolution spectral domain optical coherence tomography findings in multifocal vitelliform macular dystrophy. Surv Ophthalmol 2009;54:311–316.

13 Arnold JJ, Sarks JP, Killingsworth MC, Kettle EK, Sarks SH: Adult vitelliform macular degeneration: a clinicopathological study. Eye (Lond) 2003;17:717–726.

14 Petrukhin K, Koisti MJ, Bakall B, Li W, Xie G, Marknell T, et al: Identification of the gene responsible for Best macular dystrophy. Nature Gen 1998;19:241–247.

15 Querques G, Zerbib J, Santacroce R, Margaglione M, Delphin N, Querques L, et al: The spectrum of subclinical Best vitelliform macular dystrophy in subjects with mutations in BEST1 gene. Invest Ophthalmol Vis Sci 2011;52:4678–4684.

Dr. Giuseppe Querques
Department of Ophthalmology, University of Paris Est Créteil
Centre Hospitalier Intercommunal de Créteil
40, avenue de Verdun, FR–94010 Créteil (France)
E-Mail giuseppe.querques@hotmail.it

Coscas G, Loewenstein A, Bandello F (eds): Optical Coherence Tomography.
ESASO Course Series. Basel, Karger, 2014, vol 4, pp 62–75 (DOI: 10.1159/000355918)

Optical Coherence Tomography in the Management of Diabetic Macular Edema

Ali Erginay · Pascale Massin

Hôpital Lariboisière, AP-HP, Université Paris 7-Sorbonne Paris Cité, Paris, France

Abstract

Today, optical coherence tomography (OCT) has become the first imaging technique in the assessment and management of diabetic macular edema (DME). OCT can diagnose macular edema noninvasively even at a very early stage. OCT is able to demonstrate basic structural changes of the retina from DME: retinal swelling, cystoid edema, serous retinal detachment, vitreoretinal traction, photoreceptor layer status and atrophy. Especially the new-generation spectral domain (SD)-OCT with more rapid acquisition and the higher image resolution has new functions like eye tracking, summation, 3D image, segmentation, and better imaging of the choroid. It provides the better structural information of retina and also the better understanding of pathologies. It allows more precise quantitative measurements of retinal thickness, more accurate follow-up of DME and assessment of treatment efficacy. So it plays an important role in clinical applications. SD-OCT continues progressing. The prototypes of the ul-trahigh-resolution OCT are already available. ultrahigh-resolution OCT allows the acquisition of an image with 2 µm resolution which is almost the resolution obtained by histopathology. So OCT prepares us still much more surprises in future. But we have time and still a lot of things to learn with SD-OCT. It is already a valuable tool in the decision-making process of DME treatment and it should always be used in monitoring the effect of therapies in clinical trials.

© 2014 S. Karger AG, Basel

Introduction

Diabetic macular edema (DME) is defined as a retinal thickening involving or threatening the center of the macula. It is a major cause of visual loss in patients with diabetes. Until recently, however, the methods available for detecting and evaluating diabetic macular edema were slit-lamp

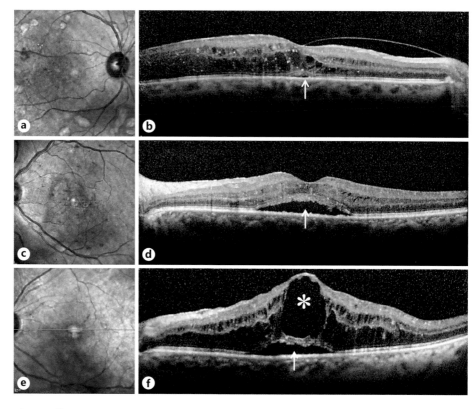

Fig. 1. Different patterns of SRD. **a** Infrared fundus photography of right eye. **b** A slight SRD which could be detected only by OCT (arrow). Mild foveal thickening with small intraretinal cysts. **c** Infrared fundus photography of left eye. **d** SRD is more important (arrow). **e** Infrared fundus photography of left eye. **f** SRD (arrow) and important foveal thickening with a big central cyst (asterisk).

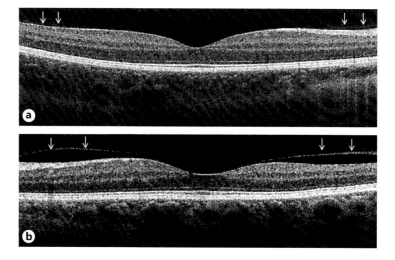

Fig. 2. Perifoveolar hyaloid detachment. **a** The posterior hyaloid is slightly detached from the macular surface in the periphery (arrows). **b** Perifoveolar hyaloid detachment is more evident (arrows).

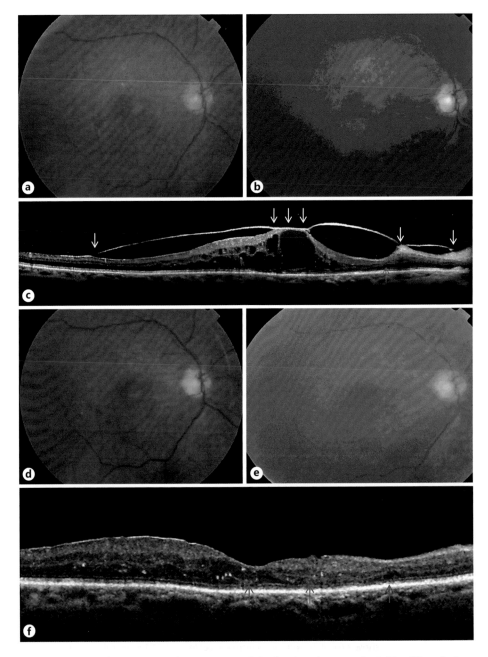

Fig. 3. Vitreomacular traction and vitrectomy. **a** Color fundus photography. **b** Blue filter photography shows better the epiretinal membrane. **c** Photomontage of the horizontal OCT scan shows a taut posterior hyaloid adherent to the retinal surface in multiple points (white arrows) generating a tractional macular edema with multiple intraretinal cysts and a big foveal cyst. There is an alteration in external layers of retina due to the traction (red arrow). **d, e** Color and blue fundus photography after vitrectomy: a few hemorrhages. **f** Macular thickness diminished after vitrectomy but the preexisting irregularities in the IS/OS persist (red arrows).

Erginay · Massin

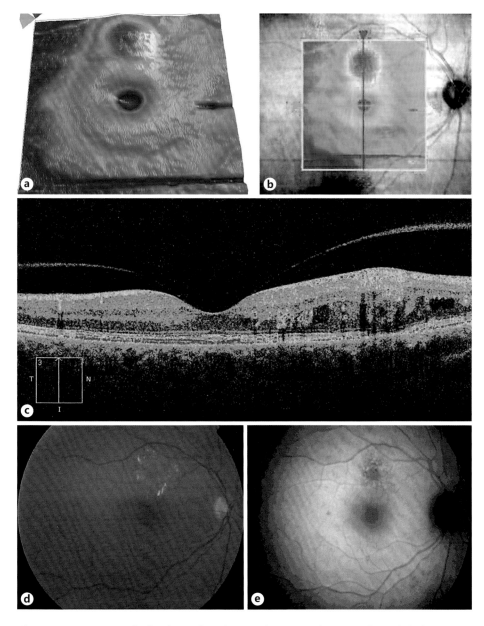

Fig. 4. Laser treatment for focal macular edema. **a, b** 3D retinal topography and thickness map show a focal thickening in right eye. **c** Vertical OCT scan: micro cystic retinal thickening with juxta foveolar exudates (red dots) in upper part of macula and a perifoveolar hyaloid detachment. **d** Color fundus photography taken immediately after focal laser treatment. **e** Autofluorescent control photography show laser scars.

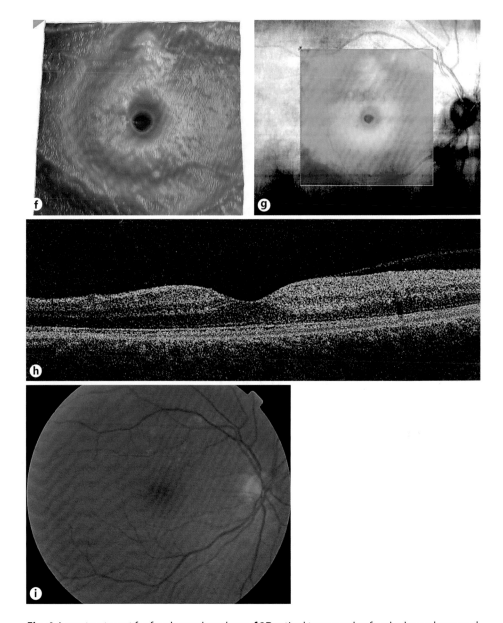

Fig. 4. Laser treatment for focal macular edema. **f** 3D retinal topography: focal edema decreased. **g** Autofluorescent control photography show laser scars. **h** Macular profile became normal. **i** There are less exudates on color fundus photography.

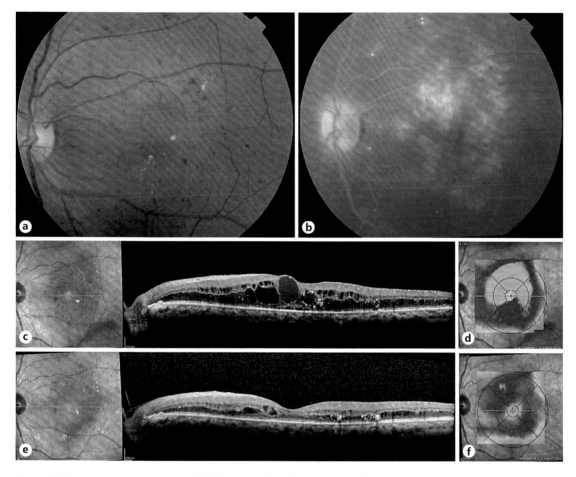

Fig. 5. OCT follow-up: intravitreal anti-VEGF injection for diffuse macular edema. **a** Color fundus photography: numerous hemorrhages and exudates. **b** Fluorescein angiography shows a diffuse leakage. **c, d** 9-mm OCT scan and mapping: Cystoid macular edema and a slight SRD. Macular thickness is 578 μm. Patient's visual acuity is 54 letters. **e, f** Control after 3 monthly anti-VEGF injections: a few intraretinal cysts persist but the macular thickness decreased to 290 μm and the patients visual acuity went up to 63 letters.

biomicroscopy and stereoscopic photography, both of which are limited in detecting earlier retinal changes.

Optical coherence tomography (OCT) provides high-resolution, cross-sectional images of the eye [1]. It is an accurate tool for the early diagnosis, analysis and monitoring of retinopathy, with high repeatability and resolution. It allows not only the qualitative DME, but also the quantitative assessment of edema. One of the first ap-

plications of OCT has been to quantify the amount of macular edema by measuring macular thickness [2].

OCT progressed rapidly and has advanced from time domain (TD) to spectral domain (SD) systems in 2006.

Compared to TD-OCT, SD-OCT has several advantages:
– Faster image acquisition (3D images, less motion artifacts).

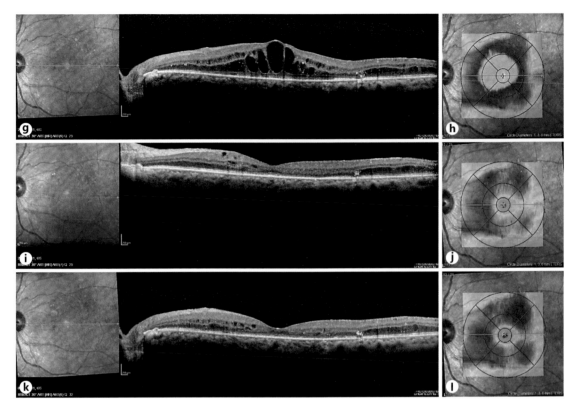

Fig. 5. g, **h** Worsening one month later. The macular thickness is 649 μm and the visual acuity is 57 letters. It is decided to realize 2 more monthly anti-VEGF injections. **i, j** Control 2 months later: Macular thickness decreased to 250 μm and the patients visual acuity went up to 61 letters. Patient had one more injection. **k, l** Control 3 months after last treatment: macular thickness stable at 242 μm and the patients visual acuity improved to 65 letters.

– Higher axial and transverse resolution (finer retina details).

OCT can detect early changes in retinal thickness, despite normal biomicroscopy. It allows diagnosis of macular edema even in very early stage [3]. It is valuable in detecting serous retinal detachment (SRD) that is not detectable on biomicroscopy (fig. 1).

SRD appears as a shallow elevation of the retina, with an optically clear space between the retina and the RPE, and a distinct outer border of the detached retina. Its pathogenesis and functional consequence, associated with DME are still unknown. But, the presence of serous retinal detachment was not correlated with poorer visual acuity [4].

OCT is particularly relevant to the analysis of the vitreous and vitreomacular relationship. In fact, OCT is much more precise than biomicroscopy in determining the status of the posterior hyaloid when it is only slightly detached from the macular surface (fig. 2). In this case, the posterior hyaloid is slightly reflective, detached from the retinal surface in the perifoveolar area and attached at the fovea center. This aspect is quite common, and corresponds to early posterior vitreous detachment [5].

In some cases, the posterior hyaloid on OCT is thick and hyper-reflective; it is partially detached from the posterior pole and taut over it, but remains attached to the disc and to the top of the

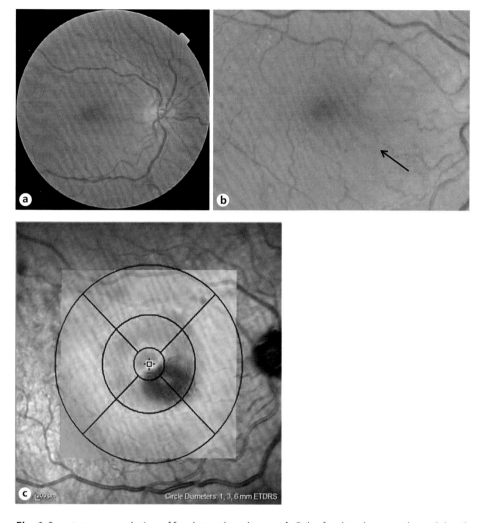

Fig. 6. Spontaneous evolution of focal macular edema. **a, b** Color fundus photography and detail: small hemorrhages juxta foveolar on nasal inferior. **c** Mapping shows a focal thickening.

raised macular surface, on which it exerts a traction (fig. 3), indicating an evident vitreomacular traction. In these cases, vitrectomy can be beneficial [6].

A number of studies have demonstrated good reproducibility of OCT measurements of single scans and retinal mapping in normal eyes and in eyes with DME [7, 8]. The scanning protocol of TD-OCT uses six radial lines of 6 mm (B-scan),

each containing 512 A-scans, with a total of 768 A-scans.

Mean macular retinal thickness is displayed as a two-dimensional false color-coded map. SD-OCT images are obtained by scanning multiple parallel lines in a rectangular scan pattern, providing a more homogeneous distribution of measured points within the macular area. But, the number of A-scans per line varies among

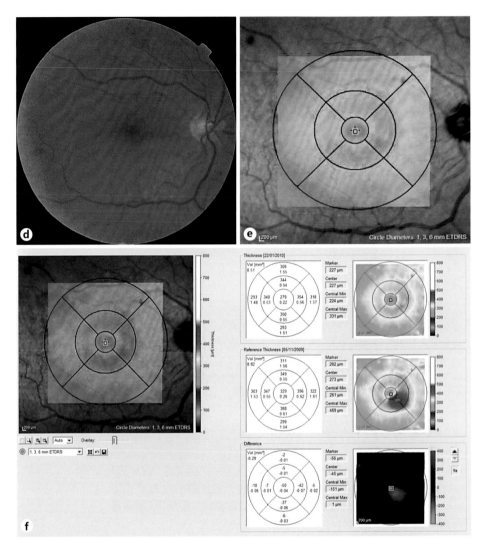

Fig. 6. Spontaneous evolution of focal macular edema. **d** Control 3 months later: hemorrhages disappeared. **e** Macular edema resorbed spontaneously. **f** Automatic mapping comparison of macular thickness change.

different OCT models (a total of 65536 A-scans for Cirrus®). The retinal thickness is displayed as a three-dimensional image of macula. So, SD-OCT seems then able to delineate more accurately the areas or retinal thickening and their location regarding the foveal center and helps to perform laser photocoagulation [9] (fig. 4).

Most of the SD-OCT is equipped with new 'eye-tracking' function which tracks eye movement and guides the OCT scanning to the previous examination position. High-contrast SLO fundus image and eye-tracking function allow repeat scans at exact same location with best precision and excellent reproducibility in follow-up examination of DME. OCT is a very use-

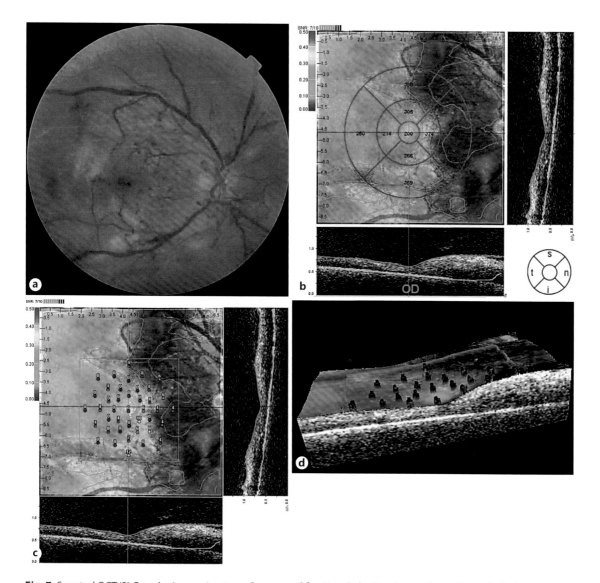

Fig. 7. Spectral OCT/SLO and microperimetry. **a** Severe proliferative diabetic retinopathy and macular ischemia mostly in temporal area. **b** Mapping obtained by OCT/SLO (Optos®) shows the reduction of retinal thickness in ischemic temporal macula. **c** Microperimetry finds a decreased sensitivity and microscotomas in the same area. **d** Same values shown on the 3D volume image.

ful tool for assessment of treatment efficacy (laser, intravitreal injections, vitrectomy…) (fig. 5) and also the spontaneous evolution of DME (fig. 6).

The change in macular profile and internal retinal structure after laser or surgical treatment are well visible with OCT. The reduction of macular edema in the course of therapeutic measures can be documented objectively with OCT. OCT has become increasingly utilized in most of the clinical management and in research protocols in the approach to DME.

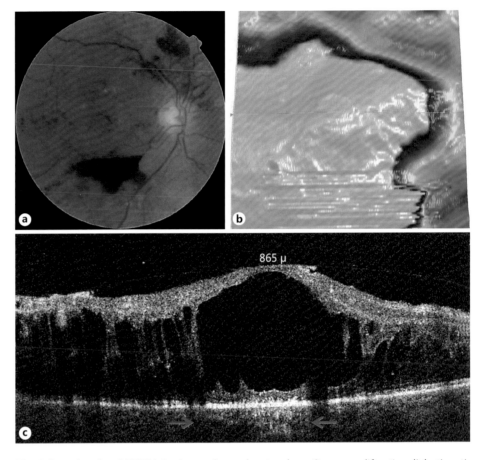

Fig. 8. Intravitreal anti-VEGF injection and macular atrophy. **a** Severe proliferative diabetic retinopathy accompanied by a pre retinal hemorrhage. **b** 3D mapping shows an important macular thickening of 865 μm. **c** 6-mm horizontal OCT scan: a large cystic cavity and an extended schisic retinal thickening. The subfoveal hyper-reflectivity (red arrows) is due to the retinal thinning by atrophy.

Some OCT devices combine angiography, high-resolution color fundus photographs and micro perimetry. OCT allows placing a scan on a simultaneously acquired angiography or microperimetry and contributing in better understanding the anatomy and structure of DME (fig. 7).

A new imaging modality for enhanced visualization of deeper tissue structures with enhanced depth imaging-OCT (EDI-OCT), such as the outer retinal layers, the choroid or the lamina cribro-

sa showed an overall thinning of the choroid in diabetic eyes [10, 11].

OCT may be used to predict visual acuity in patients with DME. The correlation between photoreceptor layer status following resolution of DME by intravitreal injection and final visual acuity has been shown [12, 13]. The integrity of the photoreceptor inner and outer segments (IS/OS) line in the fovea can be evaluated by using OCT before DME treatment (fig. 8).

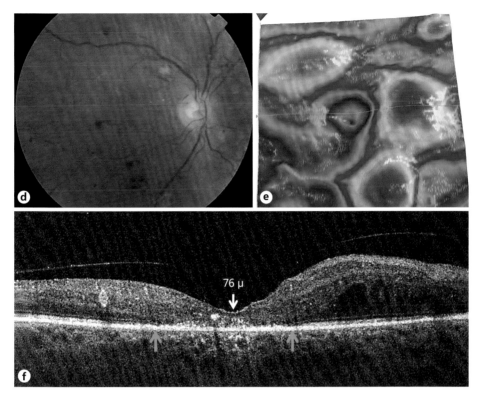

Fig. 8. Intravitreal anti-VEGF injection and macular atrophy. **d** Color fundus photography after intravitreal anti-VEGF treatment reveals the diminution of hemorrhages. **e** 3D mapping shows resorption of macular edema. **f** But the macula is completely atrophic and measures only 76 μm. The IS/OS interface and external limiting membrane are not visible (green arrows).

The quantity of retinal tissue between the plexiform layers correlates well with current VA and the amount of retinal tissue in the central area may be a prognostic factor for visual acuity after intravitreal injection in eyes with diabetic macular edema [14] (fig. 9).

OCT cannot detect nonperfusion which may explain the vision loss in some cases. Fluorescein angiography is still an important method to evaluate macular nonperfusion. It provides important information about retinal perfusion, blood-retinal barrier integrity and macular ischemia [15]. So, it should be performed if treatment of DME is being considered. It shows localization of focal or diffuse leakage areas and can be used complementary to OCT for guiding laser photocoagulation.

OCT is an accurate devise for the early diagnosis, analysis and monitoring of retinopathy, with high repeatability and resolution. It allows not only the qualitative diagnosis of DME, but also the objective and quantitative assessment of edema. Probably, OCT is the most important diagnostic and prognostic tool in the management of DME.

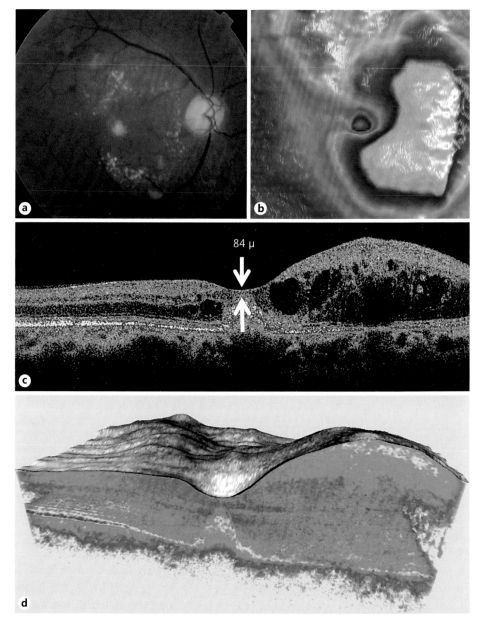

Fig. 9. Intravitreal anti-VEGF injection and macular hard exudate. **a** Color photography: retinal hemorrhages and exudates. A large macular hard exudate. **b** 3D mapping: a focal macular thickening in nasal to the macula. **c, d** OCT scan and 3D fundus image: the exudate occupy hole foveal thickness. Residual retina is atrophic and measured manually by caliper 84 μm.

References

1 Hee MR, Izatt JA, Swanson EA, et al: Optical coherence tomography of the human retina. Archf Ophthalmol 1995; 113:325–332.
2 Puliafito CA, Hee MR, Lin CP, et al: Imaging of macular diseases with optical coherence tomography. Ophthalmology 1995;102:217–229.
3 Massin P, Girach A, Erginay A, Gaudric A: Optical coherence tomography: a key to the future management of patients with diabetic macular oedema. Acta Ophthal Scand 2006;84:466–474.
4 Gaucher D, Sebah C, Erginay A, et al: Optical coherence tomography features during the evolution of serous retinal detachment in patients with diabetic macular edema. Am J Ophthalmol 2008; 145:289–296.
5 Uchino E, Uemura A, Ohba N: Initial stages of posterior vitreous detachment in healthy eyes of older persons evaluated by optical coherence tomography. Arch Ophthalmol 2001;119:1475–1479.
6 Massin P, Duguid G, Erginay A, Haouchine B, Gaudric A: Optical coherence tomography for evaluating diabetic macular edema before and after vitrectomy. Am J Ophthalmol 2003;135:169–177.

7 Massin P, Vicaut E, Haouchine B, Erginay A, Paques M, Gaudric A: Reproducibility of retinal mapping using optical coherence tomography. Arch Ophthalmol 2001;119:1135–1142.
8 Comyn O, Heng LZ, Ikeji F, Bibi K, Hykin PG, Bainbridge JW, Patel PJ: Repeatability of Spectralis OCT measurements of macular thickness and volume in diabetic macular edema. Invest Ophthalmol Vis Sci 2012;53:7754–7759.
9 Schimel AM, Fisher YL, Flynn HW Jr: Optical coherence tomography in the diagnosis and management of diabetic macular edema: time-domain versus spectral-domain. Ophthal Surg Lasers Imaging 2011;42(suppl):S41–S55.
10 Vujosevic S, Martini F, Cavarzeran F, Pilotto E, Midena E: Macular and peripapillary choroidal thickness in diabetic patients. Retina 2012;32:1781–1790.

11 Querques G, Lattanzio R, Querques L, Del Turco C, Forte R, Pierro L, Souied EH, Bandello F: Enhanced depth imaging optical coherence tomography in type 2 diabetes. Invest Ophthalmol Vis Sci 2012;53:6017–6024.
12 Shin HJ, Lee SH, Chung H, Kim HC: Association between photoreceptor integrity and visual outcome in diabetic macular edema. Graefes Arch Clin Exp Ophthalmol 2012;250:61–70.
13 Yohannan J, Bittencourt M, Sepah YJ, Hatef E, Sophie R, Moradi A, Liu H, Ibrahim M, Do DV, Coulantuoni E, Nguyen QD: Association of retinal sensitivity to integrity of photoreceptor inner/outer segment junction in patients with diabetic macular edema. Ophthalmology 2013;120:1254–1261.
14 Pelosini L, Hull CC, Boyce JF, McHugh D, Stanford MR, Marshall J: Optical coherence tomography may be used to predict visual acuity in patients with macular edema. Invest Ophthalmol Vis Sci 2011;52:2741–2748.
15 Lee DH, Kim JT, Jung DW, Joe SG, Yoon YH: The relationship between foveal ischemia and spectral-domain optical coherence tomography findings in ischemic diabetic macular edema. Invest Ophthalmol Vis Sci 2013;54:1080–1085.

Dr. Ali Erginay
Service d' Ophtalmologie, Hôpital Lariboisière
AP-HP, Université Paris 7 – Sorbonne Paris Cité
2, rue Ambroise Paré, FR–75475 Paris Cedex 10 (France)
E-Mail ali.erginay@lrb.aphp.fr

Coscas G, Loewenstein A, Bandello F (eds): Optical Coherence Tomography.
ESASO Course Series. Basel, Karger, 2014, vol 4, pp 76–92 (DOI: 10.1159/000355920)

Swept Source Optical Coherence Tomography versus Enhanced Depth Imaging-Spectral Domain Optical Coherence Tomography in Age-Related Macular Degeneration

Florence Coscas[a, b] · Gabriel Coscas[a, b]

[a]Service d'Ophtalmologie, Université Paris, Val de Marne, and [b]Centre d'Ophtalmologie de l'Odéon, Paris, France

Abstract

The introduction of spectral domain-optical coherence tomography (OCT) with combined enhanced depth imaging constitutes major technological progress. Enhanced depth imaging spectral domain-OCT provides a comprehensive and continually evolving range of imaging tools for the macula, optic disc, and anterior segment of the eye. The arrival of the swept source-OCT imaging system in 2013 represents eagerly awaited new technology. Swept source-OCT provides a large examination field, allows deeper penetration through use of an infrared wavelength of 1,050 µm, and provides a reduced masking effect on the pigment epithelium since the wavelength used can be adapted to any obstacles that are encountered.   © 2014 S. Karger AG, Basel

Imaging of the macula and fundus is of prime importance in the diagnosis and follow-up treatment of age-related macular degeneration (AMD) [1].

The different methods of investigation of the various layers of retinal and choroidal tissue based on optical coherence tomography (OCT) have been improved by the remarkable development of spectral domain (SD)-OCT combined with enhanced depth imaging (EDI) on both infrared and autofluorescence images. More recently, the use of swept source (SS)-OCT [2–4] on infrared images allows for deeper penetration by the use of an infrared wavelength of 1,050 µm.

SS-OCT versus EDI SD-OCT

A table summarizing the characteristics of the two study instruments (table 1) shows a variable infrared wavelength that can be adjusted up to 1,050 nm for SS-OCT, which is very different from the fixed wavelength of 840 nm available with EDI SD-OCT [5–7].

Table 1. Characteristics of each apparatus

Characteristics	SD-EDI-OCT	Swept source-OCT
Fundus image	IR, autofluorescence Red-free FA, ICG	IR, red-free
Wavelength	840 nm	1,050 nm
OCT scans	line, cross, star volume optical fibers iridocorneal angle, pachymetry	line, cross, star volume optical fibers
Averaging	real-time: 1–100 by eye tracking	after acquisition: fixed averaging: lines: 96 3D: 4 radial: 32
Fundus fields	15, 20, 30°	43°
Acquisition rate	40,000 A scans/s	100,000 A scans/s
Lateral resolution	14 µm	20 µm
Tissue resolution	7 µm	8 µm
Tracking	by eye tracking during acquisition from one examination to the next regardless of the initial reference scan	activation of 'autosearch' from one examination to the next

Image visualization is possible after calculation with SS-OCT and during acquisition with EDI SD-OCT.

The software in both instruments allows reconstruction of horizontal and vertical scans, 3D volumes, and radial macular scans.

Material and Methods

Our consecutive series conducted June 2012–November 2012, comprises 50 patients with AMD, examined by the same operator using the Atlantis SS-OCT (Topcon, Japan) and the Blue peak EDI SD-OCT (Heidelberg Engineering, Heidelberg, Germany).

The A-scan acquisition rate of the SS-OCT was 100 kHz with overlay (but without eye tracking); fixed image averaging after image reconstruction allowed scan acquisition in less than one second in patients with a stable fixation point (80% of cases). The A-scan acquisition rate of EDI SD-OCT was 40 kHz, compensated by real-time Eye-Tracking and adjustable image averaging; images were acquired within several seconds in all cases of AMD in our study.

Results

Using the optimized mode, these 2 instruments were able to visualize the vitreous, neurosensory retina, and choroid. The choroid and Sattler and Haller layers were visible in all cases of this series. The hyporeflective suprachoroid space was identified in more than one-third of cases.

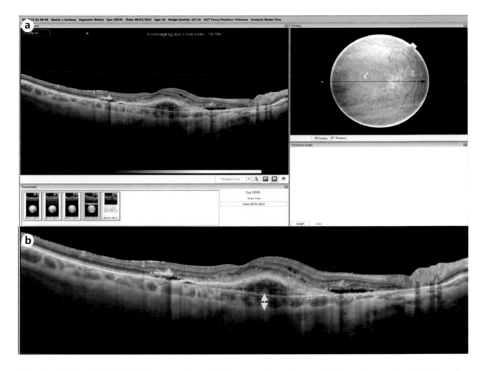

Fig. 1. a 12 µm SS-OCT with averaging of 96 scans, showing exudative pigment epithelium detachment (with SRD and intraretinal fluid). The bright spots and the blurred dense zone are visible anterior to the PED, masking the outer layers. The choroid is thinned (194 µm) with a rarefied blood supply. More posteriorly, only the choroid/sclera junction is visible. **b** Magnification (same patient as in figure 12).

The sclera/choroid junction and sclera were more clearly visible with EDI SD-OCT, while interstitial tissues between choroidal vessels were more clearly visible with SS-OCT.

Figures 1–8 illustrate the high-resolution scans obtained with each instrument on the same patients.

Swept Source-OCT

Horizontal and Vertical Scans
Horizontal and vertical 3-, 6-, 9- and 12-µm scans were rapidly obtained by fixed averaging of 96 scans; the software calculates the number of images averaged (fig. 1). These scans cover an

angle of 43°, visualizing the whole macula on a large examination field. Acquisition (screen size: 8 inches) was performed by funduscopy (slightly dilated pupil), with infrared or red-free filter; scan lines can be displaced by touch (fig. 1–4). A fluorescein angiography or indocyanine green image (JPEG file) can be imported and overlaid by recognition and alignment of retinal vessels.

Cross Lines
On SS-OCT, the masking effect on the retinal pigment epithelium was reduced after final B-scan reconstruction, since the wavelength is adapted to the obstacles that were encountered. The cross line (cross composed of 5 vertical and horizontal

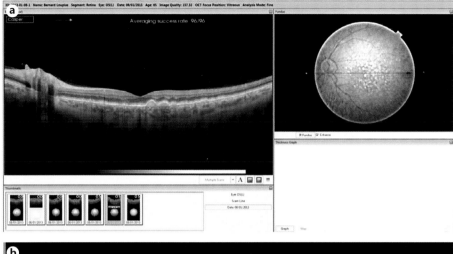

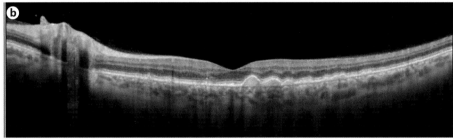

Fig. 2. a 12 nm SS-OCT scan of macular soft drusen. Moderate alteration of the outer nuclear layer, without exudation. Integrity of the retrofoveal IS/OS interface. Sattler's and Haller's layers of the choroid and, more posteriorly, the choroid/sclera junction are clearly visible. **b** Magnification (same patient as figure 13).

lines) was obtained by fixed averaging of 32 scans for a resolution of 1,024 pixels over a maximum of 12 mm (fig. 5, 6).

Radial Scans
Twelve 12-mm radial scans were acquired with fixed averaging of 32 scans per meridian, providing high-resolution images (fig. 7, 8).

Volumes
Volumes with the Early Treatment Diabetic Retinopathy Study (ETDRS) grid and virtual colors were programmed on 64 lines at intervals of 94 μm averaging only 4 images and a resolution of 512 pixels. Lower averaging

cubes of 128 or 256 lines, with interline spaces of 46 and 23.5 μm, respectively, are also available [1].

Calculation of Retinal Thickness and Retinal Volume
The seven markers for the various retinal layers (i.e. inner limiting membrane, ganglion cell fibers, outer limiting membrane, inner segment/outer segment interface, retinal pigment epithelium (RPE), Bruch membrane (BM), and choroid) were visible. Lines 2, 3 and 4, corresponding to ganglion cell fibers, outer limiting membrane, and inner segment/outer segment interface, were nonmodifiable (algorithm problem especially in

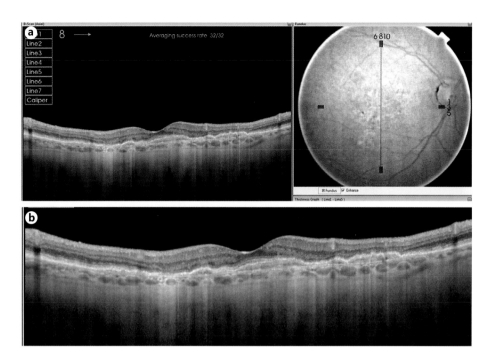

Fig. 3. a, b 12 nm SS-OCT of flat drusenoid PED. Integrity of the retrofoveal IS/OS interface. Thinning of Sattler's and Haller's layers of the choroid and the choroid/sclera junction are clearly visible. Note that the hyporeflective suprachoroidal space is well defined and corresponds to this junction. **b** Magnification (same patient as figure 14).

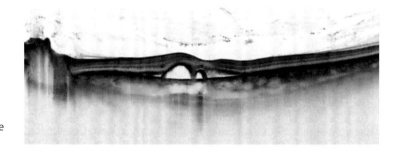

Fig. 4. The vitreous and choroid are visible on a white background.

the presence of exudative pigment epithelial detachment; PED). Lines corresponding to the outer limiting membrane, RPE, and choroid can be modified easily by hand and must be checked on all scans (fig. 9a, b).

The ETDRS target cannot be displaced. These thickness and volume measurements are visible after calculation and are presented in 2 different and distinct reports.

The originality and performance of the SS-OCT relate to automatic determination of choroid thickness and volume (fig. 10). A database and a reproducibility study of these measurements are available. Thickness measurements are

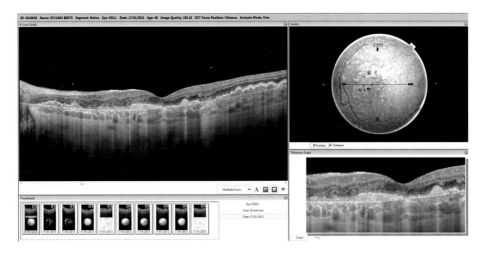

Fig. 5. Cross line composed of 5 vertical and horizontal lines. The magnification demonstrates the good image definition.

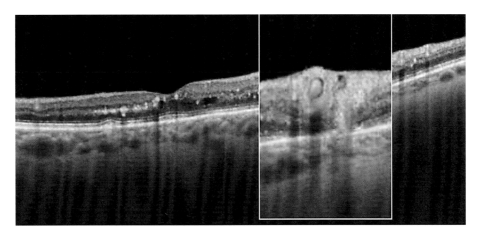

Fig. 6. Intraretinal macroaneurysm causing posterior masking. After averaging 24 images, the wavelength is adjusted to reconstitute visibility of the RPE.

also obtained with radial scans. Some markers can be modified and specific measurements can be performed with the 'caliper' function.

Automatic Follow-Up
Automatic follow-up with image alignment on retinal vessels ('auto-search' function) is possible on 3D volume, radial, and isolated line scans on 2 successive examinations (fig. 11).

Other Possible Examinations
(1) Transverse or 'en face' OCT provides disappointing results due to image averaging, which is limited to 4 images.

(2) Stereo photographs of the fundus can be obtained with a green filter.

(3) The 3D SS-OCT system allows visualization of the whole retina in a 12 × 9 mm cube (not currently tested).

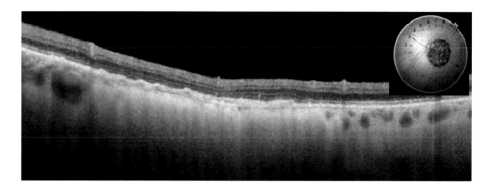

Fig. 7. Choroidal nevus on IR image, showing thinning of the choroid with loss of the choroidal vascular layers, with no visible demarcation from the sclera.

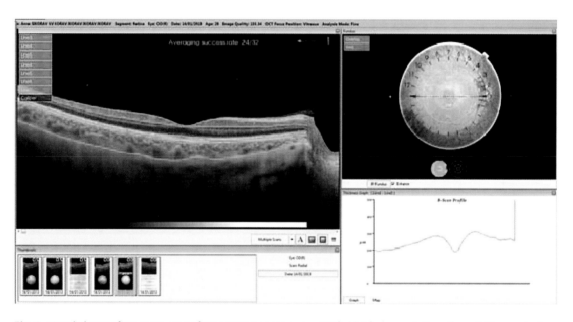

Fig. 8. 12 radial scans from averaging of 32 × 12 mm scans over a 40° field. After completion of acquisition and calculation, the software displays the real averaging number (24/32). The markers for each retinal layer can be very easily corrected.

EDI SD-OCT

Line and Cross Line Scans
(1) Horizontal and vertical scans can vary from 4 to 9 μm with adjustable averaging up to 100 scans in several seconds, without inducing any functional discomfort for the patient as a result of permanent eye tracking. These scans cover an angle of 30°, visualizing a real-time center of the macular area (nondilated pupil).

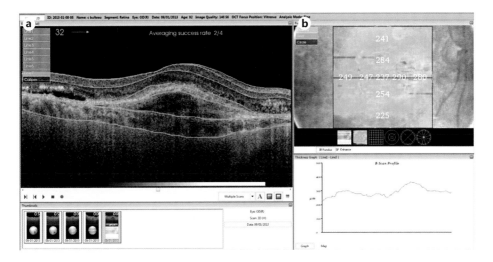

Fig. 9. a, b Retinal thickness and volume are selected separately and are displayed on various reports after manual correction of all scans.

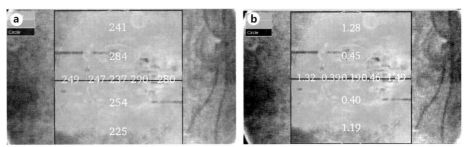

Fig. 10. a, b Choroid mapping with automatic determination of choroid thickness and volume. b Magnification. Manual verification of volume must be performed on each scan.

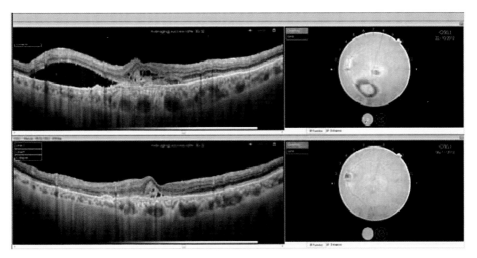

Fig. 11. Follow-up by auto-search on a preselected scan of the course of classic CNV during treatment. Courtesy of Dr. Sam Razavi.

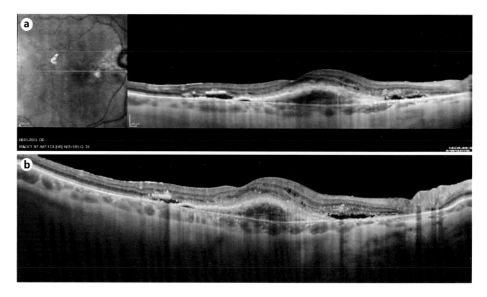

Fig. 12. a, **b** 6 μm SD-EDI-OCT averaging 100 scans showing exudative pigment epithelium detachment sub- and intra retinal fluid accumulation with a partly fibrotic cavity. The bright spots and the blurred dense zone are visible anterior to the PED, masking the outer layers. The choroid is thinned with a rarefied blood supply in both layers. More posteriorly, the choroid/sclera junction and the posterior limit of the sclera are visible. Same clinical case as in figure 1.

(2) The acquisition window is large with fundus imaging and OCT displayed on the same screen. Scan lines can be specifically and precisely displaced with the mouse. The EDI mode can be preselected on demand (fig. 12–14). OCT acquisition is performed with infrared and autofluorescence, as with color scans.

Another version of the instrument can be linked to fluorescein angiography and ICG angiography in the scanning laser ophthalmoscope mode.

(3) Examination of the vitreous in standard mode with real-time averaging of 50 images provides high-resolution images of the vitreous. Full Depth Imaging (FDI-OCT) (mode: 50 scans with EDI and 50 scans without EDI) allows OCT examination of the vitreous and choroid (fig. 15).

(4) The caliper function can also be used to detect variations in autofluorescence, or an abnormality on infrared or OCT scans, by means of the 'dual laser' process.

Automatic Follow-Up
Radial scans and averaging can be adjusted according to a cross of two 90° meridians and up to 48 meridians with an angle of 4°, over fields of 15, 20 and 30° (fig. 16).

Volumes
Volumes with ETDRS grid and virtual colors are adjustable from 19 lines separated by intervals of 240 μm in a volume of 20 × 15° and up to 591 lines separated by intervals of 11 μm in a volume of 20 × 25°, with variable averaging ranging from 1 to 100 images (fig. 17). This mode allows simultaneous calculation of retinal thickness and retinal volume in the same report for follow-up or for 2 eyes. The markers of the various retinal layers are visible (internal limiting membrane, BM) and can be manually modified point-by-point.

(1) A database and reproducibility study of these measurements is available (fig. 18). Calcu-

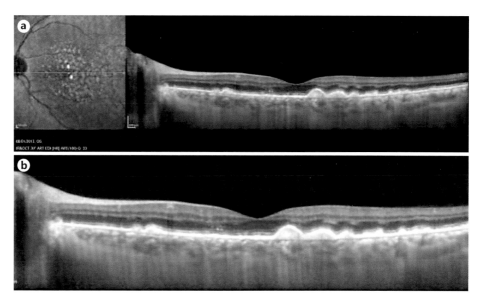

Fig. 13. a 6 µm SD-EDI-OCT of macular soft drusen. Moderate alteration of the outer nuclear layer without exudation. Integrity of the retrofoveal IS/OS interface. Sattler's and Haller's layers are clearly visible, as well as the choroid/sclera junction and the sclera more posteriorly. **b** Magnification. Same clinical case as in figure 2.

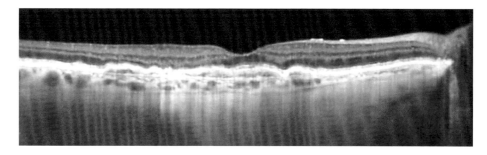

Fig. 14. 6 µm SD-EDI-OCT of a flat PED caused by confluence of drusen. Integrity of the retrofoveal IS/OS interface. Thinning of Sattler's and Haller's layers of the choroid and the choroid/sclera junction are clearly visible. Note that the hyporeflective suprachoroidal space is well defined and corresponds to this junction. The sclera is visible more posteriorly (magnification). Same clinical case as in figure 3.

lation of choroidal thickness is reproducible. The manual method places the caliper every 500 µm on the posterior surface of the BM at the choroid/sclera junction or in the suprachoroidal space when it is visible (fig. 19). By means of a series of 3 clicks, the internal limiting membrane line can be moved to the RPE, and the BM line can be moved to the choroid to automatically obtain choroidal thickness and choroidal volume [1, 3].

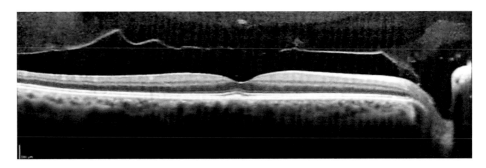

Fig. 15. Visualization of the vitreous and an operculum on SD-OCT without EDI and FDI-OCT.

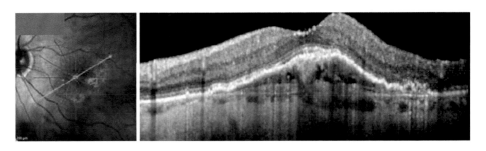

Fig. 16. Raster of 12 real-time adjustable radial scans with a field of 30° averaging 6 mm.

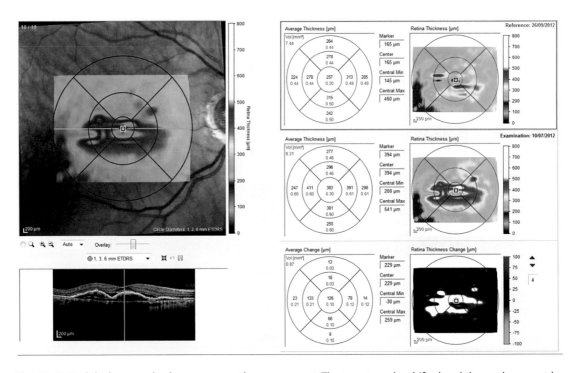

Fig. 17. Retinal thickness and volume maps on the same report. The target can be shifted and the markers must be corrected, when necessary, on 19 scans in the case presented here.

Coscas · Coscas

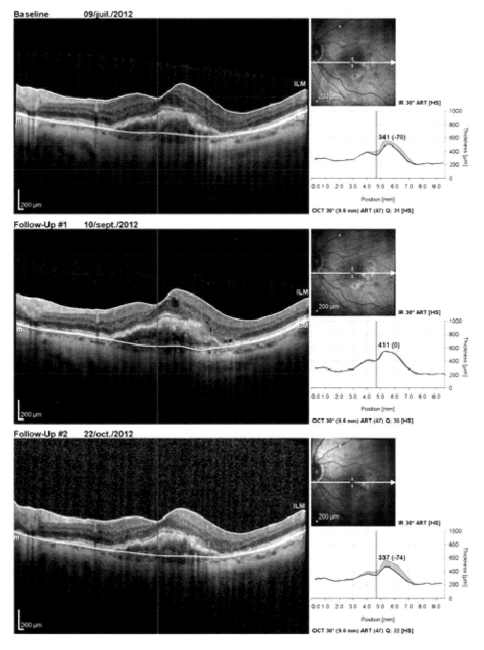

Fig. 18. Eye tracking follow-up of all previous examinations based on the reference examination (qualitative and quantitative appearance).

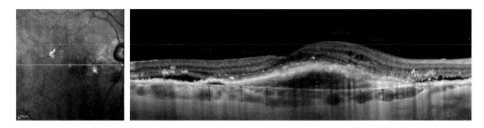

Fig. 19. Choroidal thickness is not measured automatically, but is reproducible and allows very precise selection of Bruch's membrane and the choroid/sclera junction or suprachoroidal space, when visible.

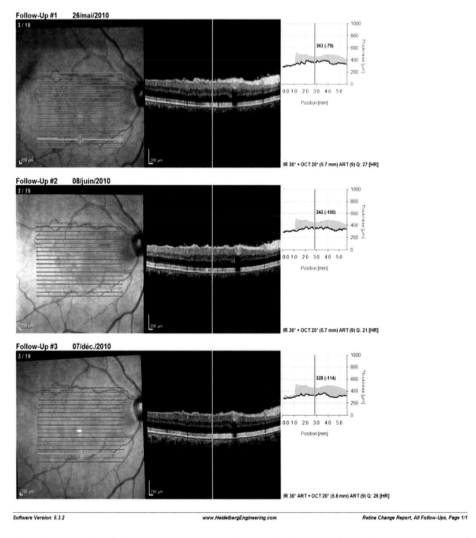

Fig. 20. Eye tracking follow-up on the raster with quantitative and color-coded determination of thickness variations (green corresponds to a reduction).

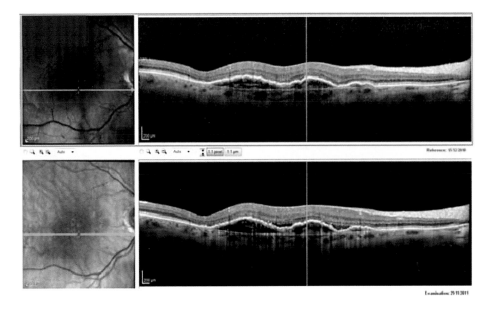

Fig. 21. Follow-up of recurrence of a PED with deterioration of SRD.

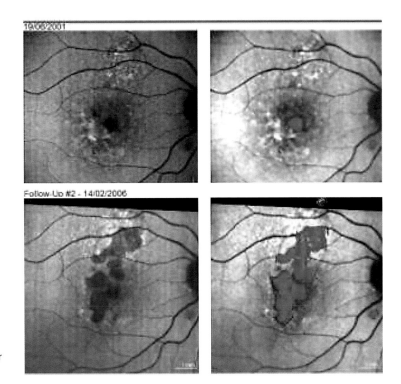

Fig. 22. Automatic calculation of the course of the lesion. The progression rate over 4 years was 1.04 mm²/year with extension and confluence of 1.768 mm²/year over the last year.

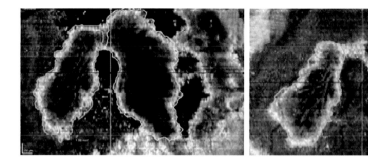

Fig. 23. 'Follow-up' of area, selected manually but with automatic alignment on OCT or infrared.

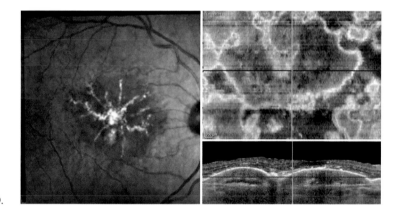

Fig. 24. Stereo photograph and 'en face' OCT of drusenoid PED. No SRD.

(2) Choroidal volume can be determined after modifying the markers, giving statistically reproducible results.

Other Possible Examinations
The EDI SD-OCT is the only OCT instrument that allows:

(1) Automatic eye tracking follow-up on 3D, radial, and isolated line scans on all successive examinations, regardless of the reference OCT (infrared, autofluorescence) in the form of a map, profiles, or lines (fig. 20, 21).

(2) Automatic follow-up of autofluorescence (fig. 22).

(3) 'Follow-up' of area calculations performed on OCT or fundus imaging and vice versa and on transverse 'en face' OCT (fig. 23).

(4) Stereo fundus photographs by selecting this mode (fig. 24).

(5) High-resolution transverse frontal or C scans with video or printable frozen image visualization of the corresponding B scan (fig. 25).

Conclusion

Both the SS-OCT and the EDI SD-OCT instruments studied allow for rigorous follow-up of the clinical course of the patient's disease.

After a positive multimodal diagnosis, the decision in favor of retreatment or conservative management, detection of complications or a new differential diagnosis, early detection of involvement of the fellow eye, and repeated and

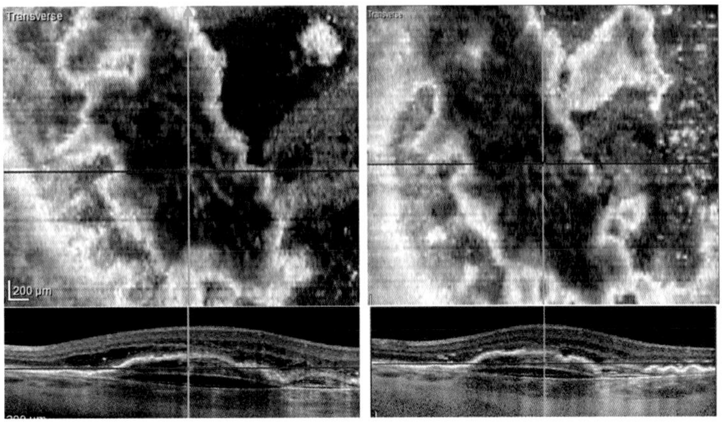

Fig. 25. Stereo photograph and 'en face' OCT of Vascularized PED with visible neovascular network without dye injection (High-resolution transverse frontal or C scans with video or printable frozen image visualization of the corresponding B scan.

verified patient education are facilitated by the technological progress provided by these instruments in combination with clinical examination. The journey from time domain-OCT to SD-OCT has constituted major technological progress.

EDI SD-OCT provides a comprehensive and continually evolving range of imaging tools for the macula, optic disc, and anterior segment of the eye.

The arrival of the SS-OCT represents new technology. Further development allowing simultaneous autofluorescence and angiographies is eagerly awaited.

References

1 Pierro L, Gagliardi M, Iuliano L, Ambrosi A, Bandello F: Retinal nerve fiber layer thickness reproducibility using seven different OCT instruments. Invest Ophthalmol Vis Sci 2012;53:5912–5920.
2 Hirata M, Tsujikawa A, Matsumoto A, Hangai M, Ooto S, Yamashiro K, Akiba M, Yoshimura N: Macular choroidal thickness and volume in normal subjects measured by swept-source optical coherence tomography. Invest Ophthalmol Vis Sci 2011;52:4971–4978.
3 Ikuno Y, Maruko I, Yasuno Y, Miura M, Sekiryu T, Nishida K, Iida T: Reproducibility of retinal and choroidal thickness measurements in enhanced depth imaging and high-penetration optical coherence tomography. Invest Ophthalmol Vis Sci 2011;52:5536–5540.
4 de Bruin DM, Burnes DL, Loewenstein J, Chen Y, Chang S, Chen TC, Esmaili DD, de Boer JF: In vivo three-dimensional imaging of neovascular age-related macular degeneration using optical frequency domain imaging at 1050 nm. Invest Ophthalmol Vis Sci 2008;49:4545–4952.
5 Wong IY, Koizumi H, Lai WW: Enhanced depth imaging optical coherence tomography. Ophthalmic Surg Lasers Imaging 2011;42:S75–S84.
6 Shao L, Xu L, Chen CX, Yang LH, Du KF, Wang S, Zhou JQ, Wang YX, You QS, Jonas JB, Wei WB: Reproducibility of subfoveal choroidal thickness measurements with enhanced depth imaging by spectral-domain optical coherence tomography. Invest Ophthalmol Vis Sci 2013;54:230–233.
7 Chhablani J, Barteselli G, Wang H, El-Emam S, Kozak I, Doede AL, Bartsch DU, Cheng L, Freeman WR: Repeatability and reproducibility of manual choroidal volume measurements using enhanced depth imaging optical coherence tomography. Invest Ophthalmol Vis Sci 2012;53:2274–2280.
8 Ellabban AA, Tsujikawa A, Matsumoto A, Yamashiro K, Oishi A, Ooto S, Nakata I, Akagi-Kurashige Y, Miyake M, Yoshimura N: Macular choroidal thickness measured by swept source optical coherence tomography in eyes with inferior posterior staphyloma. Invest Ophthalmol Vis Sci 2012;53:7735–7745.
9 Jirarattanasopa P, Ooto S, Nakata I, Tsujikawa A, Yamashiro K, Oishi A, Yoshimura N: Choroidal thickness, vascular hyperpermeability, and complement factor H in age-related macular degeneration and polypoidal choroidal vasculopathy. Invest Ophthalmol Vis Sci 2012;53:3663–3672.

10 Kuroda S, Ikuno Y, Yasuno Y, Nakai K, Usui S, Sawa M, Tsujikawa M, Gomi F, Nishida K: Choroidal thickness in central serous chorioretinopathy. Retina 2013;33:302–308.

11 Spaide RF, Koizumi H, Pozzoni MC: Enhanced depth imaging spectral-domain optical coherence tomography. Am J Ophthalmol 2008;146:496–500. Erratum in: Am J Ophthalmol 2009;148:325.

12 Kim SW, Oh J, Kwon SS, Yoo J, Huh K: Comparison of choroidal thickness among patients with healthy eyes, early age-related maculopathy, neovascular age-related macular degeneration, central serous chorioretinopathy, and polypoidal choroidal vasculopathy. Retina 2011;31:1904–1911.

13 Querques G, Querques L, Forte R, Massamba N, Coscas F, Souied EH: Choroidal changes associated with reticular pseudodrusen. Invest Ophthalmol Vis Sci 2012;53:1258–1263.

14 Nakayama M, Keino H, Okada AA, Watanabe T, Taki W, Inoue M, Hirakata A: Enhanced depth imaging optical coherence tomography of the choroid in Vogt-Koyanagi-Harada disease. Retina 2012;32:2061–2069.

Dr. Florence Coscas
Department of Ophthalmology, University Paris-Est Créteil
Centre Hospitalier Intercommunal de Créteil
40, avenue de Verdun, FR–94010 Créteil (France)
E-Mail coscas.f@gmail.com

Coscas G, Loewenstein A, Bandello F (eds): Optical Coherence Tomography.
ESASO Course Series. Basel, Karger, 2014, vol 4, pp 93–100 (DOI: 10.1159/000355967)

'En Face' Optical Coherence Tomography with Enhanced Depth Imaging of Different Patterns of the Choroidal Neovascular Network in Age-Related Macular Degeneration

Gabriel Coscas[a, b] · Florence Coscas[a, b]

[a]Service d'Ophtalmologie, Hôpital de Créteil, Université Paris-EST and [b]Centre d'Ophtalmologie de l'Odéon, Paris, France

Abstract

The purpose of this study was to develop a method of segmentation using 'en face' spectral domain-optical coherence tomography (SD-OCT) ('en face' C-scans) to evaluate different patterns of the choroidal neovascular network (CNV) due to age-related macular degeneration (AMD). ***Materials and Method:*** A series of 90 patients with AMD comprising 30 cases of subfoveal fibrovascular pigment epithelial detachment, 15 cases of classic CNV and 35 cases of polypoidal choroidal vasculopathy. Fluorescein angiography, indocyanine green angiography and OCT (Spectralis, Heidelberg, Germany) images were analyzed. Volume acquisition of 97 enhanced depth imaging sections at 30-µm intervals was obtained, with a sum of 9 images for each retrofoveal scan. The image was superimposed on infrared and SLO ICG images to confirm the neovascularization. ***Results:*** Conventional SD-OCT only provides anteroposterior planes that only visualize the exudative reaction of the neovascular network. This new 'en face' SD-OCT technology allows analysis of not only the contours and the shape of the detachment but also, and most importantly, visualizes the choroidal neovascular network in different patterns due to AMD. This imaging is obtained by means of an 'en face' frontal mode with dynamic analysis in video or on frozen images, section by section, compared to standard SD-OCT or ICGA images with point-by-point correspondence. ***Conclusion:*** Until now, the CNV itself was not precisely detectable on conventional SD-OCT but only suggested by an exudative reaction. This new 'en face' SD-OCT technology with dynamic segmentation of the macula allows to visualize the contours and the shape of the fibrovascular pigment epithelial detachment as well as the CNV in fibrovascular pigment epithelial detachment. SD-OCT can demonstrate direct signs of CNV within a pigment epithelial detachment and their localization, seen for the first time on OCT, without injection of dye in patients with a stable fixation point 'en face' and will bring help for the easy detection of CNV and the decision for retreatment easier. 'En face' OCT of classic CNV in AMD also allows to determine the origin of the CNV at the level of the choriocapillaris, the precise location of the 'effraction' of the retinal pigment epithelium layer, the hyper-reflective course of type 2 CNV, in front of the retinal pigment epithelium and the correspondence between the CNV and the 'intraretinal dense zones', and between 'en face' OCT images and angiograms. 'En face' OCT imaging of polypoidal choroidal vasculopathy allows analysis of the contours and number of polyps, visualization and localization of the abnormal choroidal network and their localization inside the (thickened) choroid, choriocapillaris and Bruch's membrane without the injection of a dye.

Recently, different techniques have been developed to improve imaging by optical coherence tomography (OCT), either enhanced depth imaging (EDI), or 'en face OCT'. This new approach to OCT imaging produces simultaneous longitudinal (B-scans) and frontal (C-scans) images of the macular area with high pixel-to-pixel correspondence.

The purpose of this study was to develop a method of segmentation using 'en face' C-scans to evaluate the choroidal neovascular network in different patterns due to AMD. Posterior pole concavity should not be forgotten when carrying out the analysis of a retinal frontal section. Around any lesion, elevated or depression, the retinal layers will appear as concentric hypo- or hyper-reflective and easily recognizable bands (fig. 1).

Methods

The images were obtained with a volume acquisition of 97 EDI sections, each comprised of 9 averaged EDI-OCT B-scans, at 30-μm intervals, within a 15° × 10° automatically obtained rectangle, in about 60 s. The resulting images were reconstructed to obtain en face (frontal) sections, visible either on video or 'frozen' images, or selected from a special segment.

The images were superimposed and compared on infrared and/or on SLO ICG images, to confirm the neovascularization.

Different Patterns of the Choroidal Neovascular Network due to Age-Related Macular Degeneration

(1) Fibrovascular Pigment Epithelial Detachment

Until now, CNV were not directly visible in OCT and detected only on 'indirect' signs, mainly a moderately hyper-reflective layer, back to the retinal pigment epithelium (RPE) band, suggestive of the presence of sub-RPE CNV (type 1 or 'occult') (fig. 2). The multimodal imaging of a fibrovascular pigment epithelial detachment (FV-PED), with fluorescein angiography, ICG-A and SD-OCT (B-scan) is now well known (fig. 3).

Analyzing an 'en face' OCT video imaging of FV-PED, it is possible to recognize successively, the retinal vessels, the foveal depression, the dome of the FV-PED, the upper part of the cavity of the FV-PED, the hyper-reflective course of CNV, and, at a deeper level behind the FV-PED, the fluid beside CNV, and, finally, the choroid.

The 'frozen' images at different levels will demonstrate these patterns (fig. 4).

The hyper-reflective course of type 1 CNV was confirmed by comparative analysis on 'en face' OCT and on ICG-A, in all 30 eyes (fig. 5). Concordance between observers was very high (intraobserver 97%, interobserver 98%).

Comments on 'En Face' OCT in Fibrovascular Pigment Epithelium Detachment

Until now, CNV themselves were not precisely detectable in conventional SD-OCT but were only suggested by an exudative reaction.

This new 'en face' SD-OCT technology with dynamic segmentation of the macula allows to visualize the contours and the shape of the FV-PED and the choroid neovascular network in the FV-PED.

'En face' SD-OCT demonstrates for the first time direct signs of CNV, without any dye injection allowing for easy detection of CNV and easy decision for retreatment [1].

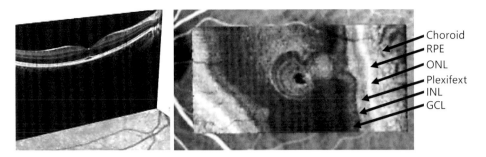

Fig. 1. Posterior pole concavity. Around any lesion, elevated or depression, the retinal layers will appear as concentric hypo- or hyper-reflective and easily recognizable bands.

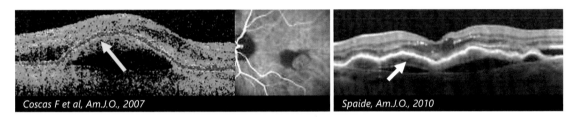

Fig. 2. CNV: not directly visible in OCT and detected only by 'indirect' signs, mainly a moderately hyper-reflective layer, back to the RPE band [2].

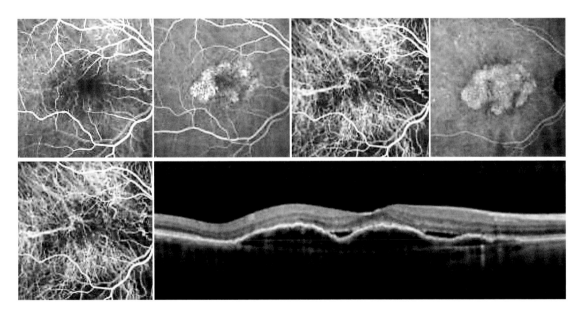

Fig. 3. Well-known multimodal imaging of a FV-PED with FA, ICG-A and SD-OCT (B-scan).

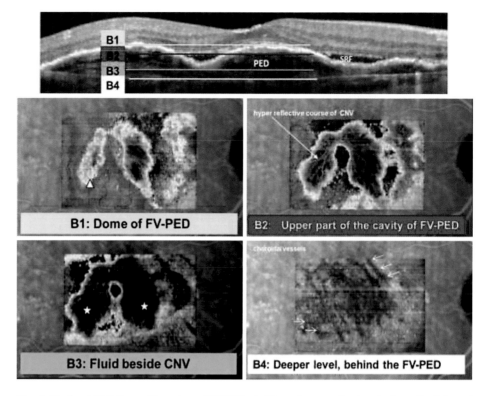

Fig. 4. 'En face' OCT 'frozen' imaging of FV-PED at different successive levels, from the internal layers to the choroid.

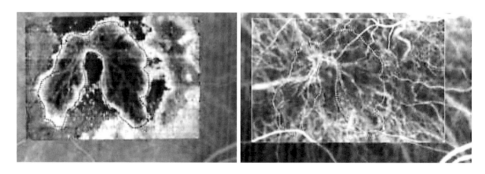

Fig. 5. Comparative analysis between 'en face' OCT and ICG-A.

(2) 'En Face' OCT and Classic CNV (Type 2)

Classic CNV are so-called 'visible' in fluorescein angiography, due to the characteristic leakage (fig. 6). They remain difficult to analyze in B-scan OCT imaging, suggested only by the presence of 'intra-retinal dense areas', but without a specific localization [2, 3].

OCT B-scans may show a localized break in the RPE layer, allowing the course of the hyper-reflective pedicle (CNV) from the inner choroid layers and choriocapillaris through Bruch's mem-

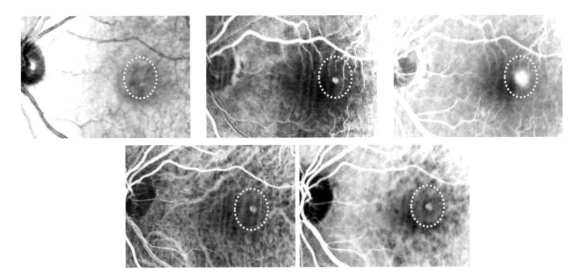

Fig. 6. Classic CNV, so-called 'visible' on fluorescein angiography due to the characteristic leakage, and on ICG-A.

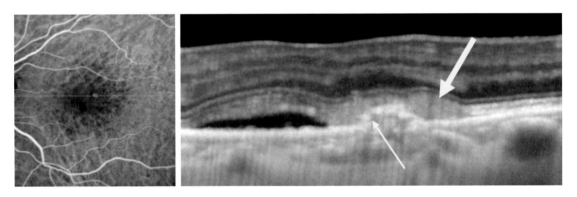

Fig. 7. Classic CNV (FA and B-scan). Localized break in the RPE layer (thin arrow) allowing the course of the hyper-reflective pedicle (CNV) from the inner choroid layers and choriocapillaris, through Bruch's membrane and RPE towards the subretinal space, associated to the sub- and intraretinal dense area (large arrow) and serous SRF. From Coscas et al. [3].

brane and the RPE towards the subretinal space, associated to the sub- and intraretinal dense area and serous subretinal fluid (SRF) (fig. 7) [4].

Analyzing an 'en face' OCT video imaging of classic CNV, it is possible to recognize, successively, the retinal vessels, the foveal depression, the dome of the CNV, the subfoveal fluid, then the CNV pedicle, the RPE hole (for CNV pedicle), the origin of CNV at the level of the choriocapillaris, and finally, at a deeper level, the choroid.

The 'frozen' images, at different level will demonstrate these patterns (fig. 8).

Comments on 'En Face' OCT of Classic Choroidal Neovascular Networks in Age-Related Macular Degeneration
In the 'en face' OCT video, the origin of the CNV at the level of the choriocapillaris, the precise location of the 'effraction' of the RPE layer, and the hyper-reflective course of type 2 CNV, in front of RPE, were clearly visible in all eyes of our series.

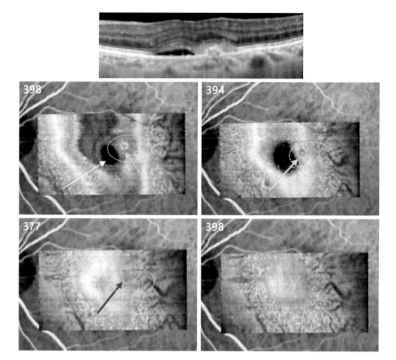

Fig. 8. 'En face' OCT 'frozen' imaging of classic CNV at different successive levels from the internal layers to the choroid. It is possible to recognize, successively, near the foveal depression, the subfoveal fluid and the CNV pedicle, then the RPE hole (for the CNV pedicle), the origin of CNV at the level of the chorio capillaris, and, at a deeper level, Bruch's membrane, the choriocapillaris, and, finally, the choroid.

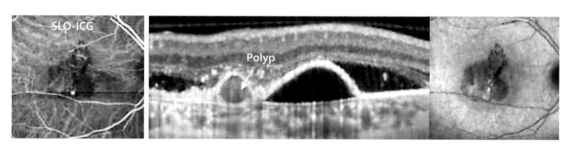

Fig. 9. Typical pattern of the PCV (ICG-A and SD-OCT).

The correspondence between the CNV and the 'intraretinal dense zones' and the exact correspondence between 'en face' OCT images and angiograms were clearly demonstrated [4].

(3) 'En Face' OCT and Polypoidal Choroidal Vasculopathy

The diagnosis of polypoidal choroidal vasculopathy (PCV) with an abnormal choroidal network and polypoidal ectasias was made on the basis of ICGA+SD-OCT (Spectralis®) in our Series of 35 consecutive patients with active PCV (13 females and 22 males, mean age 71.7 years, range 55–86) followed during more than 1 year, and treated with ranibizumab and PDT.

In SLO-ICG, the best criteria were the presence, in late images, of 1 or multiple choroidal aneurysmatic 'polyp-like' lesions associated to an abnormal choroidal network.

In SD-OCT, the presence of a typical pattern, with elevation of the RPE layer, with steep borders, and a serous (sanguineous) PED were sug-

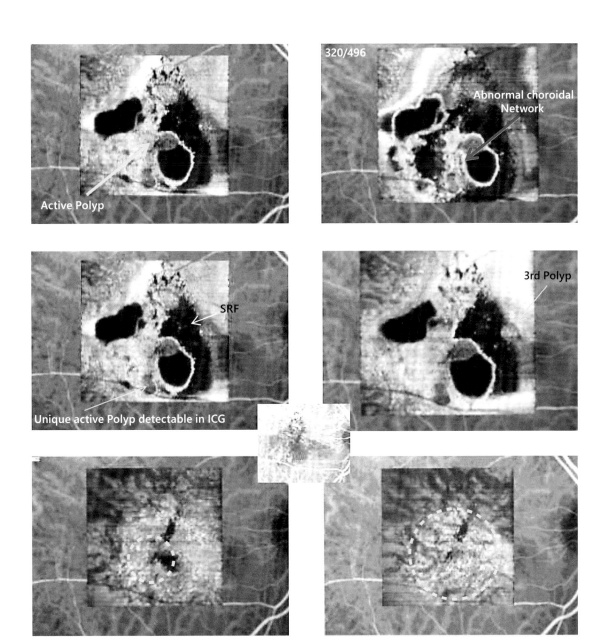

Fig. 10. 'En face' OCT 'frozen imaging' of the typical PCV pattern at different successive levels from the internal layers to the choroid. It is possible to recognize, successively, two cavities of the serous PED, surrounded by subretinal fluid and numerous hyper-reflective dots, and a first polyp. Deeper, many other polyps including the one detected on ICG can be seen. Subfoveal fluid (dark optically empty area) is visible around the serous PED. Then, deeper again, the abnormal choroidal network and an additional polyp will become visible. The polyps are disappearing at the level of the choriocapillaris and are located inner to the choroid. Large choroidal vessels are at the periphery of the lesion.

gestive of PCV. Increased choroid thickness was considered as an additional clue [5] (fig. 9).

'En face' OCT 'frozen imaging' of typical PCV at different successive levels from the internal layers to the choroid is depicted in figure 10.

Comments on 'En Face' OCT of PCV

In the 'en face' OCT video, polyps are easily recognized and detectable in 'en face' OCT.

Either in the case of pure typical VPC, or in the case of polyps associated with late AMD, they are moderately hyper-reflective and well-delimited by the RPE layer.

In our series, we found a higher number of polyps 'en face' than in SLO-ICG (12/35), not visible deeper than Bruch's membrane/choriocapillaris, and located inner to the choroid.

The polyps were associated with a PED (25/35) either in (10–35) or out (15/35) of the cavity. The abnormal choroidal network was usually visible (25/35), associated with SRF, hyper-reflective dots, and increased choroid thickness (28/35).

Conventional SD-OCT provides mainly anterior-posterior sections that essentially visualize the serous or sero-hemorrhagic exudative reaction due to the PCV network.

This new 'en face' SD-OCT imaging allows analysis of the contours and number of polyps, the visualization and localization of the abnormal choroidal network without dye injection.

The localization of the polyps is inner to the (thickened) choroid, choriocapillaris and Bruch's membrane. Large choroid vessels are placed at the periphery of the lesion. Finally, 'en face' EDI OCT will help evaluate prognosis.

References

1 Coscas F, Coscas G, Querques G, Massamba N, Querques L, Bandello F, Souied EH: En face enhanced depth imaging optical coherence tomography of fibrovascular pigment epithelium detachment. Invest Ophthalmol Vis Sci 2012;53:4147–4151.

2 Coscas F, Coscas G, Souied E, Tick S, Soubrane G: Optical coherence tomography identification of occult choroidal neovascularization in age-related macular degeneration. Am J Ophthalmol 2007;144:592–599.

3 Coscas G, Coscas F, Vismara S, Zourdani A, Li Calzi CI: OCT in AMD. 2008 Annual Report of French Ophthalmology Societies. Heidelberg, Springer, 2009.

4 Coscas F, Querques G, Forte R, Terrada C, Coscas G, Souied EH: Combined fluorescein angiography and spectral-domain optical coherence tomography imaging of classic choroidal neovascularization secondary to age-related macular degeneration before and after intravitreal ranibizumab injections. Retina 2012;32:1069–1076.

5 Imamura Y, Engelbert M, Iida T, Freund KB, Yannuzzi LA: Polypoidal choroidal vasculopathy: a review. Surv Ophthalmol 2010;55:501–515.

Prof. Gabriel Coscas, MD
Department of Ophthalmology, University Paris-Est Créteil
Centre Hospitalier Intercommunal de Créteil
40, avenue de Verdun, FR–94010 Créteil (France)
E-Mail gabriel.coscas@gmail.com

Coscas G, Loewenstein A, Bandello F (eds): Optical Coherence Tomography.
ESASO Course Series. Basel, Karger, 2014, vol 4, pp 101–109 (DOI: 10.1159/000356397)

'En Face' Optical Coherence Tomography Scan Applications in the Inner Retina

Bruno Lumbroso[a] · Marco Rispoli[a] · Jean Francois Le Rouic[b] ·
Maria Cristina Savastano[a]

[a]Centro Oftalmologico Mediterraneo, Rome, Italy; [b]Clinique Sourdille, Nantes, France

Abstract

Objectives: The authors describe the clinical applications, at inner retina level, of a new imaging approach: 'en face' spectral domain-optical coherence tomography (SD-OCT) of the retinal surface before and after epiretinal membrane (ERM) and internal limiting membrane (ILM) peeling. Preoperative and postoperative 'en face' SD-OCT images of the inner face of the macula were obtained from eyes undergoing vitrectomy with ILM peeling for ERM. *Results:* Preoperatively, 'en face' SD-OCT imaging of the retinal surface clearly showed plaques surrounded by radiating folds due to ERM. It could also disclose areas possibly devoid of ILM secondary to ERM contraction. A rough retinal surface was visible in the peeled area during the first postoperative month. At 3 months, various amounts of dimples were progressively observed in 85% of eyes. In all these cases, they lasted or increased in size and number at the last follow-up examination. Some residual epiretinal tissue was also detected by this technique. *Conclusion:* 'En face' SD-OCT of the retinal surface gives information completing the standard retinal OCT section which provides an easy approach to understand a global overview of the retinal surface. With software development 'en face' scan procedures are easy to perform and their interest as a teaching tool is evident. Preoperative 'en face' SD-OCT can also guide preretinal tissue peeling. It can detect and classify tiny progressive morphological changes in the texture of the retinal surface occurring after ILM peeling. En-face OCT imaging can stress small alterations of texture of the retinal surface that are not clearly seen on standard OCT scans. 'En face' scans allow us to study and classify the vitreoretinal interface postoperative evolution from smooth plaques surrounded with retinal radial folds to rough interface to dimpled surface with small craters that may or may not increase in size and depth with time. It appears to be a useful and necessary complement to the conventional cross-sectional B-scan.

© 2014 S. Karger AG, Basel

Optical coherence tomography (OCT) is essential for the diagnosis and follow-up of many retinal disorders and of vitreomacular interface pathologies such as epiretinal membrane (ERM) and vitreomacular traction [1, 2]. Software improvement allows also 'en face' three-dimensional reconstruction and segmentation of the retinal thickness [3–5]. 'En face' technology is now available in most OCT devices. It scans the retina and choroid in a coronal plane at 90° from a cross-section. It is very important in the study of the inner retina, as the specialist can select the retinal layer to control and follow the retinal surface concavity and highlight retinal folds and epiretinal membranes. 'En face' scans adapted to the concavity of the eye are important for clinical work and research on inner retina, even more than in other layers disorders.

The first 'en face' scans or C-scans, 10 years ago, gave perfectly flat sections. The flat or plane scans had the common inconvenience of cutting through different layers at different levels leaving the images difficult to understand. The 'en face' flat modality has presently been left aside and is no longer used in clinical work. As the retina is cup shaped, a flat plane section (classical C-scan) cuts through all the retinal and choroid layers leaving complex images difficult to analyze and understand. Most modern 'en face' technology gives frontal scans adapted to the concavity of the eye posterior pole. Nowadays, standard macula analysis should always include 'en face' analysis. As the retina is concave, 'en face' frontal scans that follow the ideal inner limiting membrane shape and cut through pathologic alterations are easier to understand than flat scans. 'En face' scanning procedures are easy to perform and the images are easy to analyze.

An 'en face' scan may follow either the inner limiting membrane shape or the pigment epithelium concavity. The profile is selected according to the retinal or choroid layers under study.

'En face' technology follows the irregularities of a pathologic inner limiting membrane. It will provide images that will be useful to understand the lesion's shape and dimensions. We can select scan thickness and depth according to the lesion we want to study.

– Scan thickness. By reducing the scan thickness, we can obtain a thin retinal slice. The image will be noisy but the sensitivity will be very high. If we increase the scan thickness the image will be smoother but little details may be lost.

– Scan depth, shifting the 'en face' scan forward or backward, we chose the retinal layer we wanted to study or moved to the different layers of the choroid. The device automatically indicates on the screen monitor the exact location inside the retina or the choroid.

The 'en face' frontal scan images are generally more complex than cross-section B-scans. They are more difficult to read and less intuitive but the learning curve is fast.

Clinical Applications

Vitreoretinal Interface before and after Macular Surgery

Clinical 'en face' scan applications are numerous. We have been interested particularly in the vitreoretinal interface before and after macular surgery.

'En face' analysis of the vitreoretinal interface is a relatively recent acquisition that adds precious qualitative data for the physician and the surgeon.

A bi-dimensional approach (traditional B-scan) to the vitreoretinal interface gives a limited view due to the extremely localized examination. In this way, it is very difficult to rebuild a three-dimensional structure by viewing bi-dimensional images (fig. 1a, b).

On the contrary, the raster acquisition (several parallel horizontal B-scans on the macula) allows the three-dimensional reconstruction of the macular cube from which all the main layers can be extracted based on tissue reflectivity. The instrument software is able to recognize at least the inner limiting membrane (ILM), the inner plexiform layer and the retinal pigmented epithelium (RPE) for each B-scan that composes the macular cube (retinal segmentation). All segmentation lines are put together by software on a three-dimensional virtual multilayer image. The operator may adjust the profile cut, the thickness cut and the deepness cut.

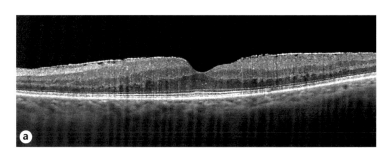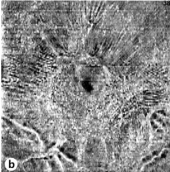

Fig. 1. Difference between a traditional B-scan (**a**) and 'en face' view (**b**) of the vitreoretinal interface. 'En face' view allows seeing the entire pucker size while B scan shows intraretinal alterations (edema).

Surgical peeling of the ILM of the retina has been proposed for different macular pathologies such as idiopathic macular hole [6], ERM [7] and macular edema [8–10]. Postoperatively, a characteristic feature of the peeled ILM area named dissociated optic nerve fiber layer (DONFL) has frequently been observed [10–14]. It consists of arcuate striae, following the direction of the optic nerve fibers, darker than the surrounding retina, and mainly visible on blue-filter frames. On traditional time domain-OCT, dimples limited to the retina nerve fiber layer thickness corresponding to retinal striae are present in the macular and perimacular regions [15].

In a series by Bovey and Uffer [16], including 268 epiretinal membrane peelings, they observed tearing and folding of the ILM in 8.6% of the patients. In this case, preoperative 'en face' spectral domain (SD)-OCT of the retinal surface was helpful in detecting areas possibly devoid of ILM. Grasping the retina with a forceps in this region would result in nerve fiber layer damage and should be avoided. Hence, preoperative 'en face' scan may guide the surgeon and inform him where he can be certain to find epiretinal tissue, and where the safer zone to grasp the ERM and begin peeling is located. 'En face' SD-OCT of the retinal surface performed within

2 weeks after surgery revealed a rough aspect of the peeled ILM area. No dimples were observed at this time.

This pattern could be due to the exposure of a rough surface composed of optic nerve fibers surrounded by Muller cell processes [10] or more probably to the early and transient swelling of the retinal nerve fiber layer [Ciardella et al., pers. commun., ARVO 2011, Fort Lauderdale] as this aspect decreased with time. Three months or more after surgery, dimples of the retinal surface were noted in 13 of 15 eyes (87%). After ILM removal, time domain-OCT studies observed dimples limited to the retinal nerve fiber layer corresponding to retinal striae on blue-filter photographs [12, 15].

In areas where the ILM has been peeled, Tadayoni et al. [10] have described the postoperative appearance of the arcuate striae in the direction of the optic nerve fibers, and appearing darker than the surrounding retina. They named this pattern the 'dissociated optic nerve fiber layer'. DONFL is not constantly observed on blue-filter photographs after ILM peeling. Its incidence has been reported to vary between 43 and 62% [10, 12–15, 17, 18]. In our study [20], the surface dotted with dimples varied greatly. Hence, it is possible that 'en face' SD-OCT may better detect small areas of dimples than blue-filter frames, which could explain the more frequent occurrence of dimples we observed.

The 'en face' study of the vitreoretinal interface is very useful before and after macular surgery. Some typical features resulting from macular peeling procedure are now well highlighted with an 'en face' view, completing and integrating the traditional B-scan. Analyzing the macular pucker before the surgery, an 'en face' cut gives a high relief of pathological structures and indicates with great accuracy dimensions, thicknesses, folds, and, going deeper, the features of tractional edema (fig. 2).

After macular pucker surgery with ILM peeling, a characteristic feature of the peeled ILM area named 'dissociated optic nerve fiber layer' has frequently been observed (fig. 3a, b). The area covered by dimples had different patterns: oval, centered by the fovea, crescent-shaped skirting the fovea or distant from the fovea.

In 15% of cases, 'en face' SD-OCT clearly shows an increasing of dimples in number and size during postoperative follow-up. Those arcuate lines develop progressively after surgery in the peeled area.

'En face' reconstruction of the retinal surface follows the concavity of the inner retinal surface, which was not possible on all commercialized SD-OCT machines so far. 'En face' SD-OCT of the retinal surface performed within a couple of weeks after surgery revealed a rough aspect of the peeled ILM area. Dimples appear rarely at this time. During the follow-up after 2 weeks, these curved dips can be observed by an 'en face' view adapted to ILM (fig. 4a–d).

This pattern could be due to the exposure of a rough surface composed of optic nerve fibers surrounded by Muller cell processes or more probably to the early and transient swelling of the retinal nerve fiber layer. Three months or more after surgery, dimples of the retinal surface were noted in 87% of the cases (fig. 5).

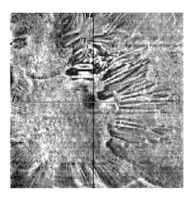

Fig. 2. 'En face' scan of a macular pucker. This scan allows studying plaque size, borders and retinal folds. Surgical interest comes from evidence of plaque detached limit, useful to start grabbing by Eckardt forceps.

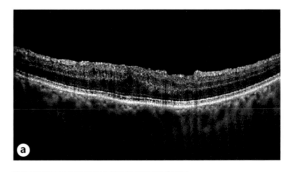

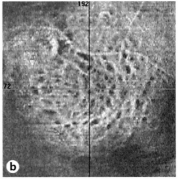

Fig. 3. a, b B-scan and ILM adapted 'en face' scan of postoperative DONFL 30 days after macular surgery with ILM removal. Several dimples (dips) appear in the area that underwent surgery.

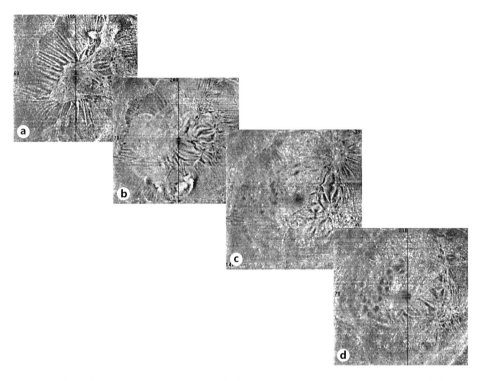

Fig. 4. a–d: 'en face' ILM study preoperatively (**a**) at 7 days (**b**), 30 days (**c**) and 90 days (**d**) after macular surgery with ILM removal. Evidence of dimples increases during OCT follow-up.

After ILM removal, several OCT studies observed dimples limited to the retinal nerve fiber layer corresponding to retinal striae on blue-light retinography. The correlation between 'en face' and blue light retinography aspects is very high (fig. 6a–c).

The Optovue RTVue® 100 is one of the few OCT devices able to analyze retina by 'en face' scans (141 horizontal parallel B-scans centered on the macula and spaced 0.49 mm). Each scan is 7 mm long on the horizontal axis. Each B-scan is made of 385 A-scans (one A-scan every 0.018 mm). System gives an analysis grid made of 54285 A-scan. The 'macular cube' is 7 × 7 mm wide by 2 mm high. Software determines automatically in each 141 B-scan the inner retinal surface. The 'en face' section can be 10 μm (or less) to 30 μm (or more) thick as need-

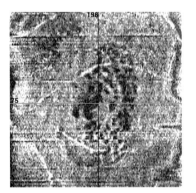

Fig. 5. 'En face' ILM adapted scan of a case that underwent surgery 14 years earlier. DONFL is well defined in the peeled area. Courtesy of Cristina Savastano, MD.

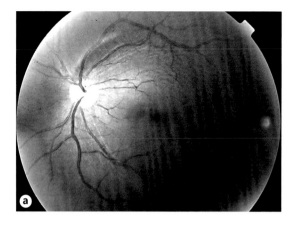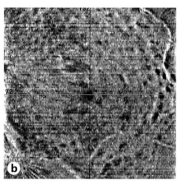

Fig. 6. Blue light retinography (**a**) and 'en face' ILM adapted (**b**), 180 days after macular surgery with ILM removal. 'En face' view seems to be more sensitive than blue light retinography in enhancing DONFL.

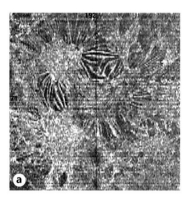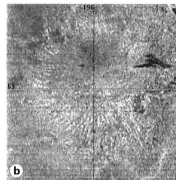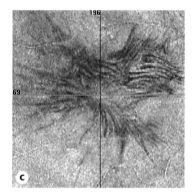

Fig. 7. a Light adherent epiretinal membrane. It is easy to evidence all the alterations as plaque and folds. **b, c** Tight adherent epiretinal membrane, surface-adapted scan (**b**). It is very difficult to enhance the density and the extension of plaque. It might be necessary to scan deeper in order to find retinal folds. This view gives an indirect image of the plaque based on fold valleys (**c**).

ed. The 'en face' slice is performed at the ILM line level.

Taking a correct 'en face' scan on the vitreoretinal interface needs some particular attention. The scanning profile must be real and adapted to the ILM profile. The best scanning thickness is about 15–20 μm, or in any case not thicker than the vertical membrane extension. A correct analysis should start from the vitreal side going towards the retina. In this way, it will be possible to observe and study some posterior vitreous relationships with the ILM. Proceeding on the surface, the entire ILM contraction will be clearly seen.

Enhancing vitreoretinal membranes will be easy for membranes that are not tightly adherent to the retinal surface (fig. 7a–c). So it will possible to study all the membrane features and, going deeper, all the retinal folds or tractional delamination (laminar holes, macular holes, schisis) (fig. 8).

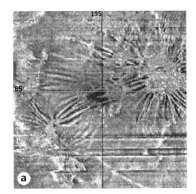 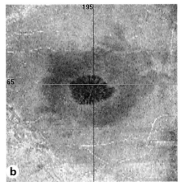

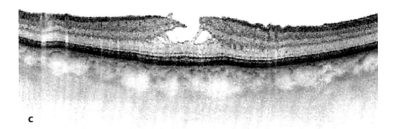

Fig. 8. Lamellar hole shape in 'en face' view. **a** 'En face' scan of the vitreoretinal interface. **b** Intraretinal 'en face' scan. **c** Cross-section scan.

DONFL morphology changes during the long-term follow-up. During the first 3 months, we can observe light dips with acute watersheds. After 6 months or more, dimples appear to be deeper and the watersheds between one dimple and another will become more flat (fig. 9).

Mechanism Leading to Retinal Surface Dimples

The mechanism leading to dimples of the retinal surface is unclear. Consistent with our study, Ito et al. [13] detected a DONFL appearance on fundus photographs between 1 and 3 months after surgery. The appearance continued to be more distinct until about 6 months; new cases did not develop DONFL 4 months after surgery. The delayed appearance of dimples suggests that the progressive morphological change of the retinal surface is not due to a true nerve fiber layer defect [12]. It could be related to a regenerative healing process initiated by the Mueller cells whose end feet are sometimes removed during ILM peeling [17].

Alkabes et al. [19] reported that inner retinal defects frequently occurred after idiopathic macular hole surgery when ILM was peeled, and it consisted of numerous dimples in the same direction of the optic nerve fibers. All patients in the study showed this typical OCT pattern 3 months after surgery. Thus, the authors suggest that this is a helpful, noninvasive technique to assess complete ILM removal in macular hole surgery if the appearance of dimples on the retinal surface is reported.

In conclusion, 'en face' OCT imaging of the macular surface is promising. With software development 'en face' scan procedures are easy to perform and their interest as a teaching tool is evident. Preoperative 'en face' SD-OCT can also guide preretinal tissue peeling.

'En face' OCT imaging can stress small alterations of texture of the retinal surface that are not

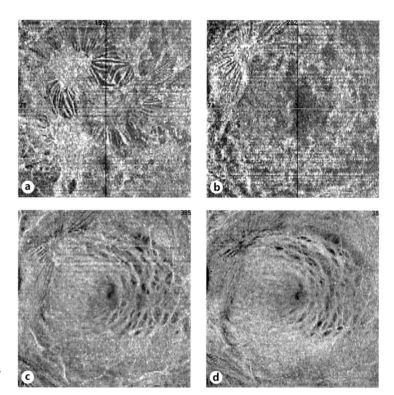

Fig. 9. DONFL progression from preoperation up to 180 days after surgery: before surgery (**a**), and 30 days (**b**), 60 days (**c**) and 180 days after surgery (**d**).

clearly seen on standard OCT scans. 'En face' scans allow us to study and classify vitreoretinal interface postoperative evolution from smooth plaques surrounded with retinal radial folds to the rough interface to dimpled surface with small craters that may or may not increase in size and depth with time.

It appears to be a useful and necessary complement to the conventional cross-sectional B-scan.

References

1 Treumer F, Wacker N, Junge O, Hedderich J, Roider J, Hillenkamp J: Foveal structure and thickness of retinal layers long-term after surgical peeling of idiopathic epiretinal membrane. Invest Ophthalmol Vis Sci 2011;52:744–750.
2 Mirza RG, Johnson MW, Jampol LM: Optical coherence tomography use in evaluation of the vitreoretinal interface: a review. Surv Ophthalmol 2007;52:397–421.
3 Lumbroso B, Savastano MC, Rispoli M, Balestrazzi A, Savastano A, Balestrazzi E: Morphologic differences, according to etiology, in pigment epithelial detachments by means of en face optical coherence tomography. Retina 2011;31: 553–558.
4 Srinivasan VJ, Wojtkowski M, Witkin AJ, et al: High-definition and 3-dimensional imaging of macular pathologies with high-speed ultrahigh-resolution optical coherence tomography. Ophthalmology 2006;113:2054.
5 Hangai M, Ojima Y, Gotoh N, et al: Three-dimensional imaging of macular holes with high-speed optical coherence tomography. Ophthalmology 2007;114: 763–773.
6 Lois N, Burr J, Norrie J, et al: Internal limiting membrane peeling versus no peeling for idiopathic full-thickness macular hole: a pragmatic randomized controlled trial. Invest Ophthalmol Vis Sci 2011;52:1586–1592.

7 Bovey EH, Uffer S, Achache F: Surgery for epimacular membrane: impact of retinal internal limiting membrane removal on functional outcome. Retina 2004;24:728–735.

8 Ma J, Yao K, Zhang Z, Tang X: 25-Gauge vitrectomy and triamcinolone acetonide assisted internal limiting membrane peeling for chronic cystoid macular edema associated with branch retinal vein occlusion. Retina 2008;28:947–956.

9 Schaal KB, Bartz-Schmidt KU, Dithmar S: Current strategies for macular hole surgery in Germany, Austria and Switzerland. Ophthalmologe 2006;103: 922–926.

10 Tadayoni R, Paques M, Massin P, Mouki-Benani S, Mikol J, Gaudric A: Dissociated optic nerve fiber layer appearance of the fundus after idiopathic epiretinal membrane removal. Ophthalmology 2001;108: 2279–2283.

11 Imai H, Ohta K: Microperimetric determination of retinal sensitivity in areas of dissociated optic nerve fiber layer following internal limiting membrane peeling. Jpn JOphthalmol 2010;54:435–440.

12 Mitamura Y, Ohtsuka K: Relationship of dissociated optic nerve fiber layer appearance to internal limiting membrane peeling. Ophthalmology 2005;112: 1766–1770.

13 Ito Y, Terasaki H, Takahashi A, Yamakoshi T, Kondo M, Nakamura M: Dissociated optic nerve fiber layer appearance after internal limiting membrane peeling for idiopathic macular holes. Ophthalmology 2005; 112:1415–1420.

14 Miura M, Elsner AE, Osako M, Iwasaki T, Okano T, Usui M: Dissociated optic nerve fiber layer appearance after internal limiting membrane peeling for idiopathic macular hole. Retina 2003;23: 561–563.

15 Mitamura Y, Suzuki T, Kinoshita T, Miyano N, Tashimo A, Ohtsuka K: Optical coherence tomographic findings of dissociated optic nerve fiber layer appearance. Am J Ophthalmol 2004;137: 1155–1156.

16 Bovey EH, Uffer S: Tearing and folding of the retinal internal limiting membrane associated with macular epiretinal membrane. Retina 2008;28:433–440.

17 Foos RY: Vitreoretinal juncture; topographical variations. Invest Ophthalmol Vis Sci 1972;11:801–808.

18 Nakamura T, Murata T, Hisatomi T, et al: Ultrastructure of the vitreoretinal interface following the removal of the internal limiting membrane using indocyanine green. Curr Eye Res 2003;27: 395–399.

19 Alkabes M, Salinas C, Vitale L, Burès-Jelstrup A, Nucci P, Mateo C: En face optical coherence tomography of inner retinal defects after internal limiting membrane peeling for idiopathic macular hole. Invest Ophthalmol Vis Sci 2011; 52:8349–8355.

20 Rispoli M, Le Rouic JF, Lesnoni G, Colecchia L, Catalano S, Lumbroso B: Retinal surface en-face optical coherence tomography. A new imaging approach in epiretinal membrane surgery. Retina 2012;32:2070–2076.

Bruno Lumbroso
Centro Oftalmologico Mediterraneo
via Brofferio 7
IT–00195 Rome (Italy)
E-Mail bruno.lumbroso@gmail.com

Coscas G, Loewenstein A, Bandello F (eds): Optical Coherence Tomography.
ESASO Course Series. Basel, Karger, 2014, vol 4, pp 110–116 (DOI: 10.1159/000355968)

Optical Coherence Tomography Findings in Acute Macular Neuroretinopathy

Maurizio Battaglia Parodi · Pierluigi Iacono · Davide Panico ·
Maria Lucia Cascavilla · Gianluigi Bolognesi · Francesco Bandello

Department of Ophthalmology, University Vita-Salute, Scientific Institute San Raffaele, Milan, Italy

Abstract

Acute macular neuroretinopathy (AMNR) is a rare retinal disorder characterized by the occurrence of wedge-shaped lesions localized at the macular region, and resulting in unilateral or bilateral macular scotomata. Although the etiology is not completely defined, vascular alterations are thought to play a possible role in the origin of morphological changes involving the outer retina. In the current study, we describe the anatomical findings associated with acute macular neuroretinopathy evaluated by mean of spectral domain-OCT and the clinical contribution of the 'en face' SD-OCT to monitoring of the retinal changes over the follow-up.

© 2014 S. Karger AG, Basel

Acute macular neuroretinopathy (AMNR) is a rare inflammatory disease characterized by unilateral or bilateral sudden onset of mild visual impairment associated with paracentral scotomata. Biomicroscopic fundus examination reveals the presence of dark reddish-brown, wedge-shaped lesions within the macular area [1–3], which can be better visualized on the infrared reflectance imaging using a confocal scanning laser ophthalmoscopy (table 1) [3–6].

The exact etiology of AMNR remains unknown, and the disease can come out as isolated, or in association with many conditions [2], as listed in table 2.

Instrumental examinations can greatly contribute to the diagnosis and clinical categorization of AMNR. Full-field electroretinogram and electroculogram are generally normal, but multifocal electroretinogram can reveal a reduced response, especially in the areas corresponding to the macular lesions. Whereas fluorescein angiography and fundus autofluorescence usually result within the normal limits, a number of abnormalities on optical coherence tomography (OCT) have been reported, including hyper-reflectivity of the outer plexiform

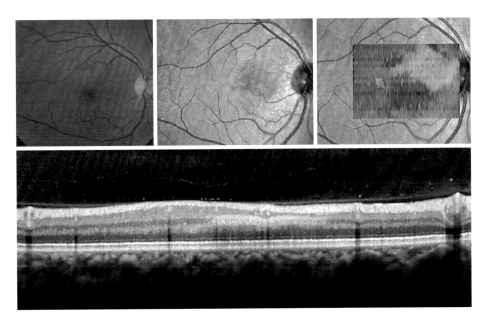

Fig. 1. AMNR in a 30-year-old woman, revealing a slightly darker macular lesion on color photograph which is far more clearly visible on infrared imaging as a dark lesion with irregular borders. 'En face' OCT unveils the large hyper-reflective area corresponding to the lesion visible on infrared imaging. SD-OCT discloses the hyper-reflectivity of the OPL with the underlying thinning of the ONL, and disruption of the OS/RPE junction.

Table 1. Clinical characteristics of acute macular neuroretinopathy

Variable visual acuity impairment
Paracentral scotomata
Darker, wedge-shaped macular lesions
Generally normal fluorescein angiography
Variable fundus autofluorescence pattern (from normal to weakly irregular)
Usually normal ERG/EOG
Visualization of lesion on infrared reflectance imaging

Table 2. Conditions associated with acute macular neuroretinopathy

Viral diseases
Intravenous sympathomimetics
Shock
Hormonal contraceptives
Postpartum
Antithymocyte globulin infusion
Subacute bacterial endocarditis
Trauma (head/chest)

Table 3. OCT signs of acute macular neuroretinopathy

Hyper-reflectivity of the OPL
Thinning of the ONL
Disruption of the IS/OS junction
Disruption of the OS/RPE junctions
Higher choroidal thickness at the level of the lesions
Hyper-reflectivity of OPL on 'en face' OCT

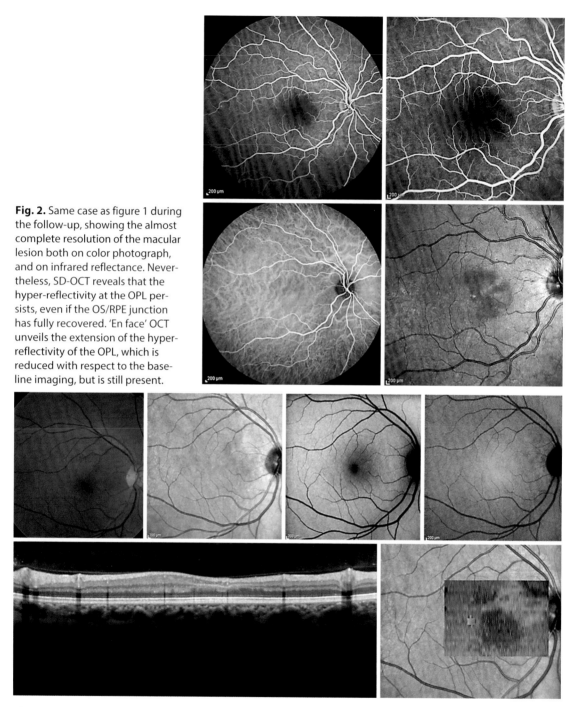

Fig. 2. Same case as figure 1 during the follow-up, showing the almost complete resolution of the macular lesion both on color photograph, and on infrared reflectance. Nevertheless, SD-OCT reveals that the hyper-reflectivity at the OPL persists, even if the OS/RPE junction has fully recovered. 'En face' OCT unveils the extension of the hyper-reflectivity of the OPL, which is reduced with respect to the baseline imaging, but is still present.

Fig. 3. AMNR in a 25-year-old woman showing slightly visible lesions at the posterior pole in both eyes. Fluorescein angiography is perfectly normal, whereas short-wavelength fundus autofluorescence and near-infrared fundus auto fluorescence show weak anomalies. Infrared reflectance imaging enables an easy identification of the macular lesions, suggesting the correct diagnosis of AMNR. SD-OCT visualizes the typical alterations, including the hyper-reflectivity at the level of the OPL, the thinning of the ONL, and the disruption of the OS/RPE in correspondence of the AMNR lesions.

Battaglia Parodi · Iacono · Panico · Cascavilla · Bolognesi · Bandello

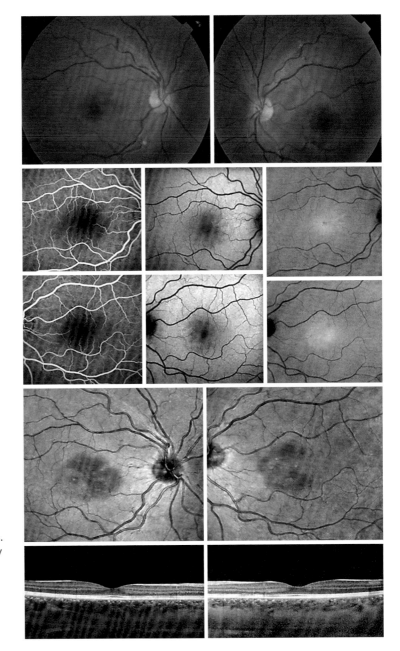

Fig. 4. Same AMNR case of figure 3. Wide-field fluorescein angiography and indocyanine green angiography in early and late phases show no alterations, whereas infrared reflectance imaging unmistakably reveals the location of the AMNR macular lesions.

layer (OPL), thinning of outer nuclear layer (ONL), disruption of the inner segment/outer segment (IS/OS) and outer segment/retinal pigment epithelium (OS/RPE) junctions (table 3) (fig. 1–4) [4, 5].

In particular, ONL thinning has been considered a long-term footprint of AMNR, whereas the RPE/OS line alterations correlate more precisely than the IS/OS junction with the extension of the lesions detectable on infrared reflec-

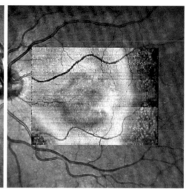

Fig. 5. 'En face' SD-OCT of the same case as in figure 4. The whole extension of the hyper-reflectivity at the OPL level is imaged by this technique, making monitoring of the disease over the follow-up period easier.

tance (fig. 5) [6]. It is of interest that the OPL hyper-reflectivity has been reported to develop within 24 h of the onset of disease, and may also predate the onset of lesions on color fundus photography or even infrared reflectance imaging [6].

The OS/RPE disruption turns out to be detectable later, as the macular lesions become more visible and darker. Thus, AMNR may start out from an inner maculopathy, to gradually evolve to an outer maculopathy involving also the RPE.

'En face' spectral domain (SD)-OCT imaging can offer immediate recognition of the whole extension of the AMNR lesion. More specifically, 'en face' SD-OCT shows a large hyper-reflective lesion at the level of the OPL, perfectly corresponding to the area affected by AMNR, as identified on infrared reflectance imaging (fig. 1, 2, 6). The representation provided by 'en face' SD-OCT allows a prompt identification and monitoring of OPL alteration, whose detection is essential for the correct diagnosis.

The measurement of the mean choroidal thickness within the area affected by AMNR shows a statistically higher value with respect to the values registered in all the macular areas not involved by the disease. This feature can hint that a choroidal vascular disturbance is associated

with the retinal modifications typical of AMNR. It is not clear whether the abnormal choroidal thickness is secondary to the retinal changes, or if it is a primary anomaly leading to subsequent alterations.

Limited information is available regarding the natural history of the disease. Although the possible resolution of AMNR lesions has been reported [2], the most refined imaging technologies, and especially SD-OCT, can reveal that alterations at OPL and ONL can still be present even in eyes showing complete resolution of the macular lesions (fig. 6).

In essence, patients affected by AMNR can show a broad pattern of choroid and retinal damages. Even though the course of the disease is generally considered favorable, and no therapy is currently advisable, the correct and timely diagnosis of the AMNR is mandatory to rule out other neurological disorders.

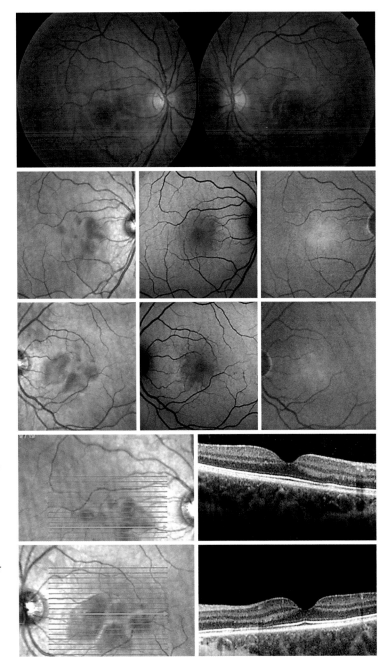

Fig. 6. Color photograph, infrared reflectance, short-wavelength fundus autofluorescence and near-infrared fundus autofluorescence of a case with bilateral AMNR. Infrared reflectance turns out to be the best imaging technique, allowing the prompt identification of multiple lesions at the posterior pole. The two fundus autofluorescence techniques provide slightly irregular images of difficult interpretation. SD-OCT clearly reveals hyper-reflectivity of the OPL, thinning of the ONL and disruption of the OS/RPE in correspondence to the AMNR lesions.

References

1 Bos PJ, Deutman AF: Acute macular neuroretinopathy. Am J Ophthalmol 1975;80:573–584.
2 Turbeville SD, Cowan LD, Gass JD: Acute macular neuroretinopathy: a review of the literature. Surv Ophthalmol 2003;48:1–11.
3 Priluck IA, Buettner H, Robertson DM: Acute macular neuroretinopathy. Am J Ophthalmol 1978;86:775–778.
4 Tingsgaard LK, Sander B, Larsen M: Enhanced visualisation of acute macular neuroretinopathy by spectral imaging. Acta Ophthalmol Scand 1999;77:592–593.
5 Corver HD, Ruys J, Kestelyn-Stevens AM, et al: Two cases of acute macular neuroretinopathy. Eye 2007;21:1226–1229.
6 Fawzi AA, Pappuru R, Saraf D, et al: Acute macular neuroretinopathy. Long-term insights revealed by multimodal imaging. Retina 2012;0:1–14.

Maurizio Battaglia Parodi
Department of Ophthalmology
University Vita-Salute, San Raffaele Scientific Institute
Via Olgettina 60, IT–20132 Milan (Italy)
E-Mail battagliaparodi.maurizio@hsr.it

Coscas G, Loewenstein A, Bandello F (eds): Optical Coherence Tomography.
ESASO Course Series. Basel, Karger, 2014, vol 4, pp 117–122 (DOI: 10.1159/000355969)

Optical Coherence Tomography in Myopic Choroidal Neovascularization

Maurizio Battaglia Parodi · Pierluigi Iacono · Gianluigi Bolognesi · Francesco Bandello

Department of Ophthalmology, Vita-Salute University, San Raffaele Scientific Institute, Milan, Italy

Abstract

Choroidal neovascularization (CNV) is one of the most important vision-threatening complications of degenerative myopia, occurring in up to 10% of highly myopic eyes. Optical coherence tomography (OCT) is a noninvasive examination technique, easy to be performed, and well accepted by the patients, which can greatly contribute to the clinical characterization of patients with myopic CNV. Many OCT features have been described in eyes affected by myopic CNV, including intraretinal cysts, subretinal fluid, alteration of the external limiting membrane, outer retinal tubulation, and modifications of the choroidal thickness. Aim of the present study is to discuss some controversial aspects about the correspondence of the fluorescein leakage and the OCT features at the onset of the CNV, and over the anti-VEGF treatment.

© 2014 S. Karger AG, Basel

Myopia is one of the leading causes of visual impairment in the world especially from 20–50 years of age [1]. The development of choroidal neovascularization (CNV) represents the most important vision-threatening complication in myopic eyes (fig. 1). The prevalence of myopic CNV has been reported to be between 5 and 10% [2–4], with the subfoveal location being quite frequent, accounting for 58–74% of cases, whereas juxtafoveal CNV has been described in 32% of the cases [5]. Myopic CNV has specific characteristics (table 1), including small size (<1 disc area), flat, greyish aspect with hyperpigmented margin and limited exudative manifestations.

Moreover, myopic CNV may occur adjacent to a lacquer crack, in an area of geographic atrophy of the retinal pigment epithelium (RPE), or also in an area of generalized attenuation of retinal pigment epithelium and choroid [6]. Among myopic patients with pre-existing CNV, more than 30% will develop CNV in the fellow eye within 8 years [7].

Fluorescein angiography (FA) may demonstrate abnormally slow choroidal and retinal blood flow in myopic patients and is helpful in identifying and locating the site of the CNV. The characteristic pattern of myopic CNV on FA is early hyperfluorescence, with little to moderate leakage in the late phases.

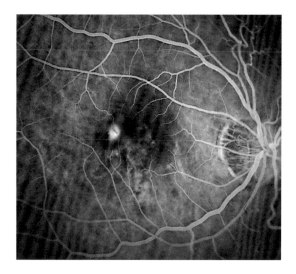

Fig. 1. Extrafoveal CNV with late fluorescein leakage and limited retinal hemorrhages.

Table 1. Clinical characteristics of myopic CNV

Small size (<1 optic disc diameter)
Minimal subretinal fluid
Limited retinal hemorrhage extension
Generally no hard exudates
Location between sensory retina and retinal
    pigment epithelium (type II CNV)

The advent of anti-vascular endothelium growth factor (VEGF) treatment has completely changed the current management of degenerative myopia-related CNV. Many studies have clinically shown that the anti-VEGF approach can halt the progression of myopic CNV, promoting a variable visual acuity improvement.

The rationale on the basis of anti-VEGF therapy is related to the histopathological evidence that myopic CNV can express VEGF [8], and also that the level of VEGF in the aqueous of eyes hosting myopic CNV can be reduced after intravitreal injection of anti-VEGF [9]. Moreover, many practical experiences have reported the positive effects of an anti-VEGF approach for myopic CNV [10–11]. However, there is no general consensus about the monitoring procedure after anti-VEGF treatment of myopic CNV. FA is generally considered the gold standard and the most efficient to detect myopic CNV activity through identification of fluorescein leakage, but being an invasive technique, it may not be so well accepted by the patients, especially if frequent monitoring is necessary. On the other hand, OCT is very practical and quick, allowing an easy identification of both the CNV and the related fluid. Nevertheless, there may be no correlation between signs of activity comparing FA and OCT (fig. 2–5).

OCT signs related to the presence of myopic CNV include both evidence of the neovascular membrane and indirect alterations (table 2).

However, in our experience there is a clear difference between OCT signs detectable at the diagnosis of the myopic CNV, and OCT signs visible after the anti-VEGF treatment. In particular, we have noticed that considering active myopic CNV on FA (i.e. CNV showing late fluorescein leakage), the intraretinal cysts can be identified in about one third of myopic CNV prior to the anti-VEGF treatment, and in less than 10% after the anti-VEGF injection. Moreover, the pure subretinal fluid turned out to be visible on OCT in half of the cases before the anti-VEGF injection, increasing up to two thirds of the cases over the subsequent follow-up. On the contrary, irregularities at the level of the external limiting membrane can be visualized in 100% of cases in leaking CNV on FA, independently of the stage of the CNV (fig. 6–8). Thus, external limiting membrane alterations directly correlate with the fluorescein leakage typical of active myopic CNV.

Outer retinal tubulation is an OCT sign which can be associated with heterogeneous disorders, including dystrophies and age-related macular degeneration. Outer retinal tubulation has been interpreted as related to alterations of the photoreceptors after injuring conditions. In-

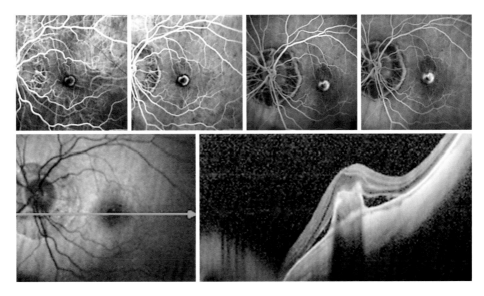

Fig. 2. Perfect correlation between FA (revealing a late leakage) and OCT (showing subretinal fluid).

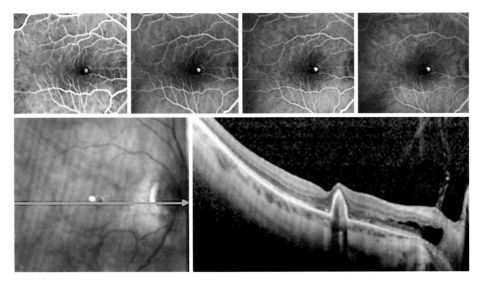

Fig. 3. Perfect correlation between FA (with no leakage) and OCT (no fluid).

frequently, outer retinal tubulation can be associated with myopic CNV (fig. 9). This alteration should be recognized in order to avoid mistakes and improperly retreat eyes requiring simply monitoring.

Another intriguing aspect is related to the alterations of the choroidal thickness which accompany the myopic CNV development [12–14]. In particular, visual acuity reduction has been linked to a decreased macular choroidal thickness, and to the de-

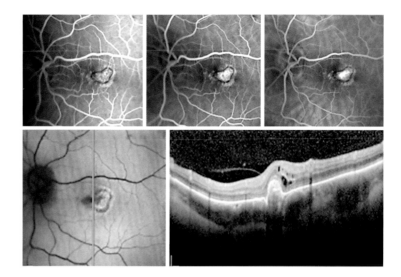

Fig. 4. Lack of correlation between FA (disclosing no leakage) and OCT (revealing intraretinal cysts).

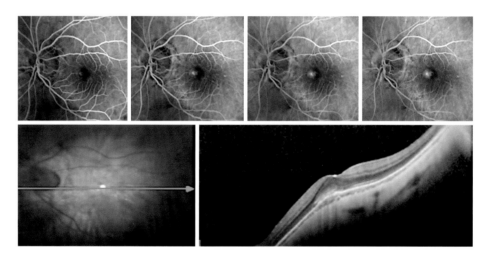

Fig. 5. Absence of correlation between FA (late leakage) and OCT (showing no fluid).

velopment of lacquer cracks which in 13% of cases precede the onset of myopic CNV [15]. A thinner subfoveal/inferior choroid at baseline indicates poor anatomic outcome for myopic CNV [12].

Moreover, the choroidal thickness is strictly related to the pattern of the lacquer cracks. Highly myopic eye without lacquer cracks have choroidal layer of normal thickness, whereas highly myopic eye with linear or stellate lacquer cracks

Table 2. OCT signs of myopic CNV

Direct identification of the CNV
  (size, location, height)
Intraretinal cysts
Subretinal fluid
Outer retinal tabulation
ELM irregularity
Choroidal thickness alterations

Battaglia Parodi · Iacono · Bolognesi · Bandello

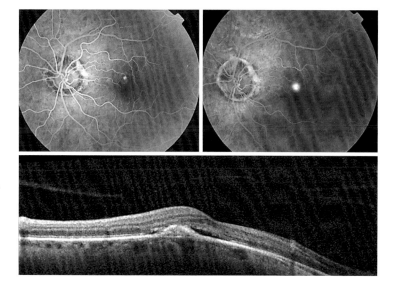

Fig. 6. Juxtafoveal myopic CNV at baseline disclosing fluorescein leakage in the late phases on FA and revealing subretinal fluid on OCT. The external limiting membrane shows an irregular profile, becoming indistinct in correspondence with the leaking side on FA.

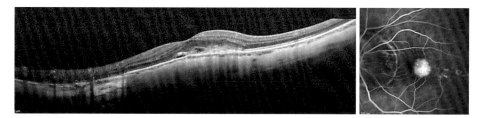

Fig. 7. Subfoveal myopic CNV at diagnosis showing a clear leakage on FA and some subretinal fluid on OCT. The external limiting membrane appears indistinguishable in comparison with the leakage site.

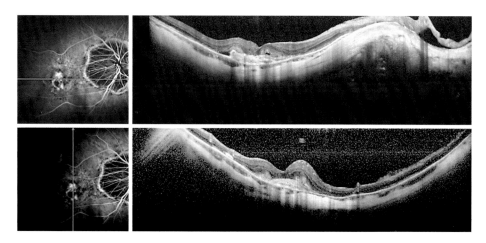

Fig. 8. Re-activation of subfoveal myopic CNV after 4 anti-VEGF injections. FA reveals the late leakage in association with the neurosensory detachment, which is visualized on OCT as subretinal fluid. There is a clear correspondence between irregular external limiting membrane and site of fluorescein leakage.

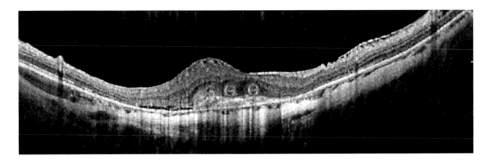

Fig. 9. Outer retinal tubulation located above a myopic CNV with no fluid.

are characterized by reduced subfoveal choroidal thickness.

In conclusion, OCT is an extremely useful tool in the diagnosis and the monitoring of myopic CNV. Nevertheless, it is not clear whether OCT can be considered sufficient for the management of myopic CNV or whether additional data from FA is sometimes needed. Further studies are necessary to find out the best OCT signs that correlate with the myopic CNV stage.

References

1 Ghafour IM, Allan D, Foulds WS: Common causes of blindness and visual handicap in the west of Scotland. Br J Ophthalmol 1983;67:209–213.
2 Curtin BJ, Karlin DB: Axial length measurements and fundus changes of the myopic eye. Am J Ophthalmol 1971;71:42–53.
3 Grossniklaus HE, Green WR: Pathologic findings in pathologic myopia. Retina 1992;12:127–133.
4 Ohno-Matsui K, Yoshida T, Futagami S, et al: Patchy atrophy and lacquer cracks predispose to the development of choroidal neovascularisation in pathological myopia. Br J Ophthalmol 2003;87:570–573.
5 Sperduto RD, Seigel D, Roberts J, Rowland M: Prevalence of myopia in the United States. Arch Ophthalmol 1983;101:405–407.
6 Gass JDM: Stereoscopic Atlas of Macular Diseases: Diagnosis and Treatment. St. Louis, Mosby-Year Book, 1997, pp 126–129.

7 Avila MP, Weiter JJ, Jalkh AE, et al: Natural history of choroidal neovascularization in degenerative myopia. Ophthalmology 1984;91:1573–1581.
8 Watanabe D, Takagi H, Suzuma K, et al: Expression of connective tissue growth factor and its potential role in choroidal neovascularization. Retina 2005;25:911–918.
9 Chan WM, Lai TY, Chan KP, et al: Changes in aqueous vascular endothelial growth factor and pigment epithelial-derived factor levels following intravitreal bevacizumab injections for choroidal neovascularization secondary to age-related macular degeneration or pathologic myopia. Retina 2008;28:1308–1313.
10 Parodi MB, Iacono P, Papayannis A, et al: Intravitreal bevacizumab for extrafoveal choroidal neovascularization secondary to pathologic myopia. Retina 2013;33:593–597.

11 Iacono P, Parodi MB, Papayannis A, et al: Intravitreal bevacizumab therapy on an as-per-needed basis in subfoveal choroidal neovascularization secondary to pathological myopia: 2-year outcomes of a prospective case series. Retina 2011;31:1841–1847.
12 Ahn SJ, et al: Association between choroidal morphology and anti-vascular endothelial growth factor treatment outcome in myopic choroidal neovascularization. Invest Ophthalmol Vis Sci 2013;54:2115–2122.
13 Wang NK, et al: Choroidal thickness and biometric markers for the screening of lacquer cracks in patients with high myopia. PLoS ONE 2013;8:e53660.
14 Wang NK, et al: Classification of early dry-type myopic maculopathy with macular choroidal thickness. Am J Ophthalmol 2012;153:669–677.
15 Hayashi K, et al: Long-term pattern of progression of myopic maculopathy: a natural history study. Ophthalmology 2010;117:1595–1611.

Maurizio Battaglia Parodi
Department of Ophthalmology
Vita-Salute University , San Raffaele Scientific Institute
Via Olgettina 60, IT–20132 Milan (Italy)
E-Mail battagliaparodi.maurizio@hsr.it

Coscas G, Loewenstein A, Bandello F (eds): Optical Coherence Tomography.
ESASO Course Series. Basel, Karger, 2014, vol 4, pp 123–126 (DOI: 10.1159/000355971)

Ganglion Cell Complex and Visual Recovery after Surgical Removal of Idiopathic Epiretinal Membranes

Luisa Pierro · Marco Codenotti · Lorenzo Iuliano

Department of Ophthalmology, Vita-Salute University, San Raffaele Scientific Institute, Milan, Italy

Abstract

The presence of ganglion cell axons in the context of surgically removed idiopathic epiretinal membranes (ERMs) was reported recently in the literature. In this prospective observational study, we used spectral domain-optical coherence tomography to investigate the change in ganglion cell complex (GCC) thickness and its possible correlation with visual recovery after vitreoretinal surgery for idiopathic ERM. We analyzed best-corrected visual acuity, mean macular thickness and mean GCC thickness 1 day before surgery, and 7 and 180 days after surgery. Internal segment/outer segment junction, external limiting membrane, cone outer segment tips defects and intra-retinal fluid were also investigated. The baseline GCC thickness was higher in patients with ERM (130 ± 13 µm) compared with healthy eyes (94 ± 5 µm; $p < 0.0001$). GCC thickness decreased after surgery to 89 ± 11 µm ($p < 0.0001$), and no difference was noted compared to controls ($p = 0.0689$). Postoperative best-corrected visual acuity gain showed direct correlation with GCC reduction ($R = 0.67$), but did not correlate with the mean macular thickness reduction ($R < 0.01$). Our data reported that mean GCC thickness is higher in eyes with idiopathic ERM, but after surgery returned to similar values of healthy eyes.

© 2014 S. Karger AG, Basel

Idiopathic epiretinal membranes (ERMs) have been identified in extensive ultrastructural studies: hyalocytes form the vitreous, glial cells in the form of both Müller cells and astrocytes, and fibroblast-like cells [1]. The presence of ganglion cell axons in the context of surgically removed idiopathic ERMs was also reported recently in the literature [1–3]. These data suggest that ganglion cells might also extend from the neural retina towards the vitreous, in association with glial cells (fig. 1).

In this prospective observational study, we used spectral domain-optical coherence tomography (SD-OCT) to investigate the change in ganglion cell complex (GCC) thickness and its possible correlation with visual recovery after vitreo-retinal surgery for idiopathic ERM.

Methods

The diagnosis of idiopathic ERM was obtained with biomicroscopy and SD-OCT examination. GCC thickness was analyzed using the SD-OCT (RTVue-100®, Optovue Inc., Freemont, Calif., USA) Optovue system.

Thirty healthy subjects, matched for age and gender, were included in this study as noninterventional controls.

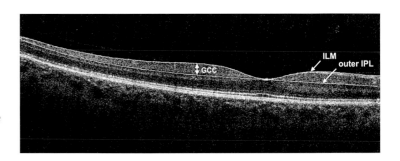

Fig. 1. SD-OCT of macular GCC of a healthy control. SD-OCT cross-section of the macula. The image was acquired using the RTVue-100 system. The GCC consists of 3 layers: the nerve fiber layer, the ganglion cell layer, and inner plexiform layer (IPL). The 2 boundaries on the image are the inner limiting membrane (ILM) and the outer IPL boundary. The GCC thickness is measured between these 2 boundaries.

Inclusion criteria were a diagnosis of idiopathic ERM in any stage and symptomatic metamorphopsia. We excluded patient with age <18 years, axial length >24 mm (myopic refractive error), BCVA <35 letters or >90 letters, any concurrent ocular disease in the study eye (e.g. diabetic retinopathy, uveitis, retinal vein occlusion, glaucoma), or any previous anterior or posterior segment surgical or laser treatment in the study eye. We decide to enroll patients with lens nuclear, posterior subcapsular or cortical cataracts >1.5 on the AREDS grading system.

Patients were visited 1 day before surgery, then 7 days and 6 months after surgery. We analyzed the changes of two variables throughout the follow-up: the GCC thickness and the total macular thickness. Furthermore, we correlated the changes of these cited variables with BCVA variation.

The presence of IS/OS disruption, ELM irregularity, COST defect and intraretinal fluid were also studied.

Three-port sutureless standard vitrectomy with inner limiting membrane peeling was successfully performed in all cases by a single experienced vitreoretinal surgeon. Phacoemulsification with intraocular lens implantation was concurrently carried out on all patients. Internal limiting membrane peeling was obtained in all patients with Brilliant Blue® staining.

The Wilcoxon test was used to compare BCVA values (number of letters of the ETDRS chart). Friedman's test for repeated measures was performed to compare total macular thickness. The Mann-Whitney test was used to compare patient age, mean GCC thickness and mean macular thickness of cases and age-matched noninterventional controls.

Results

We enrolled 30 eyes of 28 patients (15 females, 13 males). Mean age of patients and healthy age-matched noninterventional controls were, respectively, 70 ± 8 and 68 ± 8 years (p = 0.094). No patient required a vitreous substitute at the end of surgery.

All the patients had disturbing metamorphosis, which was reflected in distorted and nonuniform lines in the Amsler grid test. Average symptoms duration was 12.6 ± 2.6 months before surgery.

At baseline, 12 patients (40%) had a grade 1.5 nuclear sclerosis, 16 patients (53.5%) had a grade 1 nuclear sclerosis and 2 patients (6.5%) had a grade <1 nuclear sclerosis.

Baseline preoperative mean GCC thickness in patients affected by idiopathic ERM was 130 ± 13 μm, and significantly decreased to 114 ± 14 and 89 ± 11 μm, respectively, at the 1-week postsurgical visit and at the 6-month visit (p < 0.0001). Preoperative mean GCC thickness was significantly higher compared with that of healthy eyes (94 ± 5 μm; p < 0.0001), but at the 6-month postsurgical visit no significant difference (p = 0.0689) was noted between patients and controls.

Preoperative mean total macular thickness was 318 ± 32 μm, and significantly decreased to 304 ± 27 and 281 ± 18 μm, respectively, at the 1-week postsurgical visit and at the 6-month visit (p < 0.0001). Preoperative mean total macular

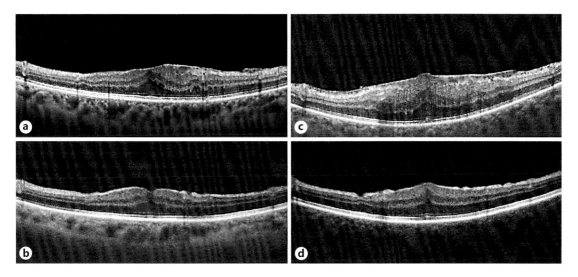

Fig. 2. SD-OCT before and after surgery for ERM. Patient 1: SD-OCT at baseline (**a**) and at the 6-month control (**b**). Patient 2: SD-OCT at baseline (**c**) and at the 6-month control (**d**).

thickness was significantly higher compared with that of healthy eyes (260 ± 8 μm; $p < 0.0001$), and the postoperative thickness value between patients and controls was still significantly different ($p < 0.0001$).

Mean BCVA significantly rose by 16 letters, from 78 ± 12 at baseline to 94 ± 6 at the 6-month visit ($p < 0.0001$). Postoperative BCVA gain showed a significant correlation with the mean GCC reduction ($R = 0.67$, $p < 0.0001$).

All our patients reported a subjective important reduction of metamorphopsia, assessed with the Amsler grid test.

Discussion

In the retinal ultrastructure, ganglion cell neurites are tightly associated with Müller cells, which are thought to play an important role in the physiology and function of the retina [4–6].

The presence of ganglion cell neurites in ERMs suggests that the adult retina might undergo a remodeling in response to various disorders or diseases [1–3]. Müller cells cannot be selectively investigated using actual clinically available equipment. We were able to study the ganglion cells using SD-OCT, the role of which is routinely employed in other diseases (diabetic retinopathy, glaucoma, central neurological disorders).

In our study, a reduction of the mean GCC thickness was evident 6 months after surgery (fig. 2), and this reduction was proportionally higher than the whole retina thinning. The postoperative mean GCC thickness changed back to similar values of healthy controls (no statistically significant difference was present), while the mean total macular thickness kept higher in pathologic subjects than in controls.

BCVA increased significantly 6 months after surgery, and was directly correlated with mean GCC thickness reduction. In the interventional group, we found minimal alterations of photoreceptors. These results might help elucidate in part the debate concerning visual recovery after ERM surgery. Our study showed that mean GCC thickness reduction turned out to have the strongest correlation with visual recovery, even more than with the total macular thickness reduction. We hypothesize that the membrane removal might possibly eliminate the ganglion cells neurites included in the ERM, leading the underlying retina to anatomical and functional restoration.

The results of the present research suggest that a decrease of the GCC layer is correlated with a visual restoration.

We believe our work opens a new debate about the crucial role of GCC in visual recovery after the removal of idiopathic ERMs and about their clinical significance in the functional outcome of surgery. Other unknown factors should be certainly considered for the correct pathophysiology interpretation, while functional research, such as electrophysiological studies, is required for a comprehensive analysis of this clinical aspect.

References

1 Lewis GP, Betts KE, Sethi CS, Charteris DG, Lesnik-Oberstein SY, Avery RL, et al: Identification of ganglion cell neurites in human subretinal and epiretinal membranes. Br J Ophthalmol 2007;91: 1234–1238.

2 Lesnik-Oberstein SY, Lewis GP, Chapin EA, Fisher SK: Ganglion cell neurites in human idiopathic epiretinal membranes. Br J Ophthalmol 2008;92:981–985.

3 Lesnik-Oberstein SY, Lewis GP, Dutra T, Fisher SK: Evidence that neurites in human epiretinal membranes express melanopsin, calretinin, rodopsin and neurofilament protein. Br J Ophthalmol 2010;95:266–272.

4 Bringmann A, Wiedemann P: Involvement of Müller glial cells in epiretinal membrane formation. Graefes Arch Clin Exp Ophthalmol 2009;247:865–883.

5 Hillenkamp J, Saikia P, Gora F, Sachs HG, Lohmann CP, Roider J, et al: Macular function and morphology after peeling of idiopathic epiretinal membrane with and without the assistance of indocyanine green. Br J Ophthalmol 2005;89: 437–443.

6 Inoue M, Morita S, Watanabe Y, Kaneko T, Yamane S, Kobayashi S, et al: Preoperative inner segment/outer segment junction in spectral-domain optical coherence tomography as a prognostic factor in epiretinal membrane surgery. Retina 2011;31:1366–1372.

Dr. Luisa Pierro, MD
Department of Ophthalmology, Vita-Salute University
San Raffaele Scientific Institute
Via Olgettina 60, IT–20132 Milan (Italy)
E-Mail pierro.luisa@hsr.it

Coscas G, Loewenstein A, Bandello F (eds): Optical Coherence Tomography.
ESASO Course Series. Basel, Karger, 2014, vol 4, pp 127–130 (DOI: 10.1159/000355973)

Choroidal Changes in Patients with Raynaud's Phenomenon Secondary to a Connective Tissue Disease: Study of Vascular Eye Involvement in Patients Affected by Raynaud's Phenomenon with in vivo Noninvasive EDI-OCT

Luisa Pierro[a] · Claudia Del Turco[a] · Elisabetta Miserocchi[a] ·
Francesca Ingegnoli[b]

[a]Department of Ophthalmology, Vita-Salute University, San Raffaele Scientific Institute and [b]Division of
Rheumatology, Instituto Gaetano Pini, Department of Clinical Sciences & Community Health, University of
Milan, Milan, Italy

Abstract

Raynaud's phenomenon (RP) is a peripheral circulatory disorder occurring in subjects exposed to cold or emotional stress. It is characterized by episodic local artery spasm, entailing exaggerated color changes of the fingers, such as pallor and cyanosis. RP is a red flag for the development of a connective tissue disease and can be accompanied by the development of systemic sclerosis-related digital ulceration. Vasospasm at the level of the capillary bed is the recognized mechanism for the development of RP. Choroid is a highly vascularized tissue composed of a choriocapillaris layer which nourishes photoreceptors and the retinal pigment epithelium. The purpose of this study was to investigate the eye vascular involvement in patients with RP secondary to a suspected connective tissue disease by measuring choroidal and macular thickness using enhanced depth imaging-spectral domain-optical coherence tomography. We found that choroidal tissue is thinned in patients suffering from vasospastic disorders of the sclerodermic spectrum disease, yet from the early phases. Choroidal imaging in these patients could represent a useful diagnostic tool for disease characterization and diagnosis.

© 2014 S. Karger AG, Basel

Raynaud's phenomenon (RP) was firstly described by the French doctor Maurice Raynaud in 1862. It has a complex pathogenesis but the contribution of blood vessel wall abnormalities interacting with altered neural control mechanism and intravascular circulating factors is well established [1].

The disturbance is defined as 'primary' RP if there is no evidence of an underlying medical illness, while 'secondary' RP occurs in association with a systemic condition, such as systemic lupus erythematosus, peripheral vascular disease or more commonly systemic sclerosis (SSc) [2]. SSc is a life-threatening condition mainly characterized by fibrosis and vasospastic ischemic phe-

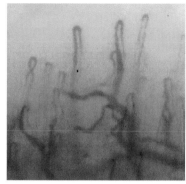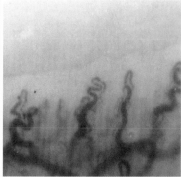

Fig. 1. Nailfold capillaroscopy patterns observed in healthy subjects with U-shaped and tortuous loops.

nomenon: it usually affects skin, cardiopulmonary system and gastrointestinal tract [3].

Primary RP is generally benign and well tolerated: the patient is recommended to keep warm the hands in order to avoid further attacks. Severe or ulcerative RP is approached with antivasospastic molecules, such as endothelin-1 receptor antagonist and oral prostanoids [4].

Autoantibodies dosing and abnormal nailfold capillary patterns (fig. 1) have shown to be helpful to distinguish between primary and secondary disease, being independent predictors of SSc, and useful tools for early diagnosis [5]. In particular, a specific capillaroscopic pattern is highly predictive for the development of SSc and may correlate with the severity of visceral involvement, while a regular capillary pattern rules out the disease with high probability.

Systemic vascular deregulation associated to SSc and CTD in general is able to induce vasospasm also in retinal vessels [3], while the behavior of the underlying choroidal circulation in these clinical conditions is mostly obscure.

Choroid is the more vascularized tissue of the eye and supplies blood to the outer retina layers, including the retinal pigment epithelium and photoreceptors. Its study could be very insightful to further investigate the vasospastic mechanism involving ocular structures in RP. With recent advance in spectral domain-optical coherence tomography (SD-OCT) imaging technology, it is now possible to explore choroidal morphology, and indirectly choroidal perfusion status by means of enhanced depth imaging-optical coherence tomography (EDI-OCT) techniques.

We decided to investigate choroidal features in subjects suffering from RP phenomenon suspected secondary to a CTD.

Methods

Twenty subjects with RP were enrolled to be studied. RP was defined as an episodic vasospastic ischemia of fingers assessed using nail fold capillaroscopy. Patients were submitted to testing for serum antinuclear antibodies increase. 26 healthy sex- and aged-matched subjects were enrolled as control group. All patients underwent complete ophthalmologic examination, including best-corrected visual acuity, slit lamp biomicroscopy, intraocular pressure measurement and fundus examination.

All subjects were submitted to macular and choroid SD-OCT examination using Zeiss Cirrus® HD-OCT implemented with the EDI scan system.

We performed scanning of central foveal thickness, central choroidal thickness and mean choroidal thickness, measured from eight perifoveal choroidal sectors (superior, inferior, nasal and temporal choroidal measurements in horizontal and vertical OCT scans at intervals of 0.5 mm up to 1 mm from the fovea) (fig. 2).

We compared the data from the RP and control groups using the Mann-Whitney test.

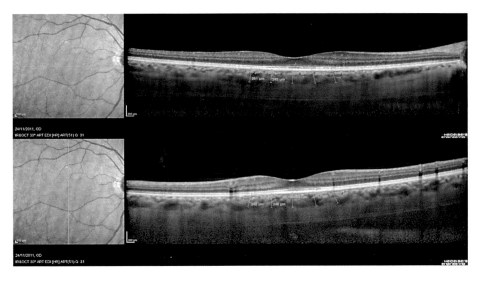

Fig. 2. EDI-OCT of horizontal and vertical scanning images of the right eye of a patient affected by RP with suspected CTD. Choroidal measurement was conducted starting from the subfoveal region up to 1 mm from the fovea at intervals of 0.5 mm in all macular sectors (superior, inferior, nasal and temporal).

Results

In the RP group (20 subjects, 18 females, mean age 51.8 years), 75% was positive for antinuclear antibodies testing and 100% showed a vasospastic ischemia at nailfold capillaroscopy, 65% of whom corresponding to a scleroderma pattern at nailfold capillaroscopy. Ocular assessment in the RP group resulted corresponding to or much similar to the ones in the control group (26 subjects, 16 females, mean age 54.2 years), the mean best-corrected visual acuity being equal to 0 logarithm of minimal angle of resolution and the mean IOP being equal to 14 mm Hg. None of the RP patients were referring ocular symptoms and all patients resulted within the normal limits at slit lamp biomicroscopy and fundus examination.

In the RP group, OCT imaging of the macular region showed a regular morphology, without any alteration concerning retinal layers. Nevertheless, in the RP group both retinal and choroidal thickness appeared as thinned. Comparing choroidal thickness measurements in the RP and control groups, we found that the subfoveal choroidal thickness was significantly thinner in the RP group than in the healthy controls (mean 256.82 vs. 313.22 µm; $p = 0.0031$). Similar results were found in the superior, temporal and nasal sectors of the retina.

Choroidal thickness was overall thinned in the inferior sectors: inner inferior (mean 258.29 vs. 293.15; $p = 0.0003$), outer inferior (mean 252.29 vs. 289.89; $p = 0.067$).

Central foveal thickness measurement also resulted significantly thinner in RP than in healthy controls (mean 257.44 vs. 275.18; $p = 0.0061$).

Discussion

Choroidal changes in terms of morphology and thickness have been already investigated with EDI-SD-OCT in various ocular pathologies, including myopia [6], diabetes [7] and uveitis [8], but not in RP and other pathologies of the CTD spectrum. The generalized thinning we found in the choroidal layers suggests an important involvement of ocular structure also in these disorders.

It is noteworthy that our patients did not complain of any visual symptom. Our results substain the hypothesis of a reduction of blood perfusion in the choroidal and retinal layers. A previous study suggested a choroidal vascular dysfunction using laser Doppler fluorometry in patients with acral vasospasms [9] and vasospastic phenomenon in retinal circulation in patient suffering from CTD [10]. It has been emphasized that prolonged vasospasm can induce retinal damage, leading to tissue damage, atrophy or even infarction [11]. Also, optic nerve head and nerve fibers are suspected to suffer from the capillary blood flow reduction correlated to vasospastic phenomenon [12]. This hypothesis is corroborated by studies reporting normal tension glaucoma to be more frequent in patients with SSc [13, 14].

With our study, we support these hypotheses and show that choroid and retinal thickness appear reduced since the early phases of CTD, when only RP is complied by patients. The importance of an early diagnosis is enforced by the demonstration that early treatment of SSc with immunosuppressive therapy led to regression of capillary rarefaction in the peripheral area [15]. EDI-OCT would be an easily reproducible in vivo reliable test for the diagnostic screening of patients with RP.

A predictive standardized use of choroidal imaging (with EDI-SD-OCT), similar to the one available for capillaroscopy, should be further investigated, in that, by facilitating the early diagnosis of SSc, it could pave the way for early treatment and new vascular protective therapies.

References

1 Herrick AL: The pathogenesis, diagnosis and treatment of Raynaud phenomenon. Nat Rev Rheumatol 2012;8:469–479.
2 Rogers M: Primary Raynaud's phenomenon. N Engl J Med 2013;368:1344.
3 Saketkoo LA, Distler O: Is there evidence for vasculitis in systemic sclerosis? Curr Rheumatol Rep 2012;14:516–525.
4 Herrick AL: Management of Raynaud's phenomenon and digital ischemia. Curr Rheumatol Rep 2013;15:303.
5 Jung P, Trautinger F: Capillaroscopy. J Dtsch Dermatol Ges 2013;11:731–736.
6 Kim M, Kim SS, Kwon HJ, Koh HJ, Lee SC: Association between choroidal thickness and ocular perfusion pressure in young, healthy subjects: enhanced depth imaging optical coherence tomography study. Invest Ophthalmol Vis Sci 2012;53:7710–7717.
7 Querques G, Lattanzio R, Querques L, Del Turco C, Forte R, Pierro L, Souied EH, Bandello F: Enhanced depth imaging optical coherence tomography in type 2 diabetes. Invest Ophthalmol Vis Sci 2012;53:6017–6024.
8 Nakayama M, Keino H, Okada AA, Watanabe T, Taki W, Inoue M, Hirakata A: Enhanced depth imaging optical coherence tomography of the choroid in Vogt-Koyanagi-Harada disease. Retina 2012;32:2061–2069.
9 Hasler PW, Orgül S, Gugleta K, Vogten H, Zhao X, Gherghel D, Flammer J: Vascular dysregulation in the choroid of subjects with acral vasospasm. Arch Ophthalmol 2002;120:302–307.
10 Salmenson BD, Reisman J, Sinclair SH, Burge D: Macular capillary hemodynamic changes associated with Raynaud's phenomenon. Ophthalmology 1992;99:914–919.
11 Grieshaber MC, Mozaffarieh M, Flammer J: What is the link between vascular dysregulation and glaucoma? Surv Ophthalmol 2007;52(suppl 2):S144–S154.
12 Guthauser U, Flammer J, Mahler F: The relationship between digital and ocular vasospasm. Graefes Arch Clin Exp Ophthalmol 1988;226:224–226.
13 Broadway DC, Drance SM: Glaucoma and vasospasm. Br J Ophthalmol 1998; 82:862–870.
14 Allanore Y, Parc C, Monnet D, Brézin AP, Kahan A: Increased prevalence of ocular glaucomatous abnormalities in systemic sclerosis. Ann Rheum Dis 2004;63:1276–1278.
15 Fleming JN, Nash RA, McLeod DO, Fiorentino DF, Shulman HM, Connolly MK, Molitor JA, Henstorf G, Lafyatis R, Pritchard DK, Adams LD, Furst DE, Schwartz SM: Capillary regeneration in scleroderma: stem cell therapy reverses phenotype? PLoS One 2008;3:e1452.

Dr. Luisa Pierro, MD
Department of Ophthalmology
Vita-Salute University, San Raffaele Scientific Institute
Via Olgettina 60, IT–20132 Milan (Italy)
E-Mail pierro.luisa@hsr.it

Subject Index

Swept source optical coherence tomography
   age-related macular degeneration imaging
      cross lines 78, 79, 81
      follow-up 81, 83
      horizontal and vertical scans 78–80
      radial scans 79, 82
      retinal thickness and volume
         calculations 79–81, 83
      volumes 79
   enhanced depth imaging optical coherence
      tomography comparison 76, 77, 90, 91

Topcon 3D OCT 2000, features 20, 21
Tubulation, outer retina 33, 118

Verhoeff's membrane, spectral domain optical
   coherence tomography 27, 28

Vitelliform macular dystrophy (VMD)
   clinical presentation 59
   preclinical stage and spectral domain optical
      coherence tomography findings 59, 60
Vitrectomy, *see* Surgical patient, optical coherence
   tomography evaluation
Vitreomacular traction syndrome
   diabetic macular edema 64, 69
   optical coherence tomography findings 15, 16
   surgical patient optical coherence tomography
      evaluation 51
Vogt-Koyanagi-Harada syndrome, choroidal
   thickness measurement 38

Zeiss Cirrus HD OCT, features 21

The Written Word   Book 2

The Written Word Book 2

A Course in Controlled Composition

Tom McArthur

Oxford University Press

Oxford University Press
Walton Street, Oxford OX2 6DP

Oxford New York
Athens Auckland Bangkok Bombay
Calcutta Cape Town Dar es Salaam Delhi
Florence Hong Kong Istanbul Karachi
Kuala Lumpur Madras Madrid Melbourne
Mexico City Nairobi Paris Singapore
Taipei Tokyo Toronto

and associated companies in
Berlin Ibadan

OXFORD and OXFORD ENGLISH are
trade marks of Oxford University Press

ISBN 0 19 451361 0

First published 1984
Sixth impression 1995

The publishers would like to thank the following for
permission to reproduce photographs.

Anglo-Australian Observatory
Elliott Erwitt/John Hillelson Agency
Christopher Hume/Camera Press
Mark Mason
Axel Poignant
Rosie Potter
Jeremy Rowland

Cover illustration by Peter Till

Typeset by Tradespools Ltd, Frome, Somerset
Printed in Hong Kong

Acknowledgements

Firstly, Basil Skinner, Head of the Department of Extra-Mural
Studies at the University of Edinburgh, Bridget Stevens, his
Administrative Assistant, and William McDowall, Head of the
Language Learning Centre. Without their help, when I was
responsible for the Department's service courses in English as a
foreign language, this course would never have come into existence.
Additionally, the hard work and interest of many students of diverse
linguistic and professional backgrounds taking the weekly courses
between 1975 and 1979 were also invaluable in helping me see where
I wanted to go. The present course owes much to them.

Secondly, Patricia Foy, Lorraine Therrien-Roy, and Claude Girard,
three English language advisers in Quebec City, who made it possible
for me to work, between 1979 and 1981, with twenty-two secondary
school teachers, all of whom I would like to thank for their interest
and inspiration.

Thirdly, colleagues at the Université du Quebec à Trois-Rivières: Ton
That Thien for his comments, and Judith Cowan, Patricia Gordon
and Gisèle Wilson, for using much of the material in their classes and
providing useful feedback from all concerned. Additionally, my
research students Lise Lachapelle, Susan MacNeil and André
Rouleau, three insightful undergraduate students France Jutras,
Cheryl Kosaka and Joane Turcotte, and many others who made
useful observations on the material when we worked with it together.

Fourthly, Keith Doyle at Three Rivers High School, for assessing the
material in relation to native and near native secondary school
students of English.

Fifthly, those who have worked with Oxford University Press in
helping me prepare the material for wider dissemination, particularly
Henry Widdowson, Professor of Education (with special reference to
speakers of other languages) University of London Institute of
Education, and those within Oxford University Press for seeing me
safely through the editorial and production stages of what remains
one of the most enjoyable – if at times frustrating – projects I have
ever worked on.

Lastly, my daughter Roshan, now fifteen, for her patient and good-
humoured services as guinea-pig, demonstrating that the material has
been comprehensible and I hope useful to at least one young native
user of the language. For her help, many thanks.

Contents

Unit 4   Revision

Unit 5

Unit 6

Unit 7

To the teacher or administrator

This is the second stage of our writing course *The Written Word*. More advanced students will be able to use Book 2 without having studied Book 1. There are, however, occasional references to material that has been covered in the first stage.

The Written Word is the product of some eight years of experimentation and practical use, first at the University of Edinburgh and later at the University of Quebec.

In Edinburgh, the course originally developed as a means of helping foreign postgraduate students – working in subjects as diverse as architecture, geology, law, medicine, language teaching and the physical sciences – to write clearly and logically in English. In Quebec, it has been adapted to cover late secondary, junior college and university work. These two very distinct areas of work proved compatible largely because the basic skills of writing are the same for most people and most purposes. Everybody has to be able to write clearly, spell adequately, punctuate consistently, follow the rules of grammar, handle stylistic differences and, importantly, be aware of the options offered within what people see as 'good written English'. This is as true today as it was a hundred years ago.

The course is, however, 'controlled'. It does not encourage the student, in the early stages, to attempt a lot of free expression. In the writer's experience over twenty years of teaching English at various levels in various parts of the world, too much freedom in writing can mean frustration. One does not say to a new learner driver: 'Get into the car and start. Anywhere will do.' In the same way, pre-analysis of the problems together with guidance throughout the work itself are prerequisites for a student's success. The discipline is often welcomed with relief.

Under guidance of the kind provided here, the student can proceed at his or her own speed, benefiting from the chance to work privately – and writing is a private art – as well as, one hopes, the opportunity to consult a tutor regularly. Additionally, the format of the units, with their detailed answer sections, enables a tutor to look after anything from one to thirty students simultaneously, without getting flooded out with material to correct. Traditional writing courses can be very hard on the tutor. This one is not.

At the same time, no limitation is placed on any teacher who wishes to supplement the graded and guided material with related free composition. This is entirely a matter between teacher and student. The important thing is that the course provides a useful framework within and around which related work can be organized.

The principle animating the course is relatively simple: to give students clearcut quantities of interrelated material through which to proceed to higher levels of skill. Intermediate and even advanced foreign users of English can benefit from the layout, the instructions and the exercises, and in one compact system are provided with core information on grammar, levels of formality, spelling, punctuation, word use and formation, composition and editing. Having taught English as a mother tongue as well as a foreign or second language, I also suspect that the course – or courses like it – will serve native users of English too.

The techniques employed combine both 'traditional' and 'modern' methodology. Texts, lists, tables, analytical and synthetic procedures, blank-filling, multiple choice, conversion exercises, pattern practice, elements of programmed learning and even the correction of deliberate mistakes all rub shoulders amicably enough. Additionally, many of the students who took the original course in Edinburgh also used it as a preparation for the Cambridge Certificate examinations, with good results. Indeed, resemblances will be found between certain procedures here and in those examinations.

Not everything in the exercises has been explained in the instructions, partly because such a procedure would have made the course too bulky, and partly because it is natural and desirable that students should induce as much as possible by themselves. Since creative expression is very much a personal thing, however, it has been assumed that teachers can encourage the free development of writing skills, and also that a professional person can divert what he or she has learnt into the channels of special interest without further help from us.

Every effort has been made to avoid an unnatural or laboured style. Consequently, grammatical and other material often appears in the model texts before it is described and practised in the exercise sections. Thus, for example, quotation and parenthesis are both used freely before the student is asked to handle them. This, it is believed, is closer to real life than a strict gradation of material so that nothing is encountered until it can be explained.

To the student

1 This is the second book of a course intended for people who have reached a reasonable level in reading and understanding the English language, the kind of level usually called 'intermediate'. Such people may or may not speak English well, but their ability to read will be much greater than their ability to write. (In practice, we have found that many 'advanced' students have benefited from doing systematic work of this kind. This includes many professional people capable of excellent written work in their own languages.)

2 The course is based on the assumption that writing well in any language is a difficult art and needs a great deal of practice. Writing adequately in a second language is often a slow, painful and frustrating experience.

3 The aim here is to make writing practice in English a pleasant, realistic and rewarding experience (at least as far as that is possible within the limits of a course of this kind). It will, however, necessitate hard work on your part.

4 The work should be done systematically. Do not, for example, start in the middle of Unit 2 because the earlier material seems too easy. It is not. It is also not a good idea to jump sections, because the units and sections are all carefully interrelated in order to provide you with the necessary repetitive practice as well as new experience.

5 If you feel at any time that the information or the answers are not in any way satisfactory, do not hesitate about consulting other sources or discussing the point in question with your tutor or a competent friend or colleague. Writing in English is an art, not part of a fixed science.

6 The language of the texts, instructions and exercises has been kept as simple as possible (especially in the earlier units), but where a choice was necessary between being simple and being natural, naturalness always won. If, consequently, you do not understand anything, consult a good dictionary (unilingual or bilingual) or grammar book. In a course of this length it is impossible (and undesirable) to try to explain everything.

7   Resist the temptation to look at the answers until you have tried an exercise at least once. Additionally, even after seeing the answers once, be prepared to do an exercise again – and again, until you achieve a satisfactory level of performance. In writing, once is almost never enough. Do rough work where necessary, before making a final version of a piece of writing. (After doing the basic material, you may also wish to 'play' with the topic, developing it in your own way. Feel free to do so.)

8   Do not accept from yourself a lower level of performance than you would accept from others:
    * Is your handwriting as clear as it might be?
    * Are you as careful about spelling and punctuation as you should be?
    * Is grammar something you want to be reasonably exact about?
    * If you type, do you take care with the organization of your page?

9   Writing must be clear and logical – and simple writing is where one begins. Complexity is often necessary, when ideas are complex, but there is no advantage in complexity when the ideas are – *or should be* – simple.

10 The basic principles of good writing are the same for all kinds of writing: story-telling, newspapers, business and scientific reports, material written for children or for adults, for general reading or for specialist purposes. This is a course in basic principles.

UNIT 1

1.1 Comprehension and composition model: 'Language'

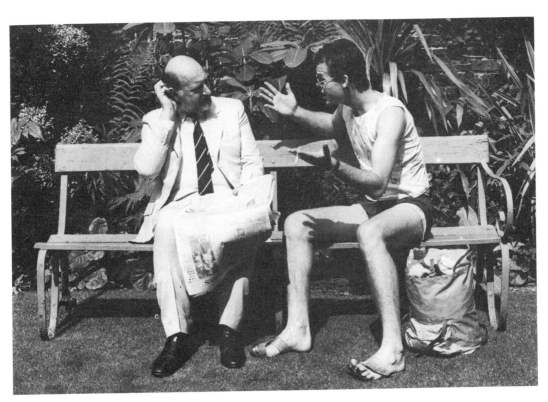

Here is a passage discussing some aspects of language. Read it twice, noting how the argument is developed, the kind of sentences used, the punctuation style and the vocabulary.

When we talk about learning a language like English, Japanese or Spanish, we speak and think as though the language in question were a fixed unchanging thing. We expect to learn it as we learned geometry or how to ride a bicycle – systematically, and with clear ultimate success. Many people subsequently give up when they discover just what a misconception this is. They have in fact embarked on an activity that could last the rest of their lives. The experience makes them realize that they are not only going to have

5

to work very hard indeed if they want to succeed, but also that they
are – in many cases – barely masters of the language they call their   10
own 'mother tongue'.

Studying any language is, in fact, an endless voyage. Each of the
thousands of languages currently used in the world is a complex
affair. Many languages do have a standard form – particularly on
paper – and this is what we learn, but they probably also have a   15
variety of regional dialects and social styles, and many are the
products of the historical mingling of other languages. The English
language is just such a hybrid. It began its career just under two
thousand years ago as a form of ancient German, collided with a
special kind of old French, was subjected to several waves of Latin   20
and a flood of Greek, and since then has acquired bits and pieces of
every other language that its users have ever been in contact with.

A second common misconception about language is that words
have fixed and clear meanings. This is – fortunately or
unfortunately – far from true. Take even the apparently simple and   25
specific English word *man*. It seems clear enough; it refers to 'an
adult male human being'. Of course it does, but just consider for a
moment the following sentences:

1) There are several men missing in that chess set.
2) The boat was manned entirely by women and children.   30

You might argue that these sentences are somewhat unnatural;
certainly, they do not represent the everyday core meaning of the
word *man*. They are, however, legitimate extensions of that core
meaning, the second being especially interesting because it is a verb
and not a noun, and suggests that we expect adult male human   35
beings to serve as the crews of ships, not women and certainly not
children. Part of the pleasure and genius of language may well arise
out of this slight 'misuse' of words. After all, if you call a person a
cat or a cabbage, no literal identification is intended, but a great
deal of meaning is nevertheless conveyed.   40

A third misconception about language claims that every language
is – or should be – equally used and understood by all its
practitioners everywhere. Certainly, users of the standard forms of
English in the United Kingdom generally understand their
equivalents in the United States; the degree of similarity between   45
these two major forms of English is great. Dialect-users in these
countries, however, have serious problems understanding each
other, to the extent that they may wonder if they are actually using
the same language. Someone from Brooklyn, New York, will have
trouble with a Cockney from London; an old-style British Army   50
colonel won't do well in discussions with a Californian flower-
child. Yet they all belong within the vast community of 20th-
century World English.

Below are some statements relating to the passage. Some are true (T) in terms of the passage, while others are false (F). Mark them appropriately, and if a statement is false, say why.

a. ☐ It is a misconception that languages are fixed unchanging things.

b. ☐ Although most people are the masters of their own mother tongues, they seldom do well in other languages.

c. ☐ Learning a foreign language is effectively a lifelong undertaking, if one takes it seriously.

d. ☐ Each of the thousands of languages currently used today has its standard form as well as regional dialects.

e. ☐ In historical terms, English cannot be called a 'pure' language.

f. ☐ A word like *man* has a clear central meaning and a range of additional meanings.

g. ☐ Calling someone a 'cat' or a 'cabbage' is a normal literal use of language.

h. ☐ The vast majority of Americans and Britons understand each other very well most of the time because they all use the same standard language.

i. ☐ In effect, distinct dialects of a language are like separate but related languages. It is reasonable to suppose that, say, a Spaniard and a Portuguese could understand each other about as well as a Brooklyner and a Cockney using their own forms of English.

j. ☐ Basically, the passage is an argument in favour of greater control over language, because if language is not controlled it is harder for people to become fluent and to understand each other satisfactorily.

1.2 Spelling:
British and American usage

Essentially, there is very little difference between British and American spelling; however, those groups of words which *are* spelled differently are quite important. The list over the page gives the major systematic differences (Nos 1–8) and a small group of special differences (No 9) that are individuals and not types.

British preferences	United States preferences
1 colour	color
labour	labor
2 centre	center
theatre	theater
3 archaeology	archeology
foetus	fetus
4 catalogue	catalog
epilogue	epilog
5 programme	program
kilogramme, kilogram	kilogram
6 organise, organize	organize
harmonise, harmonize	harmonize
7 defence	defense
pretence	pretense
8 traveller, travelling	traveler, traveling
worshipper, worshipping	worshiper, worshiping
9 aluminium	aluminum
cannon (*type of gun*)	canon
cheque	check
grey	gray
practise (*v*), practice (*n*)	practice (*n,v*)
tyre	tire

Below you will find a list of 22 words. There is a set of brackets before and after each word. In the brackets before each word, put its spelling type, whether British (Br) or United States (US), then complete the set with the alternative form. The first one is done for you as an example.

a. (*Br*) metre   (*US*) meter
b. (   ) memorize (*no option*)   (   )
c. (   ) neighbourhood   (   )
d. (   ) pretence   (   )
e. (   ) check (*money*)   (   )
f. (   ) anaemic   (   )
g. (   ) labour relations   (   )
h. (   ) saber   (   )
i. (   ) medieval   (   )
j. (   ) kilometre   (   )
k. (   ) dialog   (   )
l. (   ) systematise   (   )
m. (   ) centimeter   (   )
n. (   ) colored   (   )

o. (   ) millilitre   (   )
p. (   ) encyclopaedia   (   )
q. (   ) offense   (   )
r. (   ) aluminium   (   )
s. (   ) monologue   (   )
t. (   ) harbour   (   )

1.3 Vocabulary definitions:
Consulting dictionaries

Using any two (or, even better, three) different unilingual dictionaries
of English, look up the following words and make comparative notes
about what you find. If possible, at least one dictionary should
provide etymological information (that is, information about the
history of words, showing the languages from which they have come
into English).

a. geometry   (l.4)   f. style   (l.16)
b. misconception (l.6)   g. hybrid (l.18)
c. embark   (l.7)   h. chess   (l.29)
d. standard   (l.14) i. core   (l.32)
e. dialect   (l.16) j. genius (l.37)

1.4 Grammar:
Sentence analysis

Below you will find the sentences of the first two paragraphs of the
passage on language analysed one by one. In this analysis, each
sentence is given its sequential number (1,2,3, etc) and is labelled
simple, compound, complex or compound-complex according to its
structure. Additionally, its finite verbs (that is, those verbs that have
subjects) are underlined, and any connecting words (such as
conjunctions and relative pronouns) are in bold type. Immediately
after each compound or complex sentence the simple sentences of
which it consists are also shown. Study the analyses carefully.

1   Complex sentence

When we <u>talk</u> about learning a language like English, Japanese or Spanish, we <u>speak</u> **and** <u>think</u> **as though** the language in question <u>were</u> a fixed unchanging thing.

Simple sentences:

  i   We talk about learning a language like English, Japanese or Spanish.
  ii We speak.
  iii We think.
  iv The language in question was a fixed unchanging thing.

Note the use of *were* after 'as though'.

2   Complex sentence

We <u>expect</u> to learn it **as** we <u>learned</u> geometry **or** how to ride a bicycle – systematically, and with clear ultimate success.

Simple sentences:

  i   We expect to learn it.
  ii We learned geometry.
  iii We learned how to ride a bicycle.

Note that the phrase that completes the complex sentence after the dash goes with both ii and iii.

3   Complex sentence

Many people subsequently <u>give up</u> **when** they <u>discover</u> **just what** a misconception this <u>is</u>.

Simple sentences:

  i   Many people subsequently give up.
  ii They discover (something).
  iii What a misconception this is!
      (= This is a great misconception.)

4   Complex sentence

They <u>have</u> in fact <u>embarked</u> on an activity **that** <u>could last</u> the rest of their lives.

Simple sentences:

  i   They have in fact embarked on an activity.
  ii This activity could last the rest of their lives. (**Note** that *that* = *This activity* or something similar.)

Note also how the adverbial phrase *in fact* comes between the two parts of the finite verb 'have embarked', and also that the second finite verb is made up of the modal verb *could* and the bare infinitive *last*.

5 **Compound-complex sentence**

The experience <u>makes</u> them realize **that** they **are not only** going to have to work very hard indeed **if** they <u>want</u> to succeed, **but also that** they <u>are</u> – in many cases – barely masters of the language ∧ they <u>call</u> their own 'mother tongue'.

Simple sentences:
  i The experience makes them realize (something).
  ii They are going to have to work very hard indeed.
  iii They want to succeed.
  iv They are – in many cases – barely masters of a (particular) language.
  v They call this language their own 'mother tongue'.

Note that 'not only … but also' is a special balancing device, and that the connecting word *that* is omitted between 'language' and 'they'.

6 **Simple sentence**

Studying any language <u>is</u>, in fact, an endless voyage.

Note that it is quite common to use shorter simple sentences at the beginning of passages or paragraphs for dramatic effect.

7 **Apparent simple sentence/disguised complex sentence**

Each of the thousands of languages ∧ currently used in the world <u>is</u> a complex affair.

Simple sentences:
  i Each of the thousands of languages … is a complex affair.
  ii These languages are currently used.

Note that the sentence is, in fact, elliptical, omitting *that* or *which are*, and so turning *used* into an isolated past participle.

8 **Compound-complex sentence**

Many languages <u>do have</u> a standard form – particularly on paper – **and** this <u>is</u> **what** we <u>learn</u>, **but** they probably **also** <u>have</u> a variety of regional dialects and social styles, **and** many <u>are</u> the products of the historical mingling of other languages.

Simple sentences:
  i Many languages do have a standard form – particularly on paper.
  ii This is (something).
  iii We learn (something).

iv   They probably also have a variety of regional dialects and social styles.

v   Many are the products of the historical mingling of other languages.

Note the emphatic use of *do*; the way in which *what* is used to combine two simple sentences; and that, apart from the clause introduced by *what*, the sentence is a compounding process.

9   Simple sentence

The English language is just such a hybrid.

Note the way in which this short, simple sentence appears in the middle of longer sentences, for emphasis.

10   Compound-complex sentence

It began its career just under two thousand years ago as a form of ancient German, collided with a special kind of old French, was subjected to several waves of Latin and a flood of Greek, and since then has acquired bits and pieces of every other language **that** its users have ever been in contact with.

Simple sentences:

i   It began its career just under two thousand years ago as a form of ancient German.

ii   It collided with a special kind of old French.

iii It was subject to several waves of Latin and a flood of Greek.

iv   It has acquired bits and pieces of every other language (of a particular kind).

v   Its users have been in contact with various languages.

Note the strong list of clauses all with the same subject *It*, and the special way in which *that* and *ever* work together to create the final part of the sentence.

Having studied this analysis, proceed to a similar analysis of the remaining paragraphs of the passage.

1.5 Composition: The making of summaries

A summary is a shorter version of a text, report, book or similar piece of writing. It can also be called a précis, a resumé or a synopsis, and in the case of a book, an abridgement or abridged version. The art of making summaries is an important part of writing well.

Good summaries of a passage can be achieved by various means:

1   by looking for the main ideas in a passage, listing them, and then expressing them in a brief and simple way (often in shorter sentences and with simpler words);

2   by deliberately seeking to simplify the grammatical structure of the sentences and paragraphs, removing the less necessary parts, reducing several sentences to one, changing the order of development here and there, and generally trying, as is often said, to provide the 'bare bones' of the text;

3   by trying, in principle, to reduce complex sentences to simple sentences, simple sentences to phrases, phrases to single words, and the like;

4   any combination of these.

Someone who is good at summarizing may not consciously be aware of doing these things, but some such procedure is at the basis of most kinds of summary-writing. No two summaries are ever the same, even by the same person doing the same work on different days. There are no perfect summaries – only more or less successful ones.

How does one become a good summary-writer? The answer is simple, and like everything else in writing – by constant practice.

The technique presented below is only one possible way of approaching summary-making. It is a natural development of the preceding exercise in the analysis and simplification of sentences. Like most other things in this course, it is intended only as a guide. Study the stage-by-stage reduction of sentences carefully, then try to reduce the remainder of the passage in a similar way.

Note   The exact number of words is given as a guide in each case. Generally, summaries should be about a third the length of the original, but one cannot be rigid about this. It is also not always necessary to count every word in a text or summary. Taking the average of three lines and multiplying it by the total number of lines is a popular – and reasonably accurate – way of arriving at an approximate figure.

Some original sentences of the passage on language	Reduced versions of these sentences
1 When we talk about learning a language like English, Japanese or Spanish, we speak and think as though the language in question were a fixed unchanging thing. (27 words)	We often treat a language as though it were a simple unchanging thing. (13 words)
2 We expect to learn it as we learned geometry or how to ride a bicycle – systematically, and with clear ultimate success. (21 words)	We expect to learn it the way we learned geometry or how to ride a bicycle. (16 words)
3 Many people subsequently give up when they discover just what a misconception this is. (14 words)	This is a misconception. (4 words)
4 They have in fact embarked on an activity that could last the rest of their lives. (16 words)	Learning a foreign language is a difficult lifelong activity, . . . (9 words)
5 The experience makes them realize that they are not only going to have to work very hard indeed if they want to succeed, but also that they are – in many cases – barely masters of the language they call their own 'mother tongue'. (42 words)	. . . and makes us aware that we do not necessarily know our own mother tongue really well. (16 words)
6 Studying any language is, in fact, an endless voyage. (9 words)	**Nil** (incorporated into No 4, above)
7 Each of the thousands of languages currently used in the world is a complex affair. (15 words)	Languages are complex; . . . (3 words)
8 Many languages do have a standard form – particularly on paper – and this is what we learn, but they probably also have a variety of regional dialects and social styles, and many are the products of the historical mingling of other languages. (41 words)	. . . many of them have standard forms, regional dialects and various social styles. Many of them are the result of the mingling of other languages. (24 words)
9 The English language is just such a hybrid. (8 words)	English is just such a hybrid, . . . (6 words)
10 It began its career just under two thousand years ago as a form of ancient German, collided with a special kind of old French, was subjected to several waves of Latin and a flood of Greek, and since then has acquired bits and pieces of every other language that its users have ever been in contact with. (57 words)	. . . a form of German influenced by French, Latin, Greek and other languages. (12 words)
Total 250 words	**Total 103 words**

You may now, if you wish, write out the summary made here in continuous form, then go on to finish the whole passage.

1.6 Grammar:
Contrasts within a sentence

The table below demonstrates how the phrases *not only . . . but also* are used to express contrasts within sentences. Study it carefully, then use the examples to help you complete the sentences that follow.

Examples	Uses
1 Many languages have a standard form.	
They have a variety of regional dialects and social styles.	
▷ Many languages *not only* have a standard form, *but also* have a variety of regional dialects and social styles. OR	the commonest type, the subject not repeated in the second clause
▷ Many languages have *not only* a standard form, *but also* a variety of regional dialects and social styles.	neither the subject nor the verb repeated.
2 English is a widely-used modern language.	
It is, historically speaking, a hybrid of many other languages.	
▷ English is *not only* a widely-used modern language, *but* (is) *also*, historically speaking, a hybrid of many other languages.	with the verb *to be*: the phrase *not only* follows the verb, and the verb is optional in the second clause
3 Language students must work hard in class.	
They should read widely at home.	
▷ Language students must *not only* work hard in class, *but* should *also* read widely at home.	with modal verbs: the phrase *not only* follows the modal, and the phrase *but also* is divided by the modal

a. A language like English changes from generation to generation. It is very diverse in geographical terms.

b. Soccer is an exciting game to play. It is a great spectator sport, watched by millions throughout the world.

    c.   Enthusiastic schoolboys and university students played various kinds of football.
They began to write out rules so that these different games could be standardized.

    d.   Nordic skiing is an excellent way of keeping fit.
It can be the best way of getting from place to place in remote country areas in winter.

    e.   Skiing is a popular winter activity with a venerable history.
It is nowadays a major factor in the economies of such countries as Switzerland, Austria, Canada and the United States.

    f.   Swimming is a satisfying indoor and outdoor pastime.
It is a highly organized international sport with many forms of competition and professional opportunities.

    g.   Some people have certain general misconceptions about language and languages.
They have a deep personal conviction that, somehow, no foreign language is quite as 'real' as their own mother tongue.

Note that a variation of a more formal and emphatic nature exists, in which *not only* introduces the sentence and *but* is replaced by a semi-colon or a dash and a simple contrastive statement with *also*. Study the following examples, then re-express sentences a–g in the new form, as sentences h–n:

Example 1   Many languages not only have a standard form, but also have a variety of regional dialects and social styles.

    ▷   *Not only* do many languages have a standard form; they *also* have a variety of regional dialects and social styles.

Example 2   English is not only a widely-used modern language, but is also, historically speaking, a hybrid of many other languages.

    ▷   *Not only* is English a widely-used modern language; it is *also*, historically speaking, a hybrid of many other languages.

Example 3   Language students must not only work hard in class, but should also read widely at home.

    ▷   *Not only* must language students work hard in class; they should *also* read widely at home.

1.7 Grammar and vocabulary: Kinds of compound words

There are many kinds of compound words in English; it is, indeed, improbable that they can all be listed. This does not mean, however, that the basic principles of compounding cannot be understood fairly easily. In this section you will be introduced to a number of important factors in the making and use of compounds. Study the examples carefully, then complete the exercises appropriately.

Compound words:
First stage

The vast majority of compounds are formed on a principle of inversion. The table shows how this happens. Use it as a guide to invert the underlined words in the sentences that follow, in order to create your own compound words.

Examples	Comments
1 He is a *colonel* in the *Army*.	basic principle of inversion.
▷ He is an *Army colonel*.	
2 This is the *skin* of a *sheep*.	**Note** that the word elements of the compound are linked by ideas such as *location* ('in the') and *possession* ('of a').
▷ It is a *sheepskin*.	
3 This *area* is full of *mountains*.	**Note** that a plural word usually becomes singular when used as the first element in a compound.
▷ It is a *mountain area*.	
4 This is a *pool* for *swimming* in.	**Note** that it is not just any kind of pool. The compound is the name for a special kind of pool. Compounding is basically a name-creating process.
▷ It is a *swimming pool*.	
5 These *machines flatten snow*.	**Note** that (as in both 4 and 5) compounds may have their own special grammatical structures.
▷ They are *snow-flattening machines*.	

a.   It is a *trail* through the *snow*. It is a . . .
b.   It is a *brush* for the *teeth*. It is a . . .
c.   It is a *programme* on the *radio*. It is a . . .
d.   She is a *teacher* in a *school*. She is a . . .
e.   He *manages* a *factory*. He is a . . .
f.   They are *clerks* in a *bank*. They are . . .
g.   This is a *pot* for *flowers*. It is a . . .
h.   It is a *language* like a *hybrid* (flower). It is a . . .
i.   This is a *book* with *texts* in it. It is a . . .
j.   It is a *resort* where people can *ski*. It is a . . .
k.   These are *birds* that like living in the *snow*. They are . . .
l.   It is an *engine powered* by *steam*. It is a . . .
m.   It is a *business based* in *London*. It is a . . .
n.   This is an *agency controlled* by the *government*. It is a . . .
o.   This *machine adds* numbers. It is an . . .
p.   It is a *machine* for *sewing* clothes. It is a . . .
q.   It is a *machine* for *mixing cement*. It is a . . .
r.   It is a machine for *mixing cement*. It is a . . .
s.   He *collects stamps*. He is a . . .
t.   She *directs films*. She is a . . .
u.   It is a *factory* that *makes soap*. It is a . . .
v.   It is a *mountain covered* in/with *snow*. It is a . . .
w.   It is a *ring* that symbolizes a *wedding*. It is a . . .
x.   It is a *fish* that looks something like a *cat*. It is a . . .
y.   It is the *core* of an *apple*. It is an . . .
z.   It is a *newspaper* sold on *Sundays* only. It is a . . .

Compound words:
Second stage

It is common in English for compounds to be built up together into
'compound compounds' or 'multiple compounds'. At first this
appears strange and difficult, but is not in fact very difficult to do or
to understand. Use the examples below to help you complete the
sentences appropriately.

Example 1   The man is 29 years old and teaches in a college.
        ▷   He is a 29-year-old college teacher

Example 2   The building belongs to the government and was built in the 19th
        century.
        ▷   It is a 19th-century government building.

Example 3   She is the manager of a bank and the bank is in London.
        ▷   She is a London bank manager.

a. The man is 36 years old and works in an office. He is a . . .

b. The woman is 26 years old and teaches in a school. She is a . . .

c. He is 40 years old and manages a company that is based in Chicago. He is a . . .

d. She is 30 years old and announces (the news, etc.) on television. She is a . . .

e. The treaty is 50 years old and relates to peace. It is a . . .

f. It is a castle built in the 11th century and belonged to the Normans. It is a . . .

g. The machine weighs ten tons and is used for snow-clearing. It is a . . .

h. It is a book containing texts and dealing with the Spanish language. It is a . . .

i. It is a match between two football teams, and the match takes place on a Saturday. It is a . . .

j. It is a competition among soccer clubs to win the World Cup. It is a . . .

Compound words:
Third stage

As we have seen, the process of compounding creates special names for special things. Sometimes, while doing this, the process creates special new grammatical relationships among the elements in the compound, and may also require special punctuation. The examples below show one particular process which is very common in present-day English. Using them as a guide, complete the sentences appropriately.

Example 1   I much prefer swimming in shallow water.
      ▷   I much prefer shallow-water swimming.

Example 2   She prefers swimming in deep seas.
      ▷   She prefers deep-sea swimming.

a. Every morning he has a bath in cold water.
He has a . . .

b. She much prefers baths in hot water.
She prefers . . .

c. Some of her movements in the water were in slow motion.
They were . . .

d. The factory does operations on a small scale.
They are . . .

e.   He is a football-player of the first class.
     He is a ...

f.   He decided to have a holiday for three weeks.
     He decided to have a ...

g.   She will be here for a stay of six months.
     It will be a ...

h.   They have gone to Spain for a period of two years.
     They will be gone for a ...

i.   The club organizes swimming competitions for different age
     groups. These are called ...

j.   This is a photographic lens built to take pictures at a wide angle
     (of vision). It is a ...

1.8 Punctuation:
The colon

The colon (:) serves to carry the reader's eye quickly to the next
important thing, which may follow on the same line, or be presented
in a special display:

Material following on the same line

> Studying and using any language is an endless voyage: through
> childhood, adolescence and adulthood, in one's education, in one's
> career, and in one's general social life. It is a lifelong undertaking.

Note that this device is often used when presenting a list of items.

Material presented in a special display

> Take even the apparently simple and specific English word *man*. It
> seems clear enough; it refers to 'an adult male human being'. Of
> course it does, but just consider for a moment the following sentences:
> 1)   There are several men missing in that chess set.
> 2)   The boat was manned entirely by women and children.
>   from 'Language', lines 25–30

Note that this device in this case also presents a list, and that it can
also be used for displaying a long quotation from another writer, a
piece of poetry, a diagram, and so on.

The first letter of the word that follows a colon may or may not be capitalized, depending on whether the writer feels that what follows should be treated as a completely new sentence.

For dramatic purposes, a dash (–) may replace the colon, and some writers even combine the two (:–) for special emphatic effect.

Colons are important (along with commas and semi-colons, and sometimes brackets and dashes) in displaying lists, information in catalogues and inventories, points in systems of classification and so on. Basically, listing can be done in two ways:

Following on the same line

> He asked for: 20 pens, pencils and erasers; 100 exercise books; 200 loose sheets of notepaper; 10 textbooks, and 5 assorted dictionaries.

Note that commas serve here for minor divisions within the list, while semi-colons provide the major divisions.

Presented in a special display

> He asked for:
>   20 pens
>   20 pencils
>   20 erasers
> 100 exercise books
> 200 loose sheets of notepaper
>   10 textbooks
>   5 assorted dictionaries

Note that in this display what is technically known as 'white space' takes the place of the commas and semi-colons.

There may sometimes be a problem as regards the last comma in a list. Lists written in continuous form usually have an *and* between the last two items. Traditionally, a comma appears before that *and,* but nowadays it is usually omitted unless a serious possibility of misunderstanding may arise. Consider the following:

Traditional	He asked for some apples, oranges, bananas, pomegranates, and pears.
Present-day	He asked for some apples, oranges, bananas, pomegranates and pears.
List of phrases	I would like to visit the Castle, see the Cathedral, talk to the local people and attend a concert. **Note** that a careful traditionalist would put a comma here before the *and*.

In the following example there might be some doubt about the colour of the last item:

> She bought some books, envelopes, pens, coloured pencils and paper.

In order to ensure that no one supposed the paper was also coloured, this list could be improved in either of two ways:

By re-ordering   She bought some books, paper, envelopes, pens and coloured pencils.

By using a comma before *and*   She bought some books, envelopes, pens, coloured pencils, and paper.

Some items that go in lists normally contain an *and* (such as 'pen and ink', 'bacon and eggs', 'black and white', and so on). To avoid possible confusion in such cases, it is advisable to employ a final comma:

> Breakfast: orange juice, cereal, bacon and eggs, toast and marmalade, and coffee with cream and sugar.

Punctuation work

Below is an unpunctuated passage about words. Part of it can be presented in a special display. Punctuate the passage.

> many words in most languages have imprecise meanings even ordinary words like man run and hot such words can refer to more than one thing and have more than one use without a clear context we cannot always be sure just what they are meant to convey consider these sentences 1 the woman shouted that the house was on fire 2 the captain ordered his men to fire 3 fire sentences 1 and 2 provide enough context to show what is intended by the word fire in each case sentence 3 however presents a problem does it relate to the woman or the captain or to something else completely

1.9 Controlled composition:
Using source material

In this section you will find two things: a plan for a composition, and some source materials. Study the plan, then the source materials. Use the materials (and any other sources that you may have, including the passage on language at the beginning of this unit) in order to prepare, and then write, a composition entitled 'Some Facts about the English Language'.

Plan

1 introduction
2 historical background
3 present-day situation,
   statistics, etc
4 conclusion

Source 1

The English language belongs, historically and in terms of its basic type, to the Indo-European family of languages. It is, however, one of the younger members of this family. It is thought that the original speakers of 'Indo-European' lived somewhere in eastern Europe or western Asia, and migrated west, south and south-east. The ancient Indian language called Sanskrit is Indo-European, as are both Latin and Greek. The Slavonic languages, the Germanic languages, Armenian, Persian, Lithuanian and many other tongues share this common heritage. The common links among this great diversity of languages are easily shown in, for example, the various words for 'father': *Vater* in German, *pater* in Latin, *padre* in Spanish, *pedar* in Persian and *pita* in Sanskrit.

Source 2

449 A.D.	the first invasion of the Anglo-Saxons from northern Europe, taking over much of the island that the Romans had called Britannia, and eventually giving the name 'England' to the southern part of the island
787	the most significant date in the long period of Scandinavian or Viking raids on Britain, a process that brought many Norwegian and Danish elements into the speech of the Angles (in the middle and more northerly areas) and the Saxons (in the south)

1066	the arrival of the Norman invaders, defeating the Saxon king of England, and later spreading their influence over Wales, Scotland and Ireland as well, bringing with them Norman French as the language of the aristocracy and of government
1204	Normandy in France lost to the kings of England, forcing them to concentrate more on the development of their own kingdom
1258	the Parliament of England uses 'English' for the first time instead of French
1348	English first taught in schools, alongside Latin and French
1477	the printing press introduced into England, enabling the spread of the written form of the language
1611	the first 'authorized' version of the Bible in English, the King James's Version, named after the king who united the crowns of England and Scotland
1707	the Union of the Parliaments of England and Scotland and the creation of 'Great Britain' (the United Kingdom)
1776	the American Declaration of Independence, creating what has since become the largest English-speaking community in the world (the United States)
1857–1928	the period during which the vast *Oxford English Dictionary* was compiled, containing 414,825 entries

Source 3

The English language today is polycentric; that is, it has many distinct centres, self-governing nations with their own standards. The two most important are, of course, the United Kingdom in terms of history, and the United States in terms of population. Differences between British and American forms of English are many and varied, ranging from certain distinct forms of spelling to strong differences in vocabulary. In the United Kingdom, politicians *stand* for election; in the United States, with its faster life, they *run*. If someone says 'I'm mad about my flat', in the U.K. this would mean 'I'm delighted about my apartment', but in the U.S.A. it would mean 'I'm very angry about the puncture in my car's tyre' (spelled T-I-R-E). If a Briton says 'Come again', it may mean that he has invited you back to his home; said by an American, however, this could be a question, and mean 'Sorry, what did you say?'

Source 4

- English is currently the mother tongue of between 350 and 480 million people.
- These people live all over the world and have varied cultures, traditions and interests as well as very different environments.
- Barbara Strang (*A History of English*, Methuen, 1970) calls these people A-speakers of English.
- The original communities of A-speakers are: the U.K., the U.S.A., Ireland, Canada, Australia, New Zealand and South Africa.
- English is also used by large numbers of people as a special social and occupational language, for national and international purposes.
- Such people may live in countries that were once part of the British Empire, and may have had all or most of their education in England.
- Strang calls these people the B-speakers of English.
- They are found mainly in Asia and Africa, and are often virtually indistinguishable from native-users of English. Such countries as India and Nigeria have, more or less, their own national standards of English.
- There are also many people throughout the world who are learning or have learned English in some detail as a second or foreign language, requiring it for professional, academic, social or cultural reasons.
- To Strang, these are the C-speakers of English.
- The absolute total of people using English all or part of the time, for one purpose or another, is unknown, but it must be extremely large, and is certainly worldwide.

Final note

Sources are not intended to be used in their entirety. You should be selective, choosing what serves to develop your own particular approach to the subject.

No model answer is provided for this piece of work, because an infinite range of good compositions is possible. Your finished work should, however, be checked carefully by a suitably qualified and interested person.

UNIT 2

2.1 Comprehension and composition model: 'Examinations'

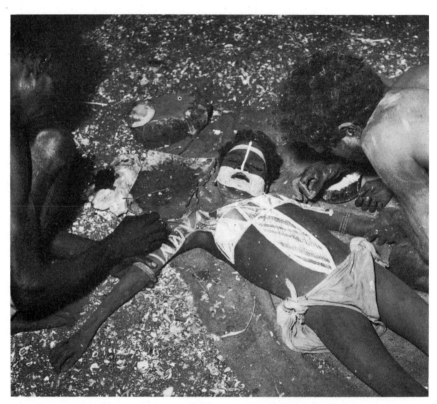

Australian aborigines prepare boy for ceremony of initiation by circumcision.

The passage below is a report on material contained in a published book. It paraphrases and summarizes the observations of the writer, with occasional elements of its own and also, at suitable points, brief quotations from the original text. Study how this is done (if possible consulting a copy of the original, if you can obtain one).

> What is an educational examination? According to the experts, it is any formal means of testing a candidate's current achievement, proficiency, aptitude or needs in a given subject area; it may be tough, but it is essentially benign.

In the view of Desmond Morris, however, author of *The Human*   5
Zoo (Jonathan Cape, 1969), it may indeed be any or all of these
things, but it is also something deeper, more primitive and even
sinister. He argues that in most – if not all – human societies
children at the age of puberty undergo important initiation
ceremonies or rites of passage. In these rites, young people are   10
taken away from their parents and kept apart in special groups
(usually boys with boys and girls with girls). They are forced to
undergo severe ordeals that often involve physical torture and
strong psychological stress, and may even result in permanent
mutilation. Their bodies may be scarred, burned, beaten or stung   15
by insects; operations may even be performed on their genitals. At
about the same time, they are instructed in the lore of the tribe
(again, often the boys by the men and the girls by the women) and,
when it is all over, are accepted – if they have passed – as adult
members of society.   20

These experiences are severe, but they should not simply be
dismissed as barbarous practices that most of the world has now
outlived. They have a certain social value. Firstly, the rites separate
the previously dependent child from its parents, requiring that it
endure pain alone and unafraid. This provides the young person   25
with a new focus of allegiance; the tribal community as a whole
replaces the family home. The adolescent not only suffers while
losing old ties, but also gains a new sense of belonging as adult
secrets are revealed to him or her. Secondly, the very violence of the
initiation ceremonies serves to fix the experiences gained at this   30
time forever in the memory. One does not forget traumatic
experiences easily, whether accidental (as in a car crash) or induced
(as in this ancient kind of education). Morris in fact calls the whole
process 'contrived traumatic teaching', and adds:

'Thirdly, it makes absolutely clear to the sub-adult that, although   35
he is now joining the ranks of his elders, he is doing so very much
in the role of a subordinate. The intense power which they
exercised over him will also be vividly remembered.'

The inevitable parallel can now be explicitly drawn: Modern
schools and colleges may not scar their students physically, but the   40
academic elders who instruct the young in the graduated 'secrets' of
society have their power outside the home and do from time to time
exert it forcefully. Public examinations are, in Morris's view, 'a
form of super-tribal initiation ceremony ... conducted in the heavy
atmosphere of high ritual, with the pupils cut off from all outside   45
assistance'. No one can help them; they must suffer on their own,
within a fixed period of time and without external aids.

The mental anguish that accompanies such tests may well be on a
par with the physical and psychological ordeals imposed on their
young by the great majority of pre-technological societies.   50

Below are some statements relating to the passage. Some are true (T) in terms of the passage, while others are false (F). Mark them appropriately, and if a statement is false, say why.

a. ☑ According to educational experts, examinations are not intended to be cruel.

b. ☑ Desmond Morris does not agree with these experts.

c. ☑ In rites of passage, parents are directly involved in the initiation of their children.

d. ☑ Adolescents are never quite the same, physically or mentally, after the rites as they were before.

e. ☑ Morris regards such rites as essentially barbarous acts with no social justification.

f. ☑ The initiation ceremonies usually help a youngster gain a larger vision of his or her place in society.

g. ☑ Morris suggests that people learn well under certain traumatic conditions.

h. ☑ He also suggests that human society has always been generally willing to inflict traumatic experiences upon its young as they reach the point of transition to adulthood.

i. ☑ The rites of passage allow an adolescent to become an adult equal to all other adults, and are therefore worth all the suffering involved.

j. ☑ The only significant difference between modern public examinations and primitive initiation rituals is the absence of physical torment directly imposed by the examiners.

2.2   Vocabulary: Word relationships

This section has five parts. Each part requires the identification of words in the passage on examinations. In each case, however, the identification is based upon a different criterion (that is, a means of judgement and selection).

1   There are four words in the paragraph that describe kinds of examinations given by educational experts. What are they, and what do you think are the differences between them?

2   Find ten words in the first two paragraphs of the passage that are opposite in meaning to the words listed below:

a. easy   f. persuaded
b. malign   g. gentle
c. sophisticated   h. temporary
d. trivial   i. rejected
e. ordinary   j. juvenile

3 Find ten words in the third and fourth paragraphs of the passage that are very similar in meaning to the words listed below:

a. rejected   f. attachments
b. behaviour   g. obtains
c. significance   h. artificial
d. demanding   i. quite
e. loyalty   j. position

4 Find ten words in the last two paragraphs of the passage which begin with the same prefix as the words listed below. When you have done this, look up all twenty words in an etymological dictionary and determine the meanings (if any) of the various prefixes.

a. intolerable   f. assertion
b. paralysis   g. suffuse
c. exceptionally   h. accommodates
d. superconscious i. impeded
e. concluded   j. pre-scientific

5 Find ten words in the first two paragraphs of the passage which end with the same suffix as the words listed below. When you have done this, look up all twenty words in an etymological dictionary and determine the meanings (if any) of the various suffixes.

a. regional   f. positive
b. population   g. urban
c. involvement   h. variety
d. efficiency   i. pressure
e. latitude   j. persistent

2.3 Grammar:
Analysis of sentences

Go through the passage on examinations, studying the structure of each sentence, deciding whether it is simple (S), complex (CX), compound (CP) or compound-complex (CC).

2.4 Grammar:
Synthesis of sentences

Below is a set of ten parts that can come together as a passage on parachuting as a military activity and also as a sport, the product of modern technology. In each part, however, it is necessary to gather the simple sentences together (in most cases) into compound and/or complex structures. This can be done by following the suggestions given to the right of each numbered part. When you have studied the possibilities, write out the full passage.

1	Every new technology seems to produce its own sports. The military use of aircraft is no exception.	**Combine with a semi-colon**
2	Parachuting is the art of jumping successfully out of aeroplanes with the aid of a special canopy. *It* began as a dangerous wartime service. Volunteer soldiers received special training and rewards *for taking part in it.*	**Combine the first and second sentences with 'and' and the second and third using 'for which'**
3	Today ∧ it is a fast-growing sport. *It has* its own unique variations. *These are* free-falling and formation sky-diving.	**Use 'however', then 'with', then a colon after 'variations'**
4	For many people, even the thought of jumping from a stationary balloon or a moving aircraft is horrifying. *It is much more horrifying than* undersea swimming or Alpine skiing.	**New paragraph. Combine the sentences with 'much more so than'**
5	It is ∧ a fact that (something). There are very few deaths and relatively few injuries in this sport.	**Use 'however' and 'that'**
6	In British parachuting ∧ only ten people died between 1968 and 1974. There is only about one injury per thousand jumps. *This ratio* compares favourably with downhill skiing.	**Use 'for example', then 'and', then 'a ratio which'**

7   A woman (did something).

She started sport-parachuting in England in 1948.

Today ∧ there are in that country many successful clubs and a number of full-time parachuting centres.

New paragraph. Begin with 'It was', then 'who', then 'and', adding in 'as a result'

8   A beginner can learn the basics of this exciting sport in one weekend training course.

Nil

9   He or she learns (something).
  ● guide a parachute
  ● deal with emergencies
  ● fall in a face-to-earth position, keeping the arms and legs spread in order to prevent the body from turning in the air.

Use 'how to' for each of the things learnt, in a list with commas and a final 'and'

10   The learner actually begins.

He or she jumps with a nylon line fixed to the balloon or plane.

The line can pull the parachute open automatically in less than three seconds.

Later the trainee jumps without the line, pulling his or her own 'ripcord' after a three-second delay, thus becoming a completely free agent.

Begin with 'when', then use 'so that', then 'but'

2.5 Punctuation, grammar and organization: Logical order

More information is provided in this section about aspects of the sport of parachuting. To obtain it, however, it is necessary first to punctuate, then to re-organize the material. Proceed.

A.   parascending has its attractions as a safe and comparatively easy introduction to parachuting generally especially for young people and may one day become the main form of the sport

B.   by such means the would be parascender can be raised into the air and set down again remarkably gently

C.   people who want to try this pastime can go for the same kind of weekend training as other more traditional parachutists

D.   bad weather is the enemy of traditional parachuting and has contributed towards a new activity called parascending

E.   on saturdays adults and teenagers learn landing rolls and safety drills and for a small sum of money are pulled off the ground on their first flights

F.   here the parachutist is attached to a car by a cable and runs behind it with open chute until he leaves the ground

G.   after a series of such flights they are allowed to release themselves and to practise steering the chute as they come down

H.   he is gradually lifted to about 1000 feet when he can release himself and do a normal descent

2.6 Grammar and vocabulary: The phrasal verb

Look at the following slightly adapted extracts from earlier passages in this course:

1   The game was in real danger of *dying out* in Western Europe.
'Football', lines *16–17* (Unit 7, Book 1)

2   The rich young men had nowhere to hunt, fish, ride or otherwise *use up* their energies.
'Football' lines *18–21* (Unit 7, Book 1)

3   Nordic skiing is essentially a way of *getting about* on snow.
'The World of Skiing', lines *14–15* (Unit 8, Book 1)

4   In 1879, when Murray succeeded Furnivall in leading the project he *took over* from him 1¾ tons of material.
'Numbers in a Text: *The Oxford English Dictionary*', lines *17–18* (Unit 8, Book 1)

5   Many people *give up* when they discover just what a misconception this is.
'Language', lines *5–6*

6   In these rites, young people are *taken away* from their parents and *kept apart* in special groups.
'Examinations', lines *10–11*

These six extracts show seven phrasal verbs at work. Such verbs differ from other verbs in English by having an adverbial particle (in these cases: *out, up, about, over, away* and *apart*) working closely with an 'ordinary' everyday verb. Verb and particle have to be regarded as a unit, and hence they are called 'phrasal verbs'. Certain important points should be remembered about the behaviour of such verbs:

1 In speech, the adverbial particle tends to be stressed, whereas ordinary prepositional particles are not usually stressed, except for purposes of contrast.

2 When a phrasal verb is transitive (that is, when it is followed by a direct object) the particle may be placed before or after the object noun without changing the meaning in any way:

Example   He used up the fuel.
    ▷   He used the fuel up.

3 When, however, the direct object is a pronoun, the particle must follow the pronoun:

Example   He used up the fuel/He used the fuel up.
    ▷   He used it up.

Practise these rules in the following sentences, the first of which is done for you:

a. He picked up the book. He picked the book up. He picked it up.
b. She took over the business. She . . .
c. They closed down the company. They . . .
d. They took away the children. They . . .
e. He cut off the water supply. He . . .
f. They broke up the old cars. They . . .
g. He chased away the dogs. He . . .
h. She will bring in the books tomorrow. She . . .
i. Hand over the money immediately. Hand . . .
j. The workmen pulled down the old building. They . . .

In most cases, phrasal verbs are simply verbs with a sense of movement plus particles indicating direction. Often, however, such particles acquire an implication of *completion*, usually psychologically linked with the direction that they represent. If a building 'blows up' the action is upwards, but the building is completely destroyed as well; if a business 'closes down', there is a strong suggestion of loss, a figurative fall; if you 'cut off' somebody's supplies, it is like a knife or a hand coming down to break a connection or to separate things. The table below summarizes to some extent the possibilities for several important particles used with verbs. Study it, then try to choose the right particles for the sentences that follow.

Adverbial particle	Examples	Probable kinds of completion
up	1 He *used up* the fuel.	until there was none left
	2 They *tidied up* the room.	as thoroughly as possible
down	1 The company lost a lot of business and had to *close down*.	never to open again (finality)
	2 The car *broke down* miles from home in the rain.	a sense of destruction, misfortune, frustration, etc.
out	1 The machine was *worn out*.	It had worked for a long time but at last could do no more.
	2 She *rubbed out* the marks.	continuous action to produce a definite result
off	They *broke off* negotiations with the enemy.	separation; clear termination

a.   She cut the vegetables _____ , making the pieces as small as possible.

b.   'Burn the building _____ !' he shouted in fury.

c.   It took him several weeks to reason the matter _____ , but he succeeded in the end.

d.   The colours slowly faded _____ in the strong sunlight.

e.   They called the meeting _____ because the date was no longer convenient and too many new problems were developing.

f.   The radio had been on all day; he grew tired of it and finally switched it _____ .

g.   She hoped that everything would turn _____ well in the end for the family.

h.   The manager could not work _____ any real enthusiasm for the new ski-resort project.

i.   The psychologist had been trying for many years to work _____ just why examinations created certain patterns of stress among the candidates.

j.   The company management was genuinely sorry that it had to turn _____ one of the scientist's best ideas, but unfortunately there just was not enough money to develop it properly.

k.   It took them twenty years to build the business _____ from almost nothing to a vast international company.

l.   After some study in the library she found _____ that skiing dated back almost 5,000 years, a fact that surprised her considerably.

m.   The parachutists decided to try _____ the new style of canopy as soon as the weather improved.

n.   The police cordoned _____ the whole area so that no one could get out or in.

o.   The meeting broke _____ not long after it started because no one could agree on the agenda.

2.7 Punctuation and layout:
Quotations and references

There are two basic uses of quotation marks (also known as quotes, inverted commas and speech marks). The first is to express conversation (as was practised in Unit 5 of Book 1 of this course); the second is to include the original words of another writer in one's own material. The quotation of another writer can also, however, be done in two distinct ways, as shown below:

Quotation continuing on the same line

---

1   Nevertheless, in 1613, King James VI of Scotland and I of England permitted himself to be entertained with 'music and a football match', and, a few decades later, the English dictator Oliver Cromwell played football when he was at university.

> from 'Football', lines *11–15*
> (Unit 7, Book 1)

2   According to the *Advanced Learner's Dictionary of Current English* (Oxford University Press, 1974), a ski is 'one of a pair of long, narrow strips of wood, strapped under the feet for moving over snow'.

> from 'The World of Skiing', lines *1–4*
> (Unit 8, Book 1)

3   Morris in fact calls the whole process 'contrived traumatic teaching' ...

> from 'Examinations', lines *33–34*

Similarly, brief uses of special words in a sentence can also be placed in quotation marks for emphasis, *as if* they were being quoted:

> A male cat gets a special name to show that he is not female. He is a 'tomcat'.
>
> from 'Cats', lines *9–10*
> (Unit 1, Book 1)

Some writers prefer *not* to place such words in quotes, and it is sometimes difficult to decide the degree of need. Writers are not always consistent in this area.

Quotation presented in a special display

> Morris . . . adds:
>> 'Thirdly, it makes absolutely clear to the sub-adult that, although he is now joining the ranks of the elders, he is doing so very much in the role of a subordinate. The intense power which they exercised over him will also be vividly remembered.'
>
> The inevitable parallel can now be explicitly drawn: Modern schools and colleges may not scar their students physically, but the . . .
>
> from 'Examinations', lines *33–40*

Note   The main idea here is to present the material as a sub-block of the main passage. It is usually introduced by means of a colon, but not always. Sometimes the writer's own sentence runs on into the quoted material. The paragraph that follows the quotation also may or may not be indented, depending on whether the writer feels the need for a proper new paragraph or not.

Quotation and reference are closely related. In the examples given above, reference is shown in the same two forms as quotation: either running on (as in the case of the reference to the dictionary published by Oxford University Press) or as a special display (as with the references saying which passage in this course the extracts come from). Brackets and dashes are variously used to make such references clearer. Sometimes, of course, a writer may not wish to have a reference embedded in the text itself. In that case there are several options: to place it at the foot of the page, as a 'footnote', or at the end of the chapter or book, article, etc., as an 'end-note'. If this is done, the writer will probably employ small superscript numbers at a suitable point in the sentence, indicating the place that the reference has in a list somewhere in the publication (usually mentioned in the introduction). The effect is as follows:

According to one important source, King James permitted himself to be entertained with 'music and a football match'[1], and, a few decades later, the English dictator Oliver Cromwell played football when he was at university.[2]

If the reader really wants to know more about the sources for these statements about King James and Oliver Cromwell, then the appropriate list of notes can be consulted.

Punctuation work:
First stage

The following material, containing quotation marks used for dialogue, is taken from an earlier part of this course. As a revision exercise, punctuate it suitably.

Note The first two lines do not need quotation marks.

everyone knows says jane austen that an unmarried man with money needs a wife mrs bennet certainly knew this and also knew that just such a young man had arrived in the neighbourhood in fact he had rented nearby netherfield park his name was bingley and he was from the north mrs bennets interest in mr bingley was simple she had five unmarried daughters it was only reasonable to assume that if he had a suitable opportunity he would fall in love with one of them which of them was not really important for this reason therefore she spoke to her husband about the interesting newcomer because after all she could not make any plans until mr bennet had called on the unsuspecting mr bingley when that was done she could invite him to their home where the young ladies could be best displayed and so my dear you must go and see him I had no plan to do so said mr bennet but you must consider your daughters he has a great deal of money so I hear and it would be a perfectly wonderful match for one of them perhaps you could just write a list of the good qualities of each girl and I could send it to him I will do nothing of the kind

Punctuation work:
Second stage

Below is an unpunctuated version of that part of the passage
'Examinations' which contains quotations. Without looking back at
the passage or the descriptions in this section, punctuate the material.
Begin with three points (...), to suggest continuation:

> secondly the very violence of the initiation ceremonies serves to fix
> the experiences gained at this time forever in the memory one does
> not forget traumatic experiences easily whether accidental as in a
> car crash or induced as in this ancient kind of education morris in
> fact calls the whole process contrived traumatic teaching and adds
> thirdly it makes absolutely clear to the sub adult that although he
> is now joining the ranks of his elders he is doing so very much in
> the role of a subordinate the intense power which they exercised
> over him will also be vividly remembered the inevitable parallel
> can now be explicitly drawn modern schools and colleges may not
> scar their students physically but the academic elders who instruct
> the young in the graduated secrets of society have their power
> outside the home and do from time to time exert it forcefully

Punctuation work:
Third stage

Below is a completely new passage. It has similar subject-matter to
the passage on examinations, and also refers to the ideas of Desmond
Morris. At one point, material quoted directly from Morris should be
put on special display. Punctuate the passage.

> in addition to the human zoo desmond morris has written several
> other popular works relating to human and animal social life these
> include the naked ape and intimate behaviour both published by
> cape the first in 1967 and the second in 1971 in the latter volume
> he considers the needs of both animals and human beings for
> physical contact he studies human social behaviour from the point
> of view of a zoologist constantly comparing our actions and needs
> with those of our natural companions on this planet he is not only
> interested in our actual capacity to touch but also in extensions of
> the idea of touching that can be found in our use of language he
> observes for example as an adult human being you can
> communicate with me in a variety of ways I can read what you
> write listen to the words you speak hear your laughter and your
> cries look at the expressions on your face watch the actions you
> perform smell the scent you wear and feel your embrace in

ordinary speech we might refer to these interactions as making contact or keeping in touch and yet only the last one on the list involves bodily contact all the others operate at a distance it is clear from what morris says that the use of words like touch and contact to describe activities like writing speaking and signalling with the body is in objective terms rather strange it is certainly however very revealing it is as if we know deep down inside us that **quote (without naming Morris)** bodily contact is the most basic form of communication morris reminds us of speakers who are said to hold their audiences of gripping experiences and touching scenes no physical contact is involved in any of the situations described by these idioms and yet the metaphor is clear to us all

2.8 Controlled composition: Writing up your notes

A great deal of professional writing is done only after the collection of notes from a variety of sources. The writer usually makes his or her own notes, but sometimes works from other people's notes. In this section we can imagine that by one means or another you have amassed the necessary background notes for an article on the history of writing. Among the notes are dates, occasional quotations and references, and so on. You may not wish to use everything in the notes, and you may even, in the end, wish to go to additional sources to increase your knowledge. Decide for yourself, and write your article, giving it whatever title you wish.

Notes

- writing historically second to speech – development of speech over 100,000 years ago – organs primarily used for survival (eating, breathing; lungs, larynx, mouth, tongue, etc) – developed whole new second set of skills
- cave paintings – about 30,000 years ago – France, Spain, etc – indicate capacity to use hand and eye in new ways – creating a secondary reality: 'pictures'
- around 15,000 years ago – Africa and elsewhere – notching of bones, evidence that people were beginning to keep tallies of things

- about 3,500 B.C. – Sumer (now southern Iraq) the earliest known 'pictographic' writing **check dictionary** – serial ordering – repeating the linearity of the spoken language but this time on surfaces
- about 3000 B.C. Egyptian 'hieroglyphics' **check dictionary, maybe use quote** – probably a separate invention, but idea may have come through culture diffusion from Sumer
- about 2,600 B.C. – Sumerians begin to use 'cuneiform' **check dictionary, especially for etymology** – lines run left to right – used baked tablets, whereas Egyptians liked walls or reeds ('papyrus', origin of word 'paper')
- many new forms of writing – Middle East, Crete, India, Iran, Turkey, China – between 2500 and 1500 B.C. – all same idea of serial ordering, but methods differed – Hittites wrote one line left to right, next right to left – Chinese used 'ideograms' **check dictionary**
- about 1400 B.C. – port of Ugarit, on Mediterranean, (Syria?) – probably linked with the Phoenicians of Byblos, Tyre and Sidon – invention of 'alphabet' – it was Greeks, however, who used vowel symbols in the modern way
- forms of writing still diverse throughout the world – historically, writing always restricted – scribes, monks, mandarins, *secret*aries (**any link with 'secret'? check etymology**) – élite groups – no universal programme of literacy till 19th century A.D.
- What about books? – papyri and clay tablets very crude – needed plenty of storage space – portability of the surface bearing the signs not initially obvious – first 'page' probably a wall, and first 'book' a whole Egyptian temple
- modern library of bound books very different from Greco-Roman library of scrolls – What will future library be like? – microfilms and projectors? computer consoles? Was writing as much of a revolution thousands of years ago as the computer is today? Did people have the same feeling of awe and incomprehension then as now?
- copying the main work of scribes – dictation a common way of teaching writing – reading and writing probably the reason for the development of schools and our modern education system – many schools began as religious institutions (training monks to copy, etc) – 'grammar' comes from a Greek word meaning 'a letter of the alphabet', so our ideas of language also stem from ideas about writing languages down rather than speaking them

- down centuries, most people learning to read traced the lines with their fingers and read aloud – same as children learning to read today – mediaeval records show that monks were surprised when some (usually to become saints) could read not only without speaking but also without even moving their lips

- modern civilization by no means 'literate' – social stigma of illiteracy – education still essentially the idea of getting, and need to get, people to read – How important *is* reading in our civilization (road signs, forms, menus, instructions on labels, etc)? – What is level of illiteracy or semi-literacy?

- **Quote:** 'In antiquity the study of language, to any extent worth mentioning, arose only among those peoples who rejoiced in the possession of an alphabetical script: among the Indians and the Greeks.' (Hans Jensen, *Sign, Symbol and Script*, George Allen and Unwin, 1970, translated from the German)

- **Quote:** 'The arts of reading and writing are not easy; this fact is demonstrated by the numbers of people who, having completed their schooling, still go out into the world insufficiently literate in their own mother tongues.' (Tom McArthur, *The Written Word*, Oxford University Press, 1984)

UNIT 3

3.1 Comprehension and composition model: 'Under the Earth'

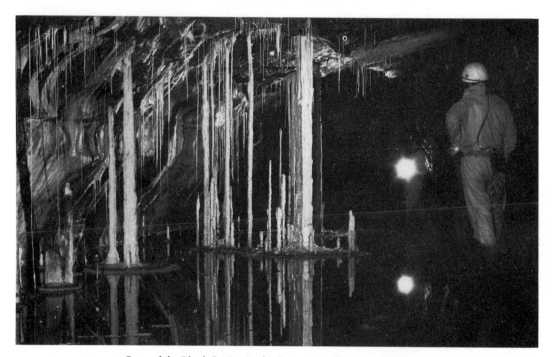

Cave of the Black Spring in the Swansea Valley, South Wales, GB.

The passage below is a detailed description, of a very factual nature, of caverns and related geological features. Its style is typical of much present-day writing in newspapers, magazines and popular scientific reports. Read it twice, studying the general organization carefully.

If you took up painting as a hobby or an occupation, where would you exhibit your work?

Would you crawl through dank subterranean passages until you could find the most inaccessible corner of a cave wall on which to work, your body uncomfortably twisted up? Anybody doing that nowadays would be considered insane, and yet that is exactly what our remoter ancestors did in the France of 20,000 years ago. If they had not done just that, we would have lost the priceless art treasures that – unintentionally – they have handed down to us.

5

Cave-explorers and geologists are usually the only people who   10
clamber down into the murky depths of caverns, but during the last
few decades they have opened up the world's great limestone
grottos to the tourist at large. Most of Europe's caverns, for
example, are today lit up by electricity, often in theatrically
wonderful colour combinations that set off to best advantage the   15
stalactites, stalagmites and cascades of snowy calcite. Steps have
been cut and wooden walkways erected where the going was once
difficult, and dangerous tunnels are sealed off. Caverns today are
proving to be big business, as people begin to appreciate that some
of the best scenery on earth lies under our feet. For example: 20

- In the foothills of the French Pyrenees, the road from St Girons to
  Mas d'Azil plunges along with the river Arize into a huge cavern.
  For 500 yards they wind together through tortuous limestone,
  electric-lit and with a large natural car park in the centre. From
  the car park one ascends with a guide into a maze of yellow sub-   25
  caves and corridors where, in a museum, the remains of early
  humans, giant cats and woolly mammoths are on display.

- One is accustomed to hearing of railways used in coal-mining,
  but in the French department of Dordogne an electric railway
  with open carriages operates inside the eerie Rouffignac Cavern.   30
  For two kilometres it rattles down into the bowels of the earth
  like a devil's chariot. When you disembark, in the dry bed of a
  prehistoric river, you find that the ceilings and walls are covered
  with a mass of animal outlines, drawn over 18,000 years ago
  with oxides of manganese – hump-backed bison, mammoths,   35
  satanic goats and mild-faced ponies, set at all angles and
  overlapping each other in an apparently meaningless profusion.
  In that unchanging atmosphere, they look as though they might
  have been drawn only yesterday.

Caves mean more to modern investigators, however, than paintings   40
and passing tourists. In January 1969, for example, two French
cavers, Jacques Chabert and Philippe Englander, came up out of the
Ollivier Cave near Nice. For about five months they had been living
– separately – down in the depths, carrying out an experiment in
underground living. They wanted to experience the effects of   45
prolonged cave-dwelling on both body and mind. Six months later,
a Yugoslav caver undertook a similar but even more arduous task;
Milutin Veljkovic went down into the Samar Cave and cut himself
off completely from the surface *for a whole year*. He then re-
established contact, talking to worried relatives from his self-   50
chosen prison, then stayed on for another three months before
coming up to the light of day.

Veljkovic had with him in the cave some cats, dogs, hens and
ducks, which adapted surprisingly well to those unfamiliar
underground conditions. He suffered badly from flies, which did   55
well in the cold, wet and dark environment, living off the fresh fruit
and vegetables that he had taken down with him. These went bad

earlier than he had expected, and the insects benefited greatly from
the processes of their decay.

The Yugoslav and the Frenchmen showed that people can live in   60
such conditions indefinitely without serious risk to their health.
They have confirmed in particular that, after a few days without
daylight and clocks, we quickly lose our sense of time, and that our
internal body clock (the regulator of all our normal bodily
activities) proceeds independently at its own speed. All three   65
investigators were convinced that time was passing more quickly
than was in fact the case.

Such findings are very interesting not only to cavers and the
general reader, but also to scientists studying the problems of
human survival in an environment far removed from caves – the   70
lifeless conditions of outer space. Although absence of gravity poses
its own special problems, the feeling of timelessness in both caves
and space is similar. Cavers, however, have their own special
interests and generally do not look towards the stars. Some cave
systems are very extensive indeed and may need long periods of   75
time for their proper exploration – weeks of living in tents or even
special cabins. It is an awesome and alien environment; there are all
the problems of mountaineers, combined with utter darkness
beyond one's own few lights, and only the little gadget on one's
wrist to speak the true passage of time.   80

Below are some statements relating to the passage. Some are true (T)
in terms of the passage, while others are false (F). Mark them
appropriately, and if a statement is false, say why.

a. ☐ Ancient cave artists often painted their pictures in parts of
      caverns that are difficult to get to.

b. ☐ The great cave paintings of France date from about 30,000
      years ago.

c. ☐ Nowadays everything possible is done to make the beauties of
      limestone grottos accessible to the general public.

d. ☐ There is a cavern in France through which a railway line passes.

e. ☐ Some caverns are so big that they contain museums and car
      parks.

f. ☐ The ancient artists seem not to have cared about keeping their
      drawings separate from each other.

g. ☐ The two French cavers worked together on their tests in the
      depths of the Ollivier Cave.

h. ☐ The Yugoslav spent a complete 12-month period in the Samar
      Cave.

i. ☐ Veljkovic's animals did not do well in the cave.

j. ☐ People's body clocks are not always in time with the rhythms of the earth, sun and moon.

k. ☐ For the cavers, the 'days' seemed shorter than they really were.

l. ☐ Outer space and deep caverns are similar because, in these environments, there are no external means of checking the passage of time.

3.2 Grammar and vocabulary: Analysis of the passage

In this section there are a variety of tasks to be done with regard to the structure and contents of the passage. Proceed.

1   Take all or any part (one or more paragraph) of the passage and analyse the sentences, deciding whether each is simple (S), complex (CX), compound (CP), or compound-complex (CC). (No analysis is provided in the answers section for this unit.)

2   Go through the passage carefully in order to write out a full list of the compound words that appear in it. You should be able to find 22 definite compounds. (**Note** that for the purposes of this course a compound is any combination of noun, verb or adjective forming a unit, but that noun-noun combinations are the commonest.)

3   Go through the passage carefully in order to write out a full list of the phrasal verbs that appear in it. You should be able to find 17 definite phrasal verbs. (**Note** that you should take care to distinguish between adverbial particles that go with verbs, and prepositional particles – or prepositions – that go with nouns or pronouns that follow them. Sometimes you will get both together, an adverbial followed by a prepositional particle. In this passage, you should interest yourself only in the adverbial particles.)

4   Below is a list of items of vocabulary used in the passage for special effect. Look each word up in at least one dictionary (but preferably two), and make notes on its relationship with the commoner word listed in brackets after it.

a. dank (damp)	(l. 3)	f. maze (mass)	(l. 25)
b. clamber (climb)	(l. 11)	g. eerie (strange)	(l. 30)
c. murky (dark)	(l. 11)	h. rattle (go; run)	(l. 31)
d. cavern (cave)	(l. 11)	i. bowels (depths)	(l. 31)
e. seal (close)	(l. 18)	j. dwell (live)	(l. 46)

3.3 Grammar:
Conditional sentences

Basically, conditional sentences in English divide into two types:

1   actual, possible and probable conditions
2   improbable and impossible conditions

The difference is expressed through different tenses, as follows:

Examples	Comments
1 If you *take* up painting, where *will* you exhibit your work?	This sentence suggests that something is possible. It therefore uses the present tense with *if*, and then the future with *will*. **Note** that *will* is not used in the *if*-clause.
2 If you *took* up painting, where *would* you exhibit your work?	This sentence suggests that something is improbable or at least a lot less probable than in 1. It therefore uses the past tense with *if*, and the hypothetical future with *would*. **Note** that *would* is not used in the *if*-clause.

Below are ten sentences. Some are Type 1; some are Type 2. By altering the tense structure, change the Type 1 sentences into Type 2, and the Type 2 into Type 1.

a.   If people travel in outer space, they will need to understand the effects of lack of gravity.

b.   If you really wanted to learn parachuting, you would take lessons in a proper club.

c.   If one wants to save money on skiing holidays, the best thing to do is to hire all the necessary clothes and equipment at the ski-resort.

d.   If X is equal to Y, then Y is also equal to Z, because X equals Z.

e.   You would watch the soccer game every Saturday if you were as enthusiastic as he is.

f.   If you do not feel at home in deep water, you will not want to try swimming with an aqualung.

g.   If you do not manage all the work satisfactorily the first time, you can always do it again.

h. If a person lives for any length of time in a cave, his or her body rhythms will change.

i. If you called a person a cat or a cabbage, no literal identification would be intended.

j. If you want to communicate with someone, you can always find a way of doing so.

In addition to the two basic types just shown, many conditional expressions are used to introduce comments, opinions, suggestions, questions, arguments and so on. The following tables and exercises show how these can be used.

3	**if** **when**	you consider one considers we consider *etc*	his her its their *etc*	age, (then)... experience,... usefulness,... wealth,... *etc*
	Considering			

Examples If you consider the age of the caverns, it is remarkable that these paintings still exist.

Considering its price, the material is not really very good.

4	**if** **when**	you take one takes we take *etc*	into	account consideration	all the facts,... the various factors,... *etc*
	Taking into		account consideration		

5	Providing (that) Provided Supposing Assuming Accepting	no one comes, (then)... nothing happens,... the information is accurate,...

<table>
<tr><td>6</td><td colspan="2">If time permits, . . .
Time permitting, . . .

If the weather permits, . . .
Weather permitting, . . .

If that is the case, . . .
That being the case, . . .

If that is so, . . .
That being so, . . .

If all goes well, . . .
All going well, . . .

If God wills, . . .
God willing, . . .</td></tr>
</table>

7	If there is In the event of	trouble, . . . an accident, . . . an explosion, . . . fire, . . . *etc*

8	On condition (that) . . . On the clear condition (that) . . .

Below are sixteen incomplete sentences. Each needs to be completed by a suitable conditional expression. At the beginning of each of the first five sentences, there is a number in a box. This directs you to the appropriate kind of conditional expression, 1 to 8, as shown in the tables. For the remainder of the sentences, you must make your own choice.

k. 5 . . . everything is done properly, we should have no difficulty getting there on time.

l. 5 . . . no one comes to help them, what will they do?

m. 6 . . . then there is no need to discuss the matter further, because we shall never agree.

n. 3 . . . all the relevant facts, it becomes clear that there are only two possibilities open to us.

o. 7 . . . major disorders, leave the city immediately.

p. 4 . . . the amount of money involved, one has no other choice but to act very carefully indeed.

q. ☐ . . ., the picnic will take place on Sunday at 12 noon.

r. ☐ . . . the winds are right, the ship can sail 200 miles in a day.

s. ☐ ..., then there is absolutely nothing to worry about; everything has clearly been taken care of.

t. ☐ ... there was nowhere else to live, would you be prepared to live in a cavern?

u. ☐ ... a volcanic eruption, the scientists in the area will undertake extensive tests.

v. ☐ ..., we should reach the sea tomorrow afternoon, but many things could prevent us getting there.

w. ☐ We shall permit you to go, but only ... you write to us every week without fail.

x. ☐ '... all the facts, and after a great deal of thought,' said the chairman of the committee slowly, 'we have decided regretfully that we have no choice but to turn your proposal down.'

y. ☐ ... the difficulties involved, it is astonishing that anyone came back from the expedition alive.

z. ☐ ... you were the attackers and not the defenders, what would *you* do?

3.4 Grammar and vocabulary: Paraphrasing compound words

Compound words are more than simply two or three words put together. There is always some kind of grammatical relationship between the elements of any compound. This relationship is best expressed by means of paraphrasing (that is, the restatement of the same material in some other way). The exercises that follow provide practice in paraphrasing compounds.

Compound work:
First stage

Many kinds of ordinary phrases can be turned into compounds by inverting the nouns, verbs or adjectives in these phrases. In this way the phrase is re-expressed in a tighter, more emphatic or concentrated way, usually providing a name for something. Study the examples, then make compounds in the same way.

Example 1   a *group* which is also a *family*

▷   a family group

Example 2   a person who *dwells* in a *cave*
    ▷   a cave-dweller

Example 3   *football* played in a *college*
    ▷   college football

Example 4   a *coach* (or trainer) for *football* played in a *college*
    ▷   a college football coach

Note, however, that this last compound can also be paraphrased as 'a coach for football, and the coach is employed by a college'.

a.   a *chair* which has *arms*
b.   a *delay* that last *two hours*
c.   *services* in a *cathedral*
d.   a *report* written in or about *London*, and the report concerns *business*
e.   a *wall* that is built of *bricks* and stands *15 feet* high
f.   the *number* of a *telephone* in *New York*
g.   a *company* that *publishes* (books, etc) in *Singapore*
h.   a *manager* of a *centre* for *tourists* in *Florida*
i.   a *box* made of *steel*, and the *box* is *8 feet square*
j.   a *strike* in a *factory* that makes *cars* in *Birmingham* in England.

Compound work:
Second stage

Effectively, when one wants to paraphrase or describe a compound, the simplest thing to do is convert back into the original fuller kind of phrase that was used in the previous exercise. This is done in the examples below. Study them carefully, then paraphrase the listed compounds in similar ways.

Example 1   a cavern waterfall
    ▷   a waterfall in a cavern
    or
    ▷   a fall of water in a cavern

Note, however, that as more is paraphrased something is lost. A 'fall of water' may only happen once, but a 'waterfall' is relatively permanent.

Example 2   soil erosion
    ▷   the erosion of soil

Note the special use of *the*

Example 3   a sheepskin

▷   the skin of a sheep

Note the special use of both *the* and *a*

Example 4   a sky-blue coffee pot

▷   a pot for coffee, and the pot is blue like the sky **or** as blue as the sky

- a.   an exploration team
- b.   a nylon line
- c.   the Mas d'Azil cave
- d.   a parachute ripcord
- e.   age barriers
- f.   a 15-foot pile
- g.   ground level
- h.   an underground river
- i.   cave artists
- j.   a 25-year-old Nice cave-explorer
- k.   a university football competition
- l.   the Queen Victoria Hospital
- m.   a diving-board accident
- n.   ski-patrol members
- o.   a 25-foot-high steel post
- p.   an Oxford University Press dictionary editor
- q.   a United States English-language program director
- r.   puberty initiation rites
- s.   river-and-lake pollution problems
- t.   a snow-clearing operation

3.5   Grammar and vocabulary: Derived words

The compounding of words is important, but the derivation of words is also important. Whereas compounds are formed by putting more or less equal elements together (nouns, verbs, adjectives), derivatives are formed by adding subordinate elements to a simple *base* – usually a noun, verb or adjective. These subordinate elements are known as *affixes*. If an affix is attached at the beginning of a base, it is a *prefix*; if it is attached at the end, it is a *suffix*. There have already been a number of sections in this course relating to prefixes and suffixes, but so far we have not considered the process of derivation as a whole. Study the following examples carefully:

1
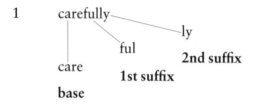

2
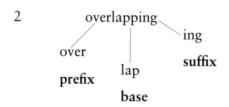

3
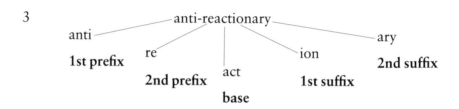

The base is naturally the principal part of the derived word, and almost always has a clear meaning. It is usually a word itself, *but not always*:

4
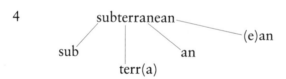

Note that the base here is *terr*, from the Latin word *terra*, meaning 'earth, land'. It is not a normal word in English, but since it 'translates' a noun, it has the value of a noun. There are many bases of this type, mostly from Latin and Greek, but sometimes also of Anglo-Saxon origin.

5
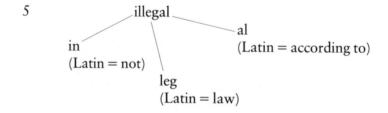

Note that this word is entirely of Latin origin and form, translatable as 'not according to the law'.

   If one removes all the apparent affixes and is left with something that seems to have no useful present-day meaning, this remainder cannot be considered a base. It is the historical *root* of the word, something that was a base long ago, perhaps in another language, but only part of the modern base on which new words can be formed. For example:

6

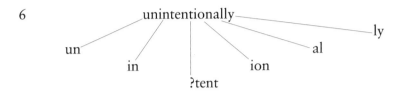

Note that the root *tent* comes from a Latin verb meaning 'to hold'. It has no present-day value; the base, therefore, has to be *intent*, a variation of the verb *intend*. If I do something unintentionally, I did not intend to do it. This means that the *in* element, though technically a prefix, has no value in modern English either. In word analysis it is necessary to distinguish constantly between bases that have a meaning and function, and roots that may be interesting but have no present-day value. The problem can be seen clearly in words like *receive*, *combat*, *prepare*, etc, where the elements 'ceive', 'bat' and 'pare' have no meaning in modern English.

   Sometimes what looks like a derived word may in fact be a disguised compound (that is, it has two bases, not one). This is common in technical words of Greek origin:

7

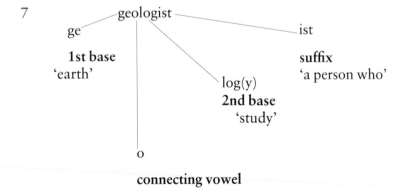

Meaning: a person who studies the earth

The accurate analysis of derivatives is a complex – though very useful – art, which can often best be practised with the help of a good etymological dictionary. In the exercises which follow, you may or may not need to use such a dictionary to gain fuller control over the words.

Derivational practice:
First stage

Analyse the following words:

a.	Mexican	k.	inspector
b.	pro-Chinese	l.	competitiveness
c.	unnatural	m.	military
d.	nationalistic	n.	pre-technological
e.	super-tribal	o.	television
f.	uncontrollable	p.	misconception
g.	readership	q.	organizational
h.	timelessness	r.	energetically
i.	re-development	s.	dissatisfaction
j.	downhill	t.	totalitarianism

Derivational practice:
Second stage

Complete the bases (etc) in the first column with the appropriate suffixes in the second column:

1	lun (*Latin = moon*)	a.	ic	(*forms adjectives*)
2	pac (*L = peace*)	b.	al	(*forms adj*)
3	mathemat (*Greek = learning*)	c.	ism	(*forms nouns*)
4	athe (*G = no god*)	d.	ite	(*forms n*)
5	concentr (*L = centre together*)	e.	ar	(*adj*)
6	urb (*L = city*)	f.	ize	(*forms verbs*)
7	mort (*L = dead, death*)	g.	ics	(*n*)
8	atom (*G, normal word*)	h.	ify	(*v*)
9	synthes (*G = put together*)	i.	ate	(*v*)
10	calc (*G = lime*)	j.	an	(*adj*)

Derivational practice:
Third stage

Below is a list of prefixes commonly used in English, with their approximate meanings in brackets. They are followed by twelve sentences that need to be completed by adapting one word in each sentence to operate with a prefix.

re- (*again*)   in-, im-, il-, ir- (*not*)
pre- (*before*)   non- (*not in any way*)
post- (*after*)   dis- (*not*, with verbs)
sub- (*under*; *less*)   mis- (*badly*; *incorrectly*)
super- (*over*; *more*)   under- (*too little*; *not enough*)
over- (*too much*)   anti- (*against*; *opposed to*)
un- (*not*)   pro- (*for*; *in favour of*)

a. She agreed with the plan, but he _____ (with it).
b. They were told to advertise the post again, so they set about _____ it.
c. He is in favour of the Americans but opposed to the British. He is therefore _____ but _____ .
d. The company works its employees too hard. It _____ them.
e. The country is badly governed. Its rulers are guilty of _____ .
f. This matter has nothing to do with science. It is completely _____ .
g. Conditions after the war were no better than before. _____ conditions and _____ conditions were pretty much the same.
h. The workmen do not use the new equipment enough. They are _____ it.
i. The upper structures of a ship are called its _____ .
j. There is no logic in that statement. It is a thoroughly _____ statement.
k. She was in no way affected by his remarks. The remarks left her completely _____ .
l. Work that is below the expected standard is quite simply _____ (work).

3.6 Punctuation:
The hyphen

Hyphenation, like the use of commas, is something of an art, and is to some extent a matter of personal preference. The most important things about a hyphen (-) is that it should not be confused with a dash (—). A hyphen occupies a single space, just like a letter, without any white space on either side; a dash, however, in writing or in print, occupies more space, and usually has some white space on each side. In typing, the same sign is normally used for both, and it is therefore particularly important to make sure that the dash gets some white space. In purely functional terms, the hyphen operates quite differently from the dash, and has two purposes:

1   to unite the elements of certain kinds of compound and derived words

2   to serve as a word-breaking device at the end of lines.

These uses are distinctly different. The first brings together various elements to make up a single new unit; the second takes apart the elements of what was already a unit. The two functions are, therefore, opposite in kind.

First function:
Uniting elements in compound and derived words

In this aspect of its work, the hyphen is like the coupling that keeps two railway carriages together; it signals that the writer recognizes a special intimacy between the elements in question. In the list below this intimacy can be seen clearly in the right-hand column, which shows the compound and derivative types that *generally* need hyphenating:

Free or open version	Hyphenated version
1 He owns land. It opens bottles.	He is a land-owner. It is a bottle-opener.
2 The aircraft flies low. The business runs smoothly.	It is a low-flying aircraft. It is a smooth-running business.
3 They make glass. He builds ships.	They engage in glass-making. His work is ship-building.
4 The company makes glass. The country produces wine.	It is a glass-making company. It is a wine-producing country.
5 The men are well trained. The group is badly led.	They are well-trained men. It is a badly-led group.
6 The mountain is covered in/ with snow. The agency is run by the government. The organization is based in London. He educated himself.	It is a snow-covered mountain. It is a government-run agency. It is a London-based organization. He is a self-educated man.
7 The woman has blue eyes. The man has red hair. The house has mud walls.	She is a blue-eyed woman. He is a red-haired man. It is a mud-walled house.
8 The shirt is blue with some green in it. The dress is green with grey. The car is blue like the sky, or as blue as the sky. The water is clear like crystal, or as clear as crystal. The area is free from accidents. The group is conscious of profits.	It is greenish-blue, a greenish-blue shirt. It is grey-green, a grey-green dress. It is sky-blue, a sky-blue car. It is crystal-clear, crystal-clear water. It is accident-free, an accident-free area. It is profit-conscious, a profit-conscious group.
9 It is a meeting between Moscow and Washington. It is a meeting of Churchill, Stalin and Roosevelt. It is an agreement between the U.S. (= United States) and Mexico.	It is a Washington-Moscow meeting (or the reverse). It is a Churchill-Stalin-Roosevelt meeting. It is a U.S.-Mexico **or** US-Mexico agreement.

Free or open version	Hyphenated version
10 They discussed relations between France and Britain.	They discussed Franco-British relations.
The warriors were both Angles and Saxons.	They were Anglo-Saxon warriors.
The differences are both social and economic.	They are socio-economic differences.
11 He likes a bath with cold water.	He likes a cold-water bath.
It was a film in slow motion.	It was a slow-motion film.
12 The man is 29 years old.	He is a 29-year-old man.
The wall is 35 feet high.	It is a 35-foot(-high) wall.
The house was built in the 19th century.	It is a 19th-century house.
13 'Never say die' is his attitude.	He has a never-say-die attitude.
This offer comes only once in a lifetime!	This is a once-in-a-lifetime offer!
Now It Can Be Told – the story of a great love!	It's a now-it-can-be-told love story.
14 This isn't what Americans do.	It is un-American.
This has nothing to do with science.	It is non-scientific.
It happened before Columbus.	It is pre-Columbian.
It happened after the war.	It is post-war.
He is against pollution.	He is anti-pollution.
She is in favour of reform.	She is pro-reform.
These materials have already been tested.	They are pre-tested materials.
Do the work again.	Re-do the work.
Discover your youth once more!	Re-discover your youth!
The committee appointed a special committee.	It appointed a sub-committee.
The sub-committee appointed a special committee.	It appointed a sub-sub-committee.

Note that only a living, meaningful prefix preceding a base has a hyphen: *ex-soldier*, but not *expect*; *pre-test*, but not *prepare*; *re-make*, but not *receive*. This difference is also generally marked in speech by stress on the hyphenated prefix, whereas the vowel in the other kind of prefix – as in *receive* – is a schwa [ə], the syllable being weak.

Second function:
Serving as a word-breaking device

The rules for breaking up words at the ends of lines are:

1   **Avoid doing it wherever possible.** It is better to have a little more
    white space than usual than too many broken words.
2   Do not do it to short words.
3   Do not break longer words too near the beginning or too near the
    end, unless the shorter pieces have a meaning (that is, they are
    common, productive prefixes or suffixes).
4   If possible, break according to the clear divisions of prefix, base,
    root, and suffix.
5   If this is not possible, break at an obvious syllable boundary, and
    in particular, if there are double letters (like *ll*, *pp*, etc), have one
    on each line.
6   *Never* have a second hyphen at the beginning of the next line.
    One at the end of a line is quite enough.

Punctuation work:
First stage

Look at a variety of textbooks, novels and magazines to see how the
printers have handled the end-of-line division of words. In this course
the lines of text are 'unjustified' (that is, they are of unequal length) in
order to avoid broken words.

Punctuation work:
Second stage

Punctuate the material which follows, dividing it into whatever
paragraphs you consider necessary, and taking care with the use of
quotation marks and hyphens.

the large underground caves called caverns are usually found in
limestone rock water from streams or from rainfall passes slowly
through cracks in the layers of limestone as this water with carbon
dioxide dissolved in it trickles through the cracks it dissolves and
carries away small amounts of the limestone so that over
thousands of years the cracks slowly widen into caves
subterranean caves may become as big as cathedrals with side
passages and chapels and even such extra marvels as underground
rivers waterfalls and lakes sometimes if a cave is not far from the

surface its roof may weaken and fall in the surface hole left by this cave in is called a sink hole or sink water often collects in these sink holes forming sink hole ponds or lakes limestone caverns often have slim icicle like stalactites hanging from their ceilings while on the ground underneath them stalagmites form as the lime laden water drips from the ends of the icicles one can remember which of these strange terms is which by associating the c of stalactite with the caves ceiling while the g of stalagmite reminds us of the ground over long periods of time the stalactites reach down and the stalagmites reach up until they join each other in beautiful pillars the largest underground chamber in the world is said to be in the carlsbad caverns new mexico in the united states of america the most extensive cave system is probably mammoth cave kentucky also in the u s a and the deepest caves are found in the pyrenees the range of mountains between france and spain in britain the largest known caves are in south wales while two of the best known caverns are gaping ghyll in yorkshire and wookey hole in somerset both in england.

3.7 Composition: Making a summary

Using any method you wish of summarizing a piece of writing (as described in Section 9.5), make a summary of the passage 'Under the Earth'. You should try to make it about one third the length of the original, and certainly not more than one half. Your summary should consist at the end of four paragraphs, each one dealing with the topics listed below:

1   prehistoric cave artists
2   caverns and tourism
3   the exploration of caverns and prolonged periods underground
4   timelessness, the body clock, caves and outer space

3.8 Editing a text: 'The Story of Lascaux'

The passage below is not quite ready for publication. It suffers from a variety of faults in layout, punctuation, spelling and grammar. Prepare it for publication.

Pre-eminent among the sights and tales of French caverns is
Lascaux, set in a hill above the town of Montignac sur-Vézère.
The caves were discovered in 1940 by a local 18 years old boy who
followed his dog into a hole beneath the roots of a tree that have
been torn down in a storm. With two companions this young man
Marcel Ravidat, discovered, in the light of there lanterns, vivid red
yellow and black paintings of massive animals that no longer walk
the earth. Since then, many books has been written on mysterious
artists who decorated the caves, and countless visitors have
entered the caverns to view these age old masterpieces.

Diaster however, struck in 1961.

After a particularly succesful year for tourists, it wss observed that
a bright green moss was spreading over the cave walls towards the
priceless paintings. By 1963 according to M. Leo Magne the
regional tourist board president the moss had advanced more in
the previous three months than in all the three preceding years,
and the progress was almost visible.

The caves were closed to the public. A comission of artists,
scientist and historians were sent from Paris to study the
phenomenon. Wearing masks and using air locks like moon
explorers, the investigators studied the fast-moving moss, seeking
to learn what it was, where it cam from, and how to stop it. Why
after 20,000 years of tranquillity, had this strange moss only
began to wander now?

The answer was simple. The moss is the work of modern man.
In all damp caves with openings to the outisde world there exists a
species of microscopic moss which grows larger where there is
light. Under normal condition it resembles slime. The introduction
of outside air, however, then electric light and heat, and finaly the
carbon dioxide breathed out by a thousand visitor a day had so
encourage this moss to grow that it had swept across the walls like
a tide.

The closing of the caves meant economic hardship for the
people of Montignac village, after their classic year of 1962 the
shop keepers had laid in large stores of photographic slides,
postcards and souvenirs, while also investing in a new road to the
site. The caves however have remained sealed off, until some
adequate solution is found to the problem of protecting the
ancient pictures which have for the time bing, returned to their
equally ancient darkness.

3.9 Composition:
Describing a locality

The passage 'Under the Earth' has its own distinctive shape. It is developed, like all the other introductory passages in this course, in a way which can make the best possible use of its content and language resources to achieve a particular effect – the willingness of the reader to continue reading. The vocabulary, grammar, punctuation and various stylistic devices all work together to achieve whatever effect it has. You, the reader, are the ultimate judge of whether or not it has achieved its effect. It is, however, only one of many possible ways of describing a geographical topic (with historical and scientific overtones). There are many other ways of doing the same kind of thing, all equally effective. Below you will find the outline of the basic structure of the passage. It is not, however, restricted to caves. This structure can be used for any place, region, city, country, mountain, river, lake or similar topic. Choose one (or more than one), using the structure shown here as a 'skeleton' on which to build your own description (drawing on whatever sources you need to do so).

Possible language items	Suggestions about the topic
1 'If you ..., where/what/how *etc* ...?'	Your introduction, a conditional statement or question, or a question alone, to arouse the reader's interest (and perhaps left as a one-sentence paragraph for dramatic effect).
2 Repetition of the questioning, conditional style, with some factual information about the topic.	Choose one of the most powerful points about the topic, in order to keep the reader interested. Is there some remarkable building in a particular city? Was something world-famous done or written or invented there? Was there some terrible disaster?
3 'Cave explorers *etc* ... **but** ...' 'Most of Europe's caverns, for example, are today ...'	Contrasts between what is expected and what is actually true, between old and new, nature and civilization, etc. Most places can be described in contrastive terms.
4 'In the foothills ...' 'One is accustomed ... **but** ...'	The use of *anecdotes* (that is, specific attractive, self-contained, stories about aspects of a place or what happens there). Two or three are enough, but while preparing your material you should collect more than you will need.
5 'Caves mean more to modern investigators, however, than ...'	Clear change of direction, interest, attitude, etc. Having provided good informative material, do not overwork it. Move on to your second main point.
6 'The Yugoslav and the Frenchmen showed that ...' 'All three investigators were convinced that time was passing more quickly than was in fact the case.' ←—	Your second point of interest also has its anecdotes, illustrating some particular point, but the time comes when a summarizing conclusion may be necessary. In this case, the last sentence of this particular paragraph is very powerful.
7 'Such findings are very interesting not only ...' '... only the little gadget on one's wrist to speak the true passage of ←— time.'	Some kind of strong general conclusion for what went immediately before (or for the whole piece). Here, the matter of cave exploration blows wide open, to include the whole universe ('outer space'), then contracts again until we are back underground with the darkness all around us – as the original cave artists must have been.

UNIT 4   Revision

4.1   Comprehension and composition model: 'The Self-Moving Boxes'

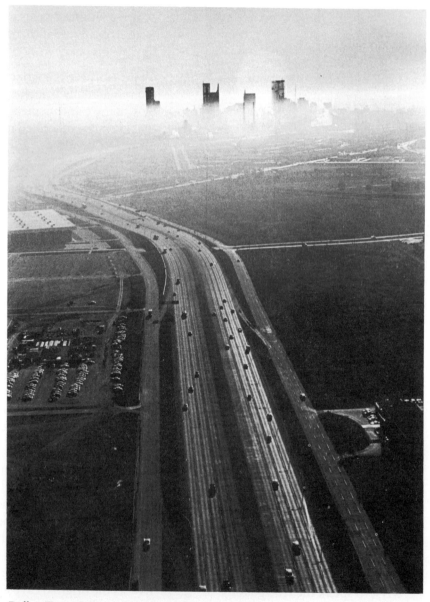

Dallas, Texas, USA.

Satire is a quiet but powerful tool. Writers use it to comment amusingly or bitterly – or both – on various things in the world around them. Earlier in this course (in Book 1, Units 4 and 5) such satirists as Aesop, Jonathan Swift and George Orwell have been mentioned. Much of the work material in this unit is centred on a piece of satirical writing, beginning with the passage below. It is set in an unspecified future time, but deals with matters that are important today. Read it twice, studying the techniques used to produce various effects, then complete the exercises based upon it.

Part of the text of a lecture delivered at a conference sponsored by the Centre for Terran Rehabilitation, the University of Mare Imbrium, Luna.

Ladies and gentlemen, colleagues and friends, when we consider the plight of our ancestors in the Middle Machine Age, we have to realize – difficult though this is – that they were not in the least aware of what they were doing to the planet Earth.

I should like to take as the focal point of my study the middle and   5
later decades of the period which they knew as the Twentieth
Century, at which time their diverse governments were engaged in a
battle of ideas known as the Cold War. In those days, they were
much more interested in ideas than in such mundane matters as
feeding and educating their populations, and had indeed – as I'm   10
sure you are aware – fought two Hot Wars already in that same
century over ideological matters.

During my period, they were divided into three camps which –
presumably viewed from the North Pole – were known as Right,
Left and South. The South was also known as 'The Third World',   15
and Right and Left spent a lot of time arguing over which of them
was entitled to be called 'The First World'.

They were in many ways at the peak of their civilization,
convinced that they were enjoying – and would go on enjoying –
the fruits of 150 years of research and invention since the start of   20
the Great Machine Revolution. Everything that in previous
centuries had been done by animal or human power was now being
done by engines, pistons, cogs, wheels, belts, cables, circuits,
transistors and micro-chips. This enabled them to spend much of
their time laying long strips of a material called 'tarmac' in spider's   25
webs across the various continents, so that their special creation,
the self-moving box, could go wherever it wanted.

The self-moving box had replaced earlier horse-drawn carriages.
The first versions were slow and clumsy, requiring men with red
flags to go before them as a warning to people to get out of the way;   30
they were for a time viewed with amused scorn by lovers of
horseflesh, while even their advocates were forced to describe their
mechanical strength in terms of 'horsepower'. These early
advocates were dedicated and resourceful people. One of them,
Henry Ford, even went so far as to promise that every family would   35
one day possess such a box.

This is where it becomes clear that the governments of the day did not realize what was happening. Despite their wars and because of their successes with medicine, the numbers of the human race were increasing like ants. The Earth's population doubled between the invention of the first 'auto-mobile' and that point in time when certain nations were beginning to change the shapes of their cities to make more room for the boxes. Henry Ford's promise now meant that in a world of some three billion souls there would be horseless carriages enough for all – and they believed him still. A point was even reached where one nation, Great Britain, measured its prosperity by the number of 'cars' rolling off the assembly lines of her Midland cities, while the United States of America asserted that Henry Ford's dream was no longer adequate, and that every family should have two, if not three, self-moving boxes in its driveway.

The possession of such a machine was a matter of prestige as well as convenience, and the type of box as well as the money spent in buying and maintaining it were an important aspect of ownership. Much of the nations' metal resources went into producing more and more and longer and longer boxes. Old-fashioned cities were clogged with them, agricultural land was swallowed up for what were called 'Super-High-Ways', and deaths from inevitable collisions and crashes equalled the casualties of a fair-sized traditional war. Despite all this, however, a popular hobby grew up of driving one's box round several countries that were not one's own, looking fleetingly at the people and scenery just beside one's strip of 'Super-High-Way'. This was called Tourism, and everybody thought of it as a good idea.

The increase in the number of self-moving boxes and similar machines had a profound effect on the international posturing of the various bickering nations. As you are probably aware, the tragedy was that their machines were powered by a fossil fuel, dug from the earth and known as the Oil-That-Comes-From-Stones, or *petroleum*. Political panics were easily started whenever anyone threatened the other fellow's supply of oil from the areas where it was brought to the surface. Once it had reached its destination, the oil was made available at special roadside sanctuaries, such refuelling points becoming one of the foremost cultural centres of the day, gaily decorated with all sorts of flags and posters.

It was in the 1970s that people began to be aware that the millions of auto-mobiles were posing more problems than just where to put them when not in use. There were, however, here and there, a few thoughtful folk who murmured warnings. Let me, for example, quote briefly from a magazine called *The Rotarian*, some copies of which we have in our microfiles. It is dated July 1965, and in it one Clifford Hicks discusses some of the problems created by all these engines with their carburettors and exhaust pipes. He observes:

'Man is now competing with his machines for breathable air.'

Below are some statements relating to the passage. Some are true (T) in terms of the passage, while others are false (F). Mark them appropriately, and if a statement is false, say why.

a. ☐ The speaker is talking about our ancestors.

b. ☐ The speaker is dealing roughly with the period 1950–1990.

c. ☐ The Right and Left were competing for the leading position in the world described.

d. ☐ It was the intention of the various governments that self-moving boxes should be able to move anywhere on the various continents, on their strips of tarmac.

e. ☐ The men with red flags were employed to stop dangerous horseless carriages.

f. ☐ The terrible wars of the 20th century did not stop the world's population from growing rapidly.

g. ☐ The growing numbers of self-moving boxes made it necessary for people to change the nature of their cities.

h. ☐ Henry Ford later said that not one but two automobiles should be available to each family.

i. ☐ The collisions and crashes on the 'Super-High-Ways' caused people to go on fewer tours in their cars.

j. ☐ Where to park an auto-mobile proved to be one of the lesser problems that it posed.

Now look in the passage for examples of the following:

k. parentheses using dashes (at least two examples)

l. capital letters at the beginnings of words used for special effect (at least four distinct examples)

m. quotation marks used for dramatic affect or to draw attention to a word or phrase (at least three examples)

n. hyphens used for normal everyday purposes (at least two examples)

o. hyphens used for satirical purposes, to emphasize words in a special way (at least two examples)

p. commas used in an unusually long list (one example)

q. an etymological explanation of a word used for dramatic effect (one example)

r. the various points in the passage where the speaker brings himself or herself into the material

s. the various points in the passage where the speaker brings his or her listeners into the material.

4.2 Spelling and organization: Alphabetic order

Ability to spell well is related to the ability to recognize patterns in words, where they are similar and where they are different. One such kind of patterning is alphabetic order. In this section there are lists of increasing length and complexity, which must all be put into proper alphabetic order, one after the other. Proceed.

1   need
    necessity
    necessary
    needy
    needless

2   receive   receptacle
    recipe   receiver
    receptive   re-cycle
    reservoir   reckoning
    reckless   reception

3   symmetry   synthetic   synchronize
    syllable   symmetrical   syntax
    sympathy   syllabic   sympathetic
    synthesis   sympathize   syllogistic
    symbolic   syllogism   symbolism

4   satyr   satirize   Saturday
    satisfy   saturate   satirical
    saturnine   Saturn   saturation
    savagery   say   satisfactory
    satanic   satellite   sadden

5   medical   mental   metal
    meditate   medicinal   medal
    mercurial   meadow   mentality
    mediation   mensuration   measure
    measles   meditation   medicine
    meditative   mermaid   mellow
    mediator   means   mediate
    measurable   medication   metallic
    meddle   mercury   mercantile
    medicare   mentalism   median

6
mechanical	success	millimetre
nature	microscope	machine
nationalist	succeed	petroleum
politician	carbolic	native
decision	million	microphone
governor	realize	successful
automobile	politics	millilitre
government	carbon	realization
destiny	microbe	mechanism
automatic	really	polite
nationality	colleague	naturally
collective	reality	mechanized
governable	petrify	destination
carburettor	political	collision
petro-chemical	micro-organism	millipede

4.3 Grammar and vocabulary: Missing words

Below are three lists. The first contains conjunctions and relative pronouns, the second contains phrasal verbs, and the third contains a number of items of general vocabulary. Below the list is a passage which continues the lecture given at the University of Mare Imbrium. It contains twenty numbered blanks. Complete the passage with the most suitable words, noting that some of the listed words are quite unconnected with the passage, and that one or two in the first list may be needed more than once.

Conjunctions and relative pronouns	Phrasal verbs	General vocabulary
as	use up	green
when	pour out	poison
which	breathe out	greatly
what	fly up	identical
that	try out	compound
although	gulp down	forceful
because	run in	cubic
so that		tankful

Clifford Hicks observed (1)_____ humankind was now competing with its machines for breathable air. The most (2)_____ example that he could offer to his readers was their own competition with their cars. '(3)_____ you drive down the highway,' he said, 'your car engine is (4)_____ 1,000 times (5)_____ much oxygen as you are consuming.' It was also (6)_____ a great cloud of mostly invisible gases (7)_____ needed to be dissipated into harmless concentrations in the atmosphere. He warned them: 'It requires from five to ten million times (8)_____ much air to dilute these (9)_____ to a safe level (10)_____ it requires to dilute your own personal air pollution each time you exhale.'

He gave his readers the statistics: A ton of air was required to burn every (11)_____ of petrol (or 'gas', as he called it). One nation, the U.S.A., was burning petrol at the rate of a billion gallons a year. Such a process of combustion was (12)_____ the oxygen in 94 trillion (13)_____ feet of air. To (14)_____ the problem, in his view, U.S. cars were discharging every day into the atmosphere some 250,000 tons of carbon monoxide, 25,000 tons of hydro-carbons, and 8,000 tons of oxides of nitrogen. Hicks asked his readers: 'Have you done your share today?'

It can be seen from this quotation (15)_____ some people understood well enough (16)_____ was happening, (17)_____ not necessarily the magnitude of the matter. They were aware that their machines were (18)'_____' into the atmosphere vast quantities of that (19)_____ gas, carbon monoxide, that was (20)_____ favoured by those among them with the urge to commit suicide. It was a peculiar age.

4.4 Grammar: Articles

Below, the comments of the Lunar lecturer continue. This time, however, the blanks in the passage relate to possible missing definite and indefinite articles. Insert articles where necessary, putting an 'X' where in your opinion no article is needed.

Many people in (1)_____ late Twentieth Century claimed to have (2)_____ great interest in (3)_____ fresh air and good health, trying to keep themselves fit by such means as running and playing (4)_____ games. Nevertheless, these same people, using their auto-mobiles, were content to turn (5)_____ air around and above their cities into canopies of pollution, (6)_____ cause of many respiratory and other illnesses. Compounding this problem, at certain times of (7)_____ day in (8)_____ cities, everybody would climb into their vehicles and take part in (9)_____ strange collective ritual. In (10)_____ morning,

people outside (11)_____ town would all try to get into
(12)_____ city centre at (13)_____ same time; in
(14)_____ evening, they would reverse (15)_____ process
and all try to get out again. (16)_____ result of this procedure
was (17)_____ miles and miles of auto-mobiles standing or
crawling in (18)_____ queues on every major road, nobody
getting anywhere for (19)_____ long time. Curiously enough,
they referred to this leisurely activity as '(20)_____ rush-hour'.

4.5 Punctuation, grammar and organization: Logical order

Below the main points in the lecture given at the Lunar Centre for
Terran Rehabilitation continue, describing the fate of those who had
so happily used the self-moving box. It is not, however, punctuated,
nor is it in logical order. Do the punctuation work, and then re-
arrange the material to make sense.

A. because it was being produced faster than it could be absorbed
    by the ocean or converted back into carbon and oxygen by
    plants the carbon dioxide began to accumulate

B. these world wide temperature changes equally inevitably set in
    motion a final unthinkable change the steady melting of the
    great polar ice caps

C. slowly scientists became concerned about the tremendous
    quantities of gas particularly carbon dioxide released into the
    atmosphere through the on going large scale burning of fossil
    fuels

D. in a single century humankind had almost casually altered both
    air and ocean more than had happened in millions of years of
    geological time

E. this not only raised the ocean levels more than ten feet but also
    effectively solved the traffic problems of the worlds great coastal
    cities by flooding them out completely

F. while doing so it produced what is called a greenhouse effect in
    the planets atmosphere

G. the inevitable result of such a blockage was an increase in
    temperatures all over the world

H. there was at least ten percent more carbon dioxide in the air by
    1980 than there had been when the century started

I. this allowed sunlight to come in but effectively blocked the heat
    generated on Earth by the suns rays from escaping back into
    space

4.6 Grammar:
Sentence synthesis

Below is a series of simple sentences, telling the story of Lascaux and other caves with paintings in them. By any means you consider suitable, combine shorter sentences into longer ones, to create a more polished piece of writing.

In the summer of 1940, a group of boys were playing near the village of Montignac, in France. Their dog got lost. One of them found it in a hole under a tree. This hole was in fact the entrance to a cave. This cave is now called the Lascaux Cave. Its main hall measures 100 feet by 30 feet. It is filled with remarkable paintings of ancient animals. Most of them are outlined in black. Some have dotted patterns. Others are coloured red or brown. The animals seem almost alive. They have true-to-life shapes. There is a very realistic scene depicting a bison. The bison has been wounded with a spear. Lascaux is not, however, the only cave in Western Europe with such paintings in it. There are more than 120 caves with paintings in them. These caves are in France, Spain and Italy. The painted caves of Europe are very interesting, but they are not unique. Paintings of ancient mammoths and cave bears have been found in the Kapova Cave in the Ural Mountains of Russia. Other caves in Australia contain paintings done by present-day aborigines. The style of these paintings is similar to the style of the ancient cave artists of Lascaux.

4.7 Vocabulary:
Nationalities

Complete the following sentences, using the national name in brackets at the beginning of each sentence in order to form appropriate nouns or adjectives.

a.   (Norway)   A _____ ship sailed into the port.
b.   (Wales)   She is studying _____ history.
c.   (Iraq)   They buy only _____ oil.
d.   (Peru)   The envelope bore several _____ stamps.
e.   (Denmark)   Her friend is a _____ .
f.   (Turkey)   Do you speak _____ ?
g.   (Portugal)   She carries a _____ passport.

h. (Netherlands) He works for a _____ company.

i. (Hungary) I like _____ wine.

j. (Sweden) _____ exports do well in this country.

k. (Sudan) He likes _____ art.

l. (Britain) Most _____ enjoy seaside holidays.

m. (Canada) The _____ flag is red and white.

n. (Egypt) The _____ pyramids are world-famous.

o. (Finland) _____ is very different from other European
    languages.

p. (Syria) The _____ capital is Damascus.

q. (Yugoslavia) His wife is _____ .

r. (Brazil) _____ coffee is very good.

s. (Mexico) The Aztecs were a _____ people.

t. (Pakistan) Most _____ are Moslems.

4.8 Vocabulary:
Word formation

In the following passage a number of words are underlined. Consider
each of these words, to see whether it is a base or a derivative, then
form as many other words as you can from that word or its base. The
first one is done for you as an example.

Many governments are concerned nowadays about the problem of
pollution. They know that industrialization is necessary, for
economic reasons and in order to develop their national resources,
but at the same time they are very much aware that waste materials
from factories and chemical plants as well as vehicles and everyday
appliances can cause serious environmental damage. The proper
disposal of such wastes is now a matter of social, political and often
legal concern.

1 government – *base*: govern
                – *other words*: governor
                               misgovern
                               misgovernment
                               governmental
                               governable
                               ungovernable
                               etc

4.9 Vocabulary:
Further word formation

Below are ten sentences containing blanks. Beside each of the
sentences are words in bold letters. Use these words as bases for the
derivation of other words that can serve to complete the sentences.

a.   Most _____ accept the theory of _____ .   **science**
                                                                 evolve

b.   Their company has _____s all over the world,   **distribute**
     engaged in large-scale _____ _____s every   **commerce**
     hour of the day.   **transact**

c.   The _____ on the stone was _____ a   **inscribe**
     _____ to an ancient king.   **appear**
                                                                 refer

d.   The work was not good enough, so the _____   **profess**
     reluctantly asked the _____ to _____ it.   **study**
                                                                 write

e.   The _____ did not want to make any   **industry**
     _____s whatever to his main business   **concede**
     _____s.   **compete**

f.   Our _____ _____ is that the _____ of   **nature**
     the project depends _____ on whether or not   **assume**
     the government will give us _____ aid.   **complete**
                                                                 entire
                                                                 finance

g.   _____ , nothing can be done until they receive a   **regret**
     clear _____ _____ on the matter.   **preside**
                                                                 decide

h.   The _____ _____ of the _____ caused a   **intend**
     great deal of _____ everywhere.   **conceal**
                                                                 inform
                                                                 resent

i.   The council made a _____ to the effect that the   **declare**
     town centre would be _____ so as to serve in   **beauty**
     future as a local _____ _____ .   **tour**
                                                                 attract

j.   As a result of his _____ _____ , the   **appal**
     company had to close down, putting four hundred   **manage**
     _____ _____ out of work.   **faith**
                                                                 employ

4.10 Composition:
The value of satire

The Lunar lecture presented in this unit takes an important present-day topic – the pollution of the environment – and handles it satirically, presenting information in an unusual and possibly arresting way. The implication of the satire is clear: the world and humanity are endangered by large-scale use (and misuse) of fossil fuels. It suggests, in fact, that our descendants might end up finding the Moon a safer place than our own planet Earth.

Two questions arise from this treatment of the issue:

1   Is such a warning necessary? (In other words, are things anywhere near as bad as the satire suggests?)

2   Whether or not it is necessary, is the satirical method *effective* in making people think afresh about such matters? Does it work better than, say, a simple presentation of factual material?

Prepare and then write an essay considering these (and related) points, making use of any other sources (books, magazines, newspaper articles, etc) that you wish. The following simple plan may serve as a skeleton for such an essay:

1   a description of the content, style and intention of the satire 'Self-Moving Boxes'

2   a parallel examination of its claims in relation to 'reality'

3   your assessment of the scale of the real problem

4   your assessment of the effectiveness of satire generally and this satire in particular as a tool for getting people to think about problems

5   your considered conclusions

UNIT 5

5.1 Comprehension and composition model: 'The Scale of Things'

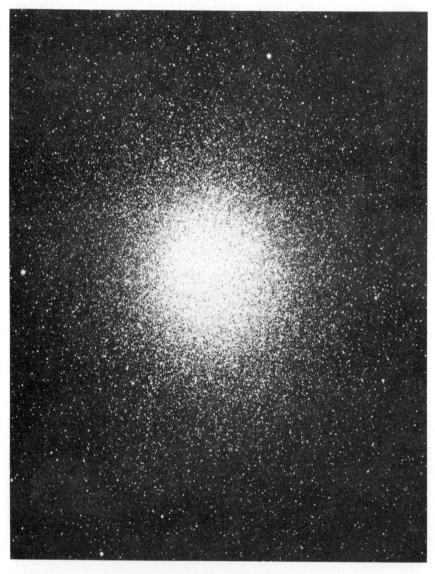

This star cluster in the constellation of Centaurus is just visible to the naked eye. It contains several million stars, all older than our sun.

Here is a passage discussing the universe, the sun, the planet Earth, its 'biosphere', and ourselves. Read it twice, noting its organization and layout, the various quotations and references, the punctuation and grammatical style, and the variety of vocabulary used. When you have done this, proceed to the various exercises and related activities based on the passage.

The sun is a star. It is not a particularly large or particularly bright star, and exists in a universe that contains literally millions of stars. Astronomers classify our small and undistinguished life-giver as a 'yellow dwarf', and point out that Capella is ten times bigger, that Antares is 300 times bigger, and indeed that the larger 'supergiants'   5
are 3,000 times bigger. These are – apparently – cosmic facts, to be accepted without argument, whatever our senses tell us about our large sun and tiny stars. Like the distances in light-years that separate stars, however, such facts are hard to digest. As Robin Kerrod observes[1]:   10

'It is difficult for anyone, even astronomers included, to view the universe in perspective. We know that it is made up of space with stars, planets, dust, and gas floating in it here and there. But empty space predominates.'

He adds that our solar system is in fact 'a comparatively crowded   15
corner of the universe', although from our point of view this is hardly credible either. By our own methods of measuring and appreciating distances Venus, the nearest planet to Earth, is more than 25 million miles (40 million kilometres) away, while our modest yellow dwarf is 93 million miles or 150 million kilometres   20
away. It is hard enough to imagine these distances; it is more difficult still when astronomers tell us that these distances are examples of crowding and are a mere nothing anyway, on the real cosmic scale of things.

Today, most people with a Western-style education accept that   25
the universe in which our earth and sun move is enormous beyond conception, yet we do not obtain this information from our normal sense impressions (which is, in effect, why we find it hard to grasp). Any conception we have of the cosmic scale of things is mediated by the intellect, not the senses: we cannot see the universe spread out   30
with all its turning galaxies; the sun does not look in any way like a twinkling star; we do not feel the earth moving either on its axis or in its orbit round the sun, or indeed in its passage along with the sun across the galaxy. On the contrary, our sensory evidence serves to contradict the findings of astronomical science. The earth seems   35
to stand still while everything else moves round it. That is immediate, practical 'reality'; yet it is also the scientifically rejected *geocentric* view of things. It prevailed for centuries, then gave way to the *heliocentric* theory of the universe – which has also in turn been rejected. The sun is the centre of its own little system and of   40
nothing else. It would appear, in fact, to be whirling out there

somewhere on the edge of things, far from the centre of our own
galaxy, and unspeakably unthinkably far from the centre of the
universe, wherever and whatever that might be.

In a sense, we have two kinds of knowledge in our 20th-century   45
brains: a scientific appreciation of how things may be, and a
practical everyday knowledge of sunrises and sunsets and flat
surfaces that aren't really flat. In broad theory we are modernists
following where Einstein leads; in everyday terms, however, we are
Flat-Earthists every one.   50

Our home planet, the Earth, is wrapped in a blanket of gases that
encompass it in several layers, and is itself structured like an onion
in its own layers of concentric shells. To our practical senses, this
blanket of gases – the atmosphere – flows in winds, while the seas
that cover so much of the planet's surface move in currents. The   55
ground beneath us, however, is solid and unchanging; the
mountains and plains have been there for ages. They will look the
same on the day we die as on the day we were born.

But is this 'really' so? Our scientific knowledge, provided by
geologists, tells us that continents move, that earthquakes and   60
floods are not the work of angry gods, but rather the results of
predictable changes in the forces of nature, obeying physical laws.
Earthquakes in Turkey and Iran and volcanoes in the United States
or Guatemala remind us that nothing necessarily stays the same,
and the dramatic appearance of a new island off Iceland is a   65
reminder that many of today's mountains were once under salt
water. The oh-so-solid crust of the earth is never quite still. The
land north and northeast of the Great Lakes in North America is
slowly rising; docks for ships, built many years ago, are now high
above water level. Columns that support an ancient temple near   70
Naples in Italy have holes bored in them – by sea animals. Clearly,
this temple was submerged and rose again from the sea by natural
processes over which you and I have no control whatsoever.

The liquids of the sea and the gases of the air move at speeds and
in ways that we understand and accept, but these changes in the   75
'solid' earth beneath us suggest that, on another time scale
altogether, there are great slow currents inside the onion-like layers
that make up the planet. Some scientists maintain that heat deep
inside our planet-spaceship causes materials to expand and move
upwards, cooling down as they approach the surface. In cooling,   80
these materials pack close together and settle down once more, but
in the process disturb the thin crust above them – what we regard as
solid rock. Such a re-settling is just the merest twitch in the planet's
long history, but for us the result might be the devastation that
visited, for example, southern Italy in 1980, destroying the homes 85
of tens of thousands of people.

Our situation is paradoxical. On our own scale of sizes and
values we have mighty cities and ancient cultures; in cosmic terms,
we are – as Arthur Conan Doyle once suggested[2] – 'tiny

animalcules' that have collected on earth during its travels round 90
the sun 'as barnacles gather on an ancient vessel'. Depending on the
scale used, we are nature's greatest achievement – or a parasitic
growth.

We live on our earthship within very strict limits. Arnold
Toynbee defines those limits as follows[3], introducing for our 95
consideration a new 20th-century term of ancient Greek
provenance:

'The biosphere is a film of dry land, water and air enveloping the
globe (or virtual globe) of our planet Earth. It is the sole present
habitat – and, as far as we can foresee today, also the sole habitat 100
that will ever be accessible – for all species of living beings,
including mankind, that are known to us.

'In terrestrial terms the biosphere is fantastically thin. Its upper
limit may be equated with the maximum altitude in the
stratosphere at which a plane can remain air-borne; its lower 105
limit is the depth, below the surface of its solid portion, to which
engineers can mine and bore. The thickness of the biosphere,
between these two limits, is minute by comparison with the
length of the radius of the globe which it coats like a delicate
skin.' 110

Within these limits, on this fragile stage, all the dramas of human
history have been performed.

Notes

1 Robin Kerrod, *The Universe*, Sampson Low, 1975
   (p. 10, in 'The Scale of Things') 115

2 Arthur Conan Doyle, *The Professor Challenger Stories*, John
   Murray omnibus edition, 1952 (p. 555, in 'When the World
   Screamed')

3 Arnold Toynbee, *Mankind and Mother Earth*, Oxford
   University Press, 1976 (p. 5, in 'The Biosphere') 120

Below are some questions about the passage. These questions
can be used for all or any of the following purposes:

1 a simple check upon your understanding of the passage
2 the basis for a group discussion of the passage
3 the basis for a brief summary of the passage, by
   answering each question in reasonable detail in the order
   given.

a. What is the sun?
b. What is Kerrod's view of the universe?
c. Can we easily understand what scientists tell us about the
    universe?
d. Why is this?

e.   What theories have been held and rejected about the position of our planet in the universe?
f.   What two kinds of knowledge do we seem to have?
g.   What is our home planet like?
h.   What do the solids, liquids and gases of our planet appear to have in common?
i.   What is the paradox about our lives on Earth?
j.   What are the limits of the biosphere?

5.2   Recall: Examining the passage

In the sections that follow, the passage 'The Scale of Things' is repeated, but with certain omissions and changes. Work through the material in order to see how well you can reconstruct the original passage from memory and logical analysis.

Recall:
First stage

In this section, certain key words have been omitted from the text. Supply in each blank the word that you think has been omitted. If you actually supply a different word, consider whether or not it is a satisfactory substitute for the original.

The sun is a star. It is not a particularly large or particularly bright star, and (1)_____ in a universe that contains (2)_____ millions of stars. Astronomers (3)_____ our small and undistinguished life-giver as a 'yellow dwarf', and (4)_____ that Capella is ten times bigger, that Antares is 300 times bigger, and (5)_____ that the larger 'supergiants' are 3,000 times bigger. These are – apparently – cosmic (6)_____, to be accepted without (7)_____, whatever our senses tell us about our large sun and tiny stars. Like the (8)_____ in light-years that separate stars, however, such facts are hard to (9)_____. As Robin Kerrod observes[1]:

'It is (10)_____ for anyone, even astronomers included, to view the universe in (11)_____. We know that it is made up of space with stars, planets, dust, and gas (12)_____ in it here and there. But empty space predominates.'

He adds that our (13)_____ system is in fact 'a comparatively (14)_____ corner of the universe', although from our point of view this is hardly (15)_____ either. By our own methods of (16)_____ and appreciating distances Venus, the nearest planet to Earth, is more than 25 million miles (40 million kilometres) away, while our (17)_____ yellow dwarf is 93 million miles or 150 million kilometres away. It is hard enough to (18)_____ these distances; it is more difficult still when astronomers tell us that these distances are (19)_____ of crowding and are a mere nothing anyway, on the (20)_____ cosmic scale of things.

Recall:
Second stage

In this section, articles have been omitted and have to be put back in. Additionally, however, some blanks have been put in where no article is needed. Mark such blanks with an × as you go along.

Today, (21)_____ most people with (22)_____ Western-style education accept that (23)_____ universe in which our earth and sun move is enormous beyond (24)_____ conception, yet we do not obtain this information from our normal sense impressions (which is, in effect, why we find it hard to grasp). Any conception we have of (25)_____ cosmic scale of (26)_____ things is mediated by (27)_____ intellect, not (28)_____ senses: we cannot see (29)_____ universe spread out with all its turning galaxies; (30)_____ sun does not look in any way like (31)_____ twinkling star; we do not feel (32)_____ earth moving either on its axis or in its orbit round (33)_____ sun, or indeed in its passage along with (34)_____ sun across (35)_____ galaxy. On (36)_____ contrary, our sensory evidence serves to contradict (37)_____ findings of (39)_____ astronomical science. (40)_____ earth seems to stand still while everything else moves round it.

Recall:
Third stage

In this section, derived words have been omitted in certain places, but a list of the base words from which they have been derived is provided immediately below. Re-construct the derived words as you go along.

(41)	practice	(46)	think
(42)	science	(47)	know
(43)	centre	(48)	real
(44)	centre	(49)	modern
(45)	speak	(50)	Earth

That is immediate (41)_____ 'reality'; yet it is also the (42)_____ rejected (43)_____ view of things. It prevailed for centuries, then gave way to the (44)_____ theory of the universe – which has also been rejected. The sun is the centre of its own little system and of nothing else. It would appear, in fact, to be whirling out there somewhere on the edge of things, far from the centre of our own galaxy, and (45)_____ (46)_____ far from the centre of the universe, wherever and whatever that might be.

In a sense, we have two kinds of (47)_____ in our 20th-century brains: a scientific appreciation of how things may be, and a practical everyday knowledge of sunrises and sunsets and flat surfaces that aren't (48)_____ flat. In broad theory we are (49)_____ following where Einstein leads; in everyday terms, we are (50)_____ every one.

Recall:
Fourth stage

In this section, twenty of the smaller (grammatical) words of the text are missing, such words as conjunctions, pronouns, prepositional and adverbial particles and adverbs. Put them in as you go along.

Our home planet, the Earth, is wrapped (51)_____ a blanket of gases that encompass it (52)_____ several layers, and is itself structured (53)_____ an onion in its own layers of concentric shells. (54)_____ our practical senses, (55)_____ blanket of gases – the atmosphere – flows in winds, (56)_____ the seas that cover (57)_____ much of the planet's surface move in currents. The ground beneath us, (58)_____, is solid and unchanging; the mountains and plains have been there (59)_____ ages. They will look the (60)_____ on the day we die as on the day we were born.

(61)_____ is this 'really' so? Our scientific knowledge, provided by geologists, tells us (62)_____ continents move, that earthquakes and floods are (63)_____ the work of angry gods, but (64)_____ the results of predictable changes in the forces of nature, obeying physical laws. Earthquakes in Turkey and Iran and volcanoes in the United States or Guatemala remind us that nothing necessarily stays the (65)_____ , and the dramatic appearance (66)_____ a new island (67)_____ Iceland is a reminder that (68)_____ of today's mountains were (69)_____ (70)_____ salt water.

Recall:
Fifth stage

In this section, twenty items in the passage have not been completely spelled out. Complete the words by spelling them fully and properly.

The oh-so-solid crust of the earth is never (71) qu_____ still. The land north and northeast of the Great Lakes in North America is (72) sl_____ rising; docks for ships, (73) b_____t many years ago, are now high above water level. (74) Co_____s that support an ancient temple near Naples in Italy have holes bored in them – by sea animals. Clearly, this temple was (75) su_____ed and rose again from the sea by natural (76) pr_____s over which you and I have no control whatsoever.

The liquids of the sea and the (77) g_____s of the air move at speeds and in ways that we understand and accept, but these changes in the 'solid' earth (78) b_____th us suggest that, on another time scale (79) al_____r, there are great slow (80) c_____ts inside the onion-like layers that make up the planet. Some scientists (81) ma_____n that heat deep inside our planet-spaceship causes (82) m_____ls to expand and move upwards, cooling down as they (83) ap_____ch the surface. In cooling, they pack close together and settle down once more, but in the process disturb the thin crust above them – what we regard as solid rock. Such a re-settling is just the merest twitch in the planet's long history, but for us the result might be the (84) dev_____n that visited, for (85) ex_____e, southern Italy in 1980, (86) d_____ing the homes of tens of thousands of (87) p_____le.

Our situation is (88) par_____l. On our own scale of sizes and values we have mighty cities and (89) anc_____ cultures; in cosmic terms, we are – as Arthur Conan Doyle once suggested[2] – 'tiny animalcules' that have collected on earth during its travels round the sun 'as (90) bar_____s gather on an ancient vessel'. Depending on the scale used, we are nature's greatest achievement – or a parasitic growth.

Recall:
Sixth stage

In this section, the punctuation of the passage has been overlooked. Punctuate it properly, taking care with quotations and references.

we live on our earthship within very strict limits arnold toynbee defines those limits as follows 3 introducing for our consideration a new 20th century term of ancient greek provenance the biosphere is a film of dry land water and air enveloping the globe or virtual globe of our planet earth it is the sole present habitat and as far as we can foresee today also the sole habitat that will ever be accessible for all species of living beings including mankind that are known to us in terrestrial terms the biosphere is fantastically thin its upper limit may be equated with the maximum altitude in the stratosphere at which a plane can remain air-borne its lower limit is the depth below the surface of its solid portion to which engineers can mine and bore the thickness of the biosphere between these two limits is minute by comparison with the length of the radius of the globe which it coats like a delicate skin within these limits on this fragile stage all the dramas of human history have been performed notes 1 robin kerrod the universe sampson low 1975 p 10 in the scale of things 2 arthur conan doyle the professor challenger stories john murray omnibus edition 1952 p 555 in when the world screamed 3 arnold toynbee mankind and mother earth oxford university press 1976 p 5 in the biosphere

5.3 Vocabulary:
Analysis of the passage

The passage contains a wide variety of kinds of words. Each of the following sections deals with one particular aspect of the vocabulary of 'The Scale of Things'. Proceed.

1   There are many words of Greek provenance in the text. Many of these contain the connecting vowel 'o', as in *biology* (bi o logy) and *geometry* (ge o metry). Find all the words containing this vowel, analysing them for the meaning of their elements (using a dictionary when necessary).

2   List the compound words in the text. When you have done this, consider how they might be classified into groups (i) according to how they are spelt and punctuated, and (ii) according to the relationships between (or among) their elements.

3   List the phrasal verbs in the text, considering whether the particle that accompanies each basic verb has a literal meaning (direction of movement) or some kind of figurative meaning (such as completion).

4   List all the words in the text that end in or contain:
   i   the suffix -*al*
   ii   the suffix -*ar*
   iii the suffix -*ic*
   iv   the combination of -*ic* and -*al*

5   Look up the meanings and histories of the following words in one or more etymological dictionary:

a.	universe	g.	enormous	m.	current
b.	dwarf	h.	normal	n.	volcano
c.	giant	i.	galaxy	o.	planet
d.	cosmic	j.	whirl	p.	twitch
e.	gas	k.	modern	q.	barnacle
f.	scale	l.	blanket	r.	fragile

5.4 Grammar:
Sentence synthesis using *that*

The connecting word *that* can be used as a relative pronoun (as practised in Unit 3.3, Book 1 of this course) or as a conjunction. Its use as a conjunction is particularly important and common in the writing of reports, surveys, reviews, critiques and all kinds of academic papers. Study the examples below and use them as a guide to create various sentences containing the conjunction *that*.

Example 1   The universe is enormous beyond imagining. Most people nowadays acept this (fact).

▷   Most people nowadays accept that the universe is enormous beyond imagining.

Note   In informal speech and writing it is possible to omit *that*, but in formal writing it should not be omitted.

Example 2   Nothing necessarily stays the same. Volcanoes in the United States and earthquakes in Italy remind us *of* this.

▷   Volcanoes in the United States and earthquakes in Italy remind us that nothing necessarily stays the same.

Note   In the combined sentence, the prepositional particle *of* is not used.

a.   The star Capella is ten times bigger than our sun. Astronomers tell us this (fact).

b.   The star Antares is 300 times bigger than our sun. Most of us are not aware *of* this (fact).

c.   The universe is made up of space with stars, planets, dust and gas floating in it. Nowadays, we know this.

d.   Earthquakes and floods do not happen because the gods are angry. Most people appreciate this.

e.   Many of today's mountains were once under salt water. The dramatic appearance of a new island off Iceland reminds us *of* this.

f.   The earth is like a spaceship travelling at high speed round the sun. Figuratively, we can say this.

g.   The temple was once submerged beneath the sea. Holes bored in its columns by sea animals are proof *of* this.

h.   On its own vast time scale the solid earth has its currents too. Slow changes in the earth's land masses suggest this.

i.   There are slow currents in the dense material under the earth's crust. A recent geological theory proposes this.

j.   Heat deep inside our planet causes material to expand and move upwards. Some scientists maintain this.

Example 3   Earthquakes happen because of changes in the earth's crust. The majority of earthquakes are tiny movements with no noticeable effect. Geologists know both these things.

▷   Geologists know that earthquakes happen because of changes in the earth's crust and also that the majority of earthquakes are tiny movements with no noticeable effect.

k.   The earth is like a spaceship travelling round the sun. It does so at a very great speed. Astronomers tell us both these things.

l.   There are slow currents in the dense material under the earth's crust. Heat deep inside the earth causes some of this material to expand and move upwards. Some geologists maintain both these things.

m.   After a few days in a cave a person loses his or her sense of time. Our body clocks work independently at their own speed. Experimenters have confirmed both these things.

n.   People can live in cold, dark and timeless environments like caverns or outer space for prolonged periods. This experience does not necessarily impair their health. This would appear to be true (= It would appear to be true...)

o. The star Capella is ten times bigger than our sun. Antares is 300 times bigger. The larger 'supergiants' are 3,000 times bigger. Astronomers are aware of all these points.

p. The universe is made up of stars, planets, dust and gas floating in empty space. The empty space is, however, predominant. Astronomical evidence forces us to accept these things. (Use *but also* rather than *and also*, and omit *however* in your answer.)

5.5 Grammar:
General sentence synthesis

Below is a set of twelve parts that can come together as a passage about the interior of the earth. In each part, however, it is necessary to gather the simple sentences together (in most cases) into compound and/or complex structures. This can be done by following the suggestions given on the right-hand side of each numbered part. When you have studied the possibilities, write out the full passage.

1   The thin outer covering of the earth ∧ is called the crust. We live *on this covering*.

Combine by using 'on which' at the caret mark (∧), replacing the italicized words.

2   It does not seem particularly thin to us. *Its thickness varies* from three miles ∧ to forty miles ∧ . *Three miles is the thickness* under the sea. *Forty miles is the thickness* under the continents.

Combine by using 'having a thickness varying', and turn the last two sentences into prepositional phrases at the caret marks.

3   This seems reassuringly thick.

Nil.

4   Our deepest mines go down about two miles. Our deepest oil wells go down about five miles. ∧ We have not yet been able to drill right through the crust.

Combine by using 'while', then use a semi-colon and 'therefore'.

5   Despite this ∧ we must accept *the following fact*. The crust is very thin. *Compare it* with the thickness of the planet itself. The distance from the surface to the centre of the earth *is* very nearly 4,000 miles.

Use 'however', then 'that', then 'when compared', then adapt the last sentence into a participial phrase with 'being'.

6	Under the crust is a layer of heavy rock. *This layer is* called the mantle. *It* goes down nearly 1,800 miles into the earth.	**Combine by using the past participle 'called' then use 'which'.**
7	The crust together with the upper part of the mantle forms ∧ the lithosphere. We call *it that*.	**Use 'what we call' at the caret mark.**
8	This rigid structure overlies the more plastic lower mantle. We call this the asthenosphere. The lithosphere drifts *on the asthenosphere*.	**Use 'which is known as' then 'on which'.**
9	The mantle in turn surrounds the earth's core. *This* is divided into inner and outer layers.	**Use 'which'.**
10	The rocks of the lower mantle or asthenosphere are probably white-hot. They meet the outer core.	**Use 'where'.**
11	This is apparently a molten or fluid mass of nickel and iron. *It is* very hot indeed. *It is* in the region of 2,500°C (4,600°F). The inner core, of course, is even hotter still.	**Combine by using 'which', then 'being' to replace 'it is', then 'while'.**
12	This central kernel of the earth ∧ seems to be squeezed solid. *It is* formed of the same substances. *The pressure is enormous*. The atoms of nickel and iron are packed together incredibly densely.	**Combine by using the past participle 'formed' (etc) at the caret mark, then a comma and 'under such enormous pressures that'.**

Note   This synthesis is only one possible way of bringing the simpler sentences together. A variety of other combinations are possible. You may wish to try some of them.

5.6 Grammar, organization and punctuation: Logical order

Below are two sections containing material which is not yet organized in its proper order. The first list is properly punctuated, but the second is not. Write out both lists as properly organized and punctuated passages.

1 Satellites

A. It is held in its orbiting position by the gravitational pull of the larger body.

B. These newcomers orbit the sun, the moon, the earth and other planets, engaged in sending back to earth information of many kinds.

C. The planets are satellites of the sun and the moon is a satellite of the earth.

D. Today, however, there are also many artificial satellites orbiting in space, man-made objects sent up for specific purposes.

E. A satellite is a body that circles – or 'orbits' – a larger body.

F. Planets and moons are natural satellites, part of the solar system from the beginning.

2 Soil

A. climate is also an important factor in determining what kind of soil develops in any particular part of the earth

B. underneath the subsoil comes the weathered bed rock its colours determined by the basic rock structure of the area

C. whatever the soil its uppermost layer is called topsoil containing animal and plant remains in various stages of decomposition

D. soils are part of the earths crust in which plants can root themselves

E. these remains are known as humus

F. underneath is the subsoil usually lighter in colour and reddish or brownish because of the minerals washed into it from above

G. it is harder for plants to grow in subsoil than topsoil due to lack of humus

H. they are made of weathered rocks and decaying animal and plant matter and differ in depth colour and mineral content

5.7 Vocabulary:
Word formation

Many technical words in English are of Latin and Greek origin (or provenance). Some are quite simple in structure; others are complex. This section provides practice in recognizing, analysing and synthesizing such words.

Word formation:
First stage

It is common to find that the same concept is expressed in English by means of several different *bases* (as explained in Section 3.5 of this book). The first and most easily recognizable base is usually a free word itself, coming from everyday English. The others may or may not be easily recognizable at first, and come from Latin and Greek. Thus, for example:

Everyday English	star
Latin base	*stell*
Greek base	*ast(e)r*

These three parallel bases provide us with a wide range of derivatives and compounds, all in some way (literally or figuratively) connected with the idea 'star'. You will find ten such words in the left-hand column below. Match them with their meanings in the right-hand column.

1	starry-eyed	a.	a small star-like body in space
2	constellation	b.	lit or lighted by the stars
3	asteroid	c.	a small star-like symbol
4	interstellar	d.	prediction of events by means of the stars
5	starlit	e.	a group of stars in the sky
6	asterisk	f.	one who 'sails' among the stars
7	disaster	g.	a very great 'star' in films, etc
8	astrology	h.	among the stars
9	superstar	i.	with one's eyes full of stars
10	astronaut	j.	an event happening under a 'bad' star

Word formation:
Second stage

In this section you will find a table with four columns. In the first column are ten Latin bases. In the second column are their usual meanings in English, while in the third column there are examples of words derived from them. The passage contains other examples of words derived from these bases. Find them and put them in the fourth column. They appear in the passage more or less in the order that they appear in the table.

Latin bases	Meanings	Common derivatives	Derivatives from the passage
1 *liter*	'a letter'	literature	
2 *spect*	'to see/look'	inspector	
3 *cred*	'to believe'	incredulous	
4 *preci*	'price/value'	precious	a.
5			b.
6 *dict*	'to say'	diction	a.
7			b.
8 *domin*	'master'	dominant	
9 *ject*	'to throw'	projector	
10 *cent*	'one hundred'	centenary	
11 *terr*	'land/earth'	subterranean	
12 *frag*	'to break'	fragment	

Word formation:
Third stage

In this section you will find a second table with four columns. In the first column this time are eight Greek bases. Their usual meanings are in the second column, and examples of derived words in the third. Again, the passage contains other examples of words derived from these bases. Find them and put them in the fourth column. They appear in the passage more or less in the order that they appear in the table.

Greek bases	Meanings	Common derivatives	Derivatives from the passage
1 *cosm*	'world/universe'	cosmopolitan	
2 *kil*	'a thousand'	kilogram	
3 *nom*	'law/rule/ organization'	autonomy	a.
4			b.
5 *ge*	'the earth'	geometry	a.
6			b.
7 *heli*	'the sun'	helium	
8 *physi*	'nature'	physiology	
9 *bi(o)*	'life'	biology	
10 *dox*	'opinion/ convention'	orthodox	

Word formation:
Fourth stage

In making compound words in English, the elements are either put together on paper as one word (*spaceship*), hyphenated (*light-year*), or kept side by side but separate (*space dust*). These are the great majority of compounds, but English also uses many compounds of Latin and Greek provenance. Compounds in the Latin style usually have a connecting vowel 'i', while those in the Greek style usually have a connecting vowel 'o'. Such compounds can generally, however, be explained (or paraphrased, as in Section 3.4 of this book) in the same way as the normal compounds of English. Thus:

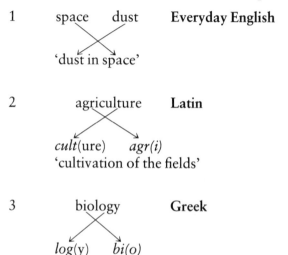

1   space   dust   **Everyday English**

'dust in space'

2   agriculture   **Latin**

cult(ure)   *agr(i)*
'cultivation of the fields'

3   biology   **Greek**

log(y)   *bi(o)*
'the study of life/living things'

For practice, cut up the following Latin and Greek compounds into their parts (bases, connecting vowels, affixes):

a.   astronomy – astronomer – astronomical
b.   geology – geocentric – geometrical
c.   heliocentric
d.   atmosphere – biosphere – lithosphere – stratosphere
e.   agriculture – viniculture – horticultural
f.   aquifer – somniferous – quadrilateral – unilateral

Word formation:
Fifth stage

Below you will find a list of twelve common Latin bases, with their approximate meanings in everyday English. They are followed by ten sentences that can be completed by studying the compounds in them, relating their elements to the Latin bases, then providing a simple English 'translation'.

aqu	'water'	*later*	'a side'
art	'art/craft/craftsmanship, etc'	*mult*	'many'
		omn	'all; total; everything; everywhere'
cult	'farming/cultivation, etc'		
fer	'carry(ing)'	*pot*	'power'
fic	'make or making/do(ing)'	*sci*	'know(ing)'
hort	'a garden'	*vin*	'vine/wine'

a. An aquifer is a stratum of rock that _____ _____ .
b. Horticulture is the _____ of _____s, especially in order to sell the produce.
c. An omniscient person is one who _____ _____ .
d. 'Artificial' originally meant _____ by _____ .
e. A multilateral agreement has _____ _____ .
f. Omnipotence is _____ _____ .
g. An artificer is a person who uses _____ to _____ things.
h. Viniculture is the _____ of _____s, for the purpose of _____-making.
i. If something is omnipresent it is present _____ .
j. A bilateral meeting involves two _____ , and a trilateral one involves _____ _____ .

Word formation:
Sixth stage

Below you will find a list of twelve common Greek bases, with their approximate meanings in everyday English. They are followed by ten sentences that can be completed by studying the compounds in them, relating their elements to the Greek bases, then providing a simple English 'translation'.

ast(e)r	'a star'	*logy*	'study'
cardi	'the heart'	*nomy*	'laws'
dem	'people'	*phot*	'light'
ge	'the earth'	*psych*	'the mind'
graphy	'writing/description/ distribution'	*spher(e)*	'globe/sphere'
		zo	'an animal/living creature'
iatr	'heal(ing)'		

a.   Geography is the subject that makes _____s of _____.

b.   A cardiologist is a doctor who _____ _____.

c.   Demography is a statistical study of the _____ of _____ in various areas.

d.   The original meaning of 'photography' is _____ in or with _____.

e.   A psychiatrist is someone who tries to _____ _____.

f.   The _____ of _____ is called zoology.

g.   A person who _____ someone's _____ story is his or her biographer.

h.   The photosphere or _____ of _____ is the bright surface layer of a star.

i.   Oceanography is the _____ of the world's oceans.

j.   Astronomy and astrology are very different subjects; the first is the scientific study of the _____ of the _____, while the second is the _____ of the _____ for purposes of prediction.

5.8 Punctuation:
The careful presentation of material

This section deals with a number of subtle points of punctuation that can be important in more advanced styles of writing. They are:

1   when to use or not to use quotation marks with single words or short phrases

2   when to use or not to use a capital letter with single words or short phrases

3   when to use quotation marks or underlining/italicization with single words or short phrases

4   when to use parenthetical commas or dashes

5   how to present the notes at the end of an article (or, indeed, at the foot of a page)

1   When to use or not to use quotation marks

Compare these extracts from the passage:

Astronomers classify our small and undistinguished life-giver as a 'yellow-dwarf', and point out that . . .   lines 3–4

... Venus, the nearest planet to Earth, is more than 25 million miles (40 million kilometres) away, while our modest yellow dwarf is 93 million miles or 150 million kilometres away.

  lines
  18–21

Why is the first *yellow dwarf* in quotation marks, while the second is not? The reason is that in the first case the phrase is being introduced as a rather strange technical term, whereas in the second case it has already been introduced and can serve in a normal way as a substitute for the word 'sun'.

2   When to use or not to use a capital letter

Compare these extracts from the passage:

... Venus, the nearest planet to Earth, is more than ...

  lines
  18–19

... the universe in which our earth and sun move ...

  line
  26

Why does *earth* begin with a capital in one place, but not in the other? The reason is that in the first case 'Earth' is the proper name of a planet, one of a set of proper names (Venus, Mars, Jupiter, etc), whereas in the second case it remains unique, but is not a proper name, in the same way that *universe* and *sun* are not proper names. If it were given a capital in the second case, then we would also need to capitalize 'Universe' and 'Sun', and would have doubts about what other nouns to capitalize. Such capitalization does occur in children's books, but should be avoided as far as possible in adult material.

3   When to use quotation marks or underlining/italicization

Consider the following extract from the passage:

The earth seems to stand still while everything else moves round it. That is immediate, practical 'reality'; yet it is also the scientifically rejected *geocentric* view of things. It prevailed for centuries, then gave way to the *heliocentric* theory of the universe – which has also been rejected.

  lines
  35–40

Why is *reality* in quotation marks, while *geocentric* and *heliocentric* are italicized? The reason is that the issue of 'What is reality?' is central to the whole passage. Which reality? The word is therefore put in quotation marks to emphasize its strangeness, the doubt attached to it. The writer, however, also wants to emphasize two technical terms, but does not want to suggest that they are in the same situation as *reality*. There is nothing strange or doubtful about either *geocentric* and *heliocentric*, except that they may be new words to the reader and slightly unusual because they are of Greek origin. They are technical terms, and belong together because they share the base *centre*, while also being contrastive. The writer therefore uses underlining (for a typescript) or italicization (for print).

4   When to use parenthetical commas or dashes

Compare these extracts from the passage:

Our home planet, the Earth, is wrapped in a blanket of gases ...	line *51*
... this blanket of gases – the atmosphere – flows in winds ...	lines *53–54*

Why is the appositional phrase *the Earth* placed between commas, while the appositional phrase *the atmosphere* is between dashes? The reason is that the first is a simple reminder that our home planet has a name (and there are no competing commas nearby), whereas the second parenthetical phrase provides a technical term that is meant to stand out clearly (and there are already enough commas nearby as it is).

5   How to present the notes at the end of an article

There are many different ways of presenting additional notes. They can be placed at the foot of the same page (as footnotes), or can be gathered together into a longer or shorter list at the end of either a chapter or the complete book or thesis as end-notes. Such notes may be combined with one's list of books consulted (one's bibliography), or kept separate. Essentially, a note of this kind is something that the writer does not, for any reason, wish to have in the flow of the actual text – although such notes *could* be incorporated into the text. Whether notes come at the foot of a page or the end of an article, chapter or book, however, they all have certain things in common, and these are indicated in the following diagrammatic analysis of the style used at the end of 'The Scale of Things':

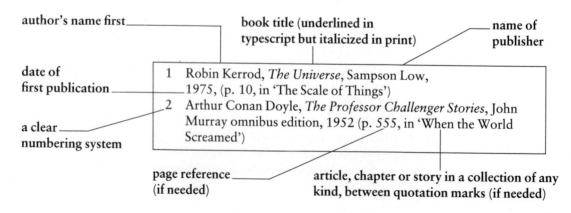

The above presentation (with minor variations) is very common. An academic variation that often appears in bibliographical lists is as follows:

1   Conan Doyle, Arthur (1952) *The Professor Challenger Stories*, John Murray omnibus edition, p. 555 (in 'When the World Screamed')

2   Kerrod, Robin (1975) *The Universe*, Sampson Low, p. 10 (in 'The Scale of Things')

Note that in such lists, alphabetical order is preferred, and the number refers to the place of the title, etc, in this list, and *not* the order of appearance in the text.

You have possibly already done Section 5.2 of this course, including 'Recall: Sixth Stage'. If you have, you may or may not have managed to reproduce successfully the last part of the passage entitled 'The Scale of Things'. Whatever the case, do 'Recall: Sixth Stage' again now.

5.9   Controlled composition: 'The Oceans'

The passage 'The Scale of Things' has a definite structure that moves from the larger and more general to the smaller and more particular, through the following stages:

1   the sun's place in the universe
2   relative distances
3   views of reality: two kinds of knowledge
4   the earth with its layers
5   the 'solidity' of the ground beneath us
6   ourselves and our biosphere

It is a text of a general scientific nature, based upon notes and ideas drawn from astronomy, geology, biology and aspects of sociology and history. Below you will find a quantity of parallel notes and ideas, this time relating to the oceans that cover so much of our home planet, the Earth. Study the notes, plan your presentation, then write a composition with a title like 'The Oceans'. If possible, get several opinions on the final result – and do not be afraid to re-write it later in order to improve it in the light of constructive criticism. Use the same kind of style, punctuation, quotation and organization of notes as in 'The Scale of Things'.

Notes for 'The Oceans'

1   **General background information**

- looking at the planet Earth from space – more water visible than land – might be better called 'Ocean' or 'Oceania' than 'Earth'

- no other planet in the solar system has as much water – **Quote** Isaac Azimov:

  'The earth is unusual among the planets of the solar system in possessing a surface temperature that permits water to exist in all three states: liquid, solid, and gas. The earth is also the only body in the solar system, as far as we know, to have oceans. Actually I should say "ocean", because the Pacific, Atlantic, Indian, Arctic and Antarctic oceans all comprise one connected body of salt water in which the Europe-Asia-Africa mass, the American continents, and smaller bodies such as Antarctica and Australia can be considered islands.' (*Guide to Science 1: The Physical Sciences*, Penguin Books, 1975, p. 138, in 'The Ocean')

- over 70% of planet's surface covered by water – 97% of this in the three great oceans (Pacific, Indian, Atlantic)

  (**Add** any other source material from elsewhere, as desired)

2   **Composition of sea water, etc**

- What is sea water? – saline; salty – one kilogram (kg) of sea water contains about 35 grams (g) of dissolved materials – sodium chloride (common salt) makes up about 30 g or 85% of total – so about 3.5% of sea water is dissolved material, 3% salt (average)

- sea water highly complex – 73 of the 93 natural chemical elements present in measurable/detectable amounts – appreciable quantities of sulphate, magnesium, potassium, calcium, 13% of total

- other elements in small quantities include gold – more gold in the sea than on land – low concentration – four-millionths of one part per million

- the salinity of sea water varies with local conditions – fresh water from large rivers dilutes coastal regions – ice in polar seas or winter and evaporation increase it – Baltic Sea low salinity with 0.7% compared with Red Sea very high at 4.1%

- the salt in world's salt mines presumably originally from sea water – accumulated in layers – very long period of time, in basins where evaporation left salt behind – salt mines of Wieliczka in Poland, layer of salt 366 metres (1,200 feet) thick – in Texas, layers up to 3,658 m (12,000 ft)

- a column of water about 305 m (1,000 ft) high would leave behind only about 4.6 m (15 ft) of salt –
  question: How explain such quantities as in Texas?

- desalination of sea water means separating out dissolved salts – can be done electrically, chemically or by 'change of phase' (means methods such as turning into steam or freezing)

- natural freezing point of sea water –2°C – results in the formation of surface ice with little salt content – long used by Eskimos (Inuit) and others in polar areas as source of fresh water

3   Oceanography

- **Quote** Isaac Asimov:

  'The founder of modern oceanography was an American naval officer named Matthew Fontaine Maury. In his early thirties, he was lamed in an accident that, however unfortunate for himself, brought benefits to humanity. Placed in charge of the depot of charts and instruments (undoubtedly intended as a sinecure), he threw himself into the task of charting ocean currents. In particular he studied the course of the Gulf Stream, which had first been investigated as early as 1769 by the American scholar Benjamin Franklin.' (same source, p 139)

- Maury made a classic remark about the Gulf Stream: 'There is a river in the ocean' – and such 'rivers' are certainly much larger than those on land

- Maury was the moving spirit behind a historic international conference in Brussels, 1853 – in 1855, he published his *Physical Geography of the Sea*, the first textbook in oceanography

- the study of oceans called 'oceanography' – wide-ranging, including and drawing on such disciplines as chemistry, biology, geology, physics

- **Quote:**

  'The study of oceans ... has become a matter of urgency, because man's future on earth may depend on his knowledge of the ocean's potential resources of food, minerals and power.'

  – *The Physical Earth*, Erik Abranson and Dougal Dixon, editors, Mitchell Beazley, 1977 (in 'The Sea and Sea Water', p. 76)

- the currents, the nature, the depths and the bed of the sea have always fascinated people – Ferdinand Magellan tried to sound the depths of the Pacific, reaching 370 m (1,200 ft) with a rope – first true sounding of its depths by James Clark Ross in 1840 – measured a depth of nearly 3,700 m (12,140 ft) with a line

- (between 1872 and 76) *HMS Challenger*, British ship (Royal Navy), famous voyage taking soundings round the world – sailed 67,000 nautical miles – samples of marine life – laboratories on board – discovered 4,417 new species of marine plants and animals – forerunner of the modern oceanographic vessels – classification of ocean's deep sediments (muds) by ship's geologist John Murray has been improved on but never discounted

- actual topography of ocean floor revealed by technique called 'echo-sounding' – uses sonic and ultrasonic signals and seismic methods (**check these terms, if necessary**) – there are, we now know, hills, mountain ranges, volcanoes, island complexes, rift valleys, etc, under the sea just as on land

- new era of marine geo-sciences 1961 – Mohole project – US drilling ship failed to drill down to the earth's mantle, but this and later investigations confirmed theory of 'continental drift' (**plate tectonics – check if necessary**) – much work still to be done

- present-day emphasis in oceanography the finding of new food and physical resources (minerals and energy) – control pollution – conserve life in seas – now an advanced science using satellite photography etc, computers on ships, large shore-based facilities – will lead inevitably to whole new industries – perhaps even cities under the sea or floating on it – certainly a new kind of investigator used to **Bathyscaphes (check?)**, aqualung equipment, etc.

- **Check:**

plankton	fish
phytoplankton	demersal fish
zooplankton	pelagic fish
crustaceans	
molluscs	

  varieties of marine life

- **Quote (all or parts of):**

  'Life in the abysmal depths of the oceans is much more difficult to observe than at comparable heights above sea level. But the greater volume of habitable, oxygen-rich room down there may make it all the more important, for the area of earth covered by water 2½ miles deep is as vast as all the continents put together, and even the scattered abysses deeper than 4 miles total almost half the area of the United States.

'It imposes more than a little strain on the imagination to visualize life in the sea-bottom world of utter and inky blackness, of passing mysterious shapes and unexpected encounters, of eternal cold (perpetually less than ten degrees above freezing) and of pressures thousands of times greater than in the air. But that there is life down there we know without doubt, for fine steel nets on cables several miles long have hauled its organisms up to the light of day and Jacques Piccard and Lieutenant Don Walsh who descended in their bathyscaph to the nadir nigritude of the Mariana trench in 1960, the deepest abyss known on Earth and more than seven miles straight down, saw flounderlike flat fish at the very bottom blithely swimming through the water under a pressure of seven tons per square inch, their carefree relaxation certainly attributable to the pressure being equalized inside and outside the body and its cells.'

– Guy Murchie, *The Seven Mysteries of Life*, Houghton Mifflin, 1978, pp. 29–30, in 'The Animal Kingdom'

- **Add material from whatever other sources seem useful**

UNIT 6

6.1 Comprehension and composition model: 'Assassination'

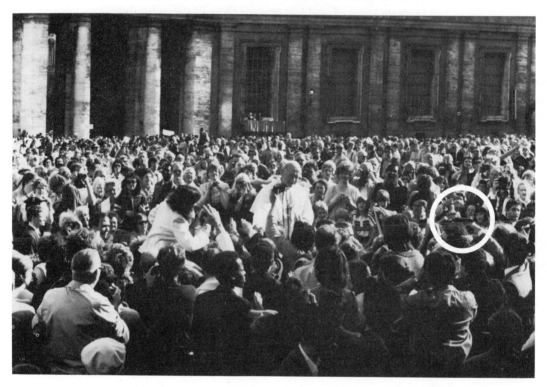

Christopher Hume, a student on holiday in Rome, took this photograph of Pope John Paul II in St. Peter's Square, May 1981. The raised gun of the would-be assassin is clearly visible.

Here is a passage dealing with the social and political topic of murder, particularly in the form that has come to be known as 'assassination'. Read it twice, noting its organization and layout, the way in which its notes and references are organized (rather differently from 'The Scale of Things'), its punctuation and grammatical style, and the vocabulary used. When you have done this, proceed to the various exercises and related activities based on the passage.

Murder is as old as the human race, whether we bedeck it in such fancy names as 'war', 'execution' or 'the final solution'[1]. We classify it for legal convenience, so that Eichmann[2] is guilty of genocide, Cromwell[3] of regicide, and Crippen[4] of homicide. Although there exist people for whom the slaughter of fellow humans is a pleasure comparable to hunting wild beasts, murder is generally a last resort. It is something compulsive to which a person is finally driven by certain circumstances. This is particularly true of the crime we call 'assassination', named after the drug-addicted killers of mediaeval Persia[5]. In this survey, the term is restricted to meaning the killing of a world figure, whether by conspiracy or isolated act, without resource to revolution, trial or warfare.

The four most significant assassinations of modern times are those of Abraham Lincoln, Archduke Franz Ferdinand of Austria, Mohandas K Gandhi and John F Kennedy. I would like to highlight aspects of each, along with some salient features of other comparable assassinations, before drawing any conclusions.

The US Civil War[6] had come to an end. It was the most devastating war of its time, wasteful of lives and material on a scale no one had anticipated. It lasted for four years (1861–65), having as its *raison d'être* the emancipation of a race from slavery. However, historians agree that this was only a superficial reason, that in truth war broke out because of economic rivalry between the largely agricultural South and the mainly industrial North, slavery being simply the convenient human symbol on which to hang a 'just cause'. This is amply proven by the subsequent failure of the North to ensure a square deal for the freed Negroes[7].

Although Lincoln was a brave and honest leader, the legend that he stood resolutely for Negro rights is misleading. In the second year of the war he stated firmly: 'My paramount object is to save the Union[8], and not to save or destroy slavery.' Emancipation was declared in the third year of the struggle, rather late if it was the cause of the conflict.

The war was over when Lincoln met his death. General Lee[9] had surrendered at Appomattox Court House on the 9th April, 1865. The South was crushed under the sheer weight of industry, manpower and naval strength assembled by the North. The assassination which took place on the 14th April must therefore be seen as a kind of last resort, foredoomed in its wider aims. Lincoln was shot dead by the actor John Wilkes Booth, a Marylander[10], while watching a comedy at Ford's Theatre in Washington. The report of the pistol was drowned in laughter. Booth cried out in Latin: 'So always with tyrants!' and fled, recalling the killing of Julius Caesar with these words. The same evening, his accomplice Paine made an attempt on the life of Secretary of State Seward, who was ill in bed.

Four vital points emerge from this farrago of violence:

1   Booth was motivated by racial feeling. He regarded Lincoln as betraying his kind, and had stated in a letter to a friend: 'The country was formed for the white, not the black man.' In his view, slavery was a blessing bestowed by God on a 'favoured people'.

2   Booth was a 'loner', as the Americans say, someone with few close friends, and a one-track mind.

3   His identification with the Southern cause was self-styled. Being from Maryland, he disagreed with the State decision to stay Northern. He regarded the South as cultured and dignified, the North as barbarous and mercenary. At no time, however, did he receive or even ask for any official help from the Confederacy[11] in his original plan to kidnap Lincoln before the war ended.

4   He was an unstable man, guilty of sexual excesses and callousness that in one instance led a young woman, Henrietta Irving, to commit suicide. As a child, he had rebelled against his father's peaceful nature and enjoyed giving him mental pain by killing animals, preferably before his eyes.

Incidentally, his vengeful act made no ultimate difference to anything. The abolition of slavery was made law by the adoption of the 13th Amendment to the Constitution of the United States on the 18th December that same year.

Booth's futile outburst resembles very closely the killing of Alexander II of Russia in 1881. Under the stress of nationalistic feelings and political repression, a Polish student threw a bomb and killed the Czar[12]. Alexander's death, however, took place on the very day that he had agreed to grant reform. This was not known to the public, and after his murder all thought of reform vanished. In consequence, the assassin had harmed his own cause. In the same way, Booth gravely damaged Southern chances after the war by eliminating the one man who could have ensured even-handed treatment of the defeated states, on the basis of his own statement of 'malice toward none, charity for all'. Lincoln's death ushered in the suppression and exploitation of the South that kept Federal troops there till 1877, fanning the bitter resentment that has lasted to some degree right up to the present time. In this negative way, these two assassins achieved a place in the history books.

The obscure Balkan[13] town of Sarajevo claimed *its* terrible place in history when, on the 28th June 1914, a Bosnian Serb[14] called Gavrilo Princip shot dead both Archduke Franz Ferdinand of Austria and Archduchess Sophia while they were riding in a motorcade. The awful paradox of this killing was that, unknown to the plotters, neither the Heir Apparent[15] to the Austro-Hungarian throne nor his wife were at all popular with the reactionaries who dominated the Viennese Court. It was for them a convenient act of slaughter in two ways: firstly, it removed a dangerously liberal heir; secondly, it gave them a chance to intimidate little independent

Serbia, the nation in which Sarajevo lay, in an ultimatum that   95
sparked off the First World War.

No doubt the war would have broken out through some other
excuse, even if Princip had not killed Franz Ferdinand. In the cause
of Bosnian nationalism, however, he had removed one man who
might well have exercised restraint over both the Austrian and   100
German war-mongers. The secret society which had planned the
killing completely failed to achieve the independence of Bosnia that
they wanted. Today, like Serbia, their land is one of the states of
Yugoslavia.

This assassination marked the fate of royalty at the turn of the   105
century. Estranged from the people by a militant aristocracy,
unable to initiate reforms even where they wanted to, the kings and
queens remained a classical target for assassins and similar violent
radicals. The plight of Franz Joseph of Austria exemplifies this,
throughout his long life. His brother, Maximilian, Emperor of   110
Mexico[16], was executed by rebels in 1867, his son Rudolf
committed suicide at Mayerling in 1889, his wife Elizabeth was
murdered by an anarchist in Geneva in 1898, and now his nephew
and heir, Franz Ferdinand, was assassinated at Sarajevo in 1914.   115
Franz Joseph, Emperor of Austria-Hungary, died himself amidst an
all-European conflagration in 1916.

Notes

1   '*the final solution*': the name given by Hitler's Nazis to the
    programme for the total extermination of the Jewish people
    during the Second World War (1939–45)

2   *Eichmann*: a leading Nazi largely responsible for organizing
    'the final solution'

3   *Cromwell*: dictator of the British Isles (1653–58), and one of
    the men responsible for the execution of King Charles I in
    1648, at the end of the English Civil War

4   *Crippen*: an English murderer (1862–1910), famous for
    having killed and cut up his wife

5   *Persia*: part of the country nowadays known as Iran

6   *The US Civil War*: the civil war in the United States of
    America, between the states in the North which were
    determined to maintain the Union or federal status of the
    nation and the seceding states of the South which wished to
    form their own looser Confederacy, known briefly as the
    Confederate States of America

(contd. over)

7   *Negroes*: with a capital 'n', a term long considered the most neutral and respectful for the inhabitants of the USA whose ancestors had been brought as slaves from Africa. Currently, the term 'blacks' is preferred.

8   *the Union*: see Note 6, above

9   *General Lee*: Robert E Lee, commander-in-chief of the Confederate forces in the US Civil War

10   *Marylander*: a native of the Atlantic coast American state of Maryland

11   *Confederacy*: see Note 6, above

12   *the Czar*: the title of the emperor of Russia

13   *Balkan*: a term referring to an area and certain countries to the north of the Mediterranean Sea, now including Greece, western Turkey, Bulgaria, Yugoslavia and Albania, collectively still known as 'the Balkans'

14   *a Bosnian Serb*: Bosnia was one of the small nations of the Balkans dominated by Austria at the turn of the century, and the Serbs were (and are) one of the ethnic groups making up the South Slavs (who now live in Yugoslavia, 'the land of the South Slavs').

15   *Heir Apparent*: the lawful heir to, or inheritor of, a throne

16   *Emperor of Mexico*: What is now the Republic of Mexico was briefly an empire between 1864 and 67, imposed upon the unwilling Mexicans by the French.

Below are some questions about the passage. These questions can be used for all or any of the following purposes:

1   a simple check upon your understanding of the passage

2   the basis for a group discussion of the passage

3   the basis for a brief summary of the passage, by answering each question in reasonable detail in the order given.

a.   How does the writer present murder and assassination?

b.   What are 'the four most significant assassinations of modern times?'

c.   What factors characterized the US Civil War?

d.   What were the facts about the 'just cause' of Negro emancipation?

e.   Under what circumstances was Lincoln assassinated?

f.   What four facts are considered important in understanding John Wilkes Booth?

g.   What similarities were there between the killing of Lincoln and the killing of Czar Alexander II of Russia?

h. What was the significance of Sarajevo for Austria and for the world?

i. What was the paradoxical result of Princip's actions?

j. How did the family of Franz Joseph of Austria typify the fate of royalty at the turn of the century?

6.2 Vocabulary: Analysis of material used in the passage

Below is a list of defining statements and blanks. Complete the blanks by finding the words in the passage that are defined here. The list is in the same order as the appearance of the items in the text. The first one is done for you as an example.

a. the unlawful killing of a human being   *murder (line 1)*

b. ornamental and perhaps deceptive   _____

c. put in groups or categories   _____

d. the destruction of a race or people   _____

e. that can be compared   _____

f. arising from an inner urge   _____

g. limited or confined   _____

h. important or noteworthy   _____

i. draw attention to or emphasize   _____

j. setting free or liberation   _____

k. appearing on the surface only   _____

l. competition, often of a serious kind   _____

m. firmly, definitely and strongly   _____

n. above all other things; principal   _____

o. fated to fail; doomed in advance   _____

p. confused nonsense   _____

q. presented as a formal gift   _____

r. having only one interest; obsessed   _____

s. willing to do anything for money   _____

t. extreme actions   _____

u. the taking of one's own life   _____

v. act of bringing (something) to an end   _____

w.	officially agreed alteration	_____
x.	balanced; fair; tolerant and just	_____
y.	causing (something) to increase by direct action	_____ _____
z.	extreme conservatives	_____

6.3 Grammar:
General sentence synthesis

Below is a set of fourteen parts that can come together as a passage about the assassination of Mohandas K Gandhi, in India, the third of the four most significant political killings of our time, as described by the writer of the text 'Assassination'. In each part, it is necessary to gather these simple sentences together (in most cases) into compound and/or complex structures. This can be done by following the suggestions given on the right-hand side of each numbered part. When you have studied the possibilities carefully, write out the whole passage.

1   *It all happened after a lifetime devoted to* human brotherhood, non-violence and national freedom. Mohandas K Gandhi was heart-broken by the Partition of British India into the new states of India and Pakistan.

Begin with 'after a lifetime devoted to', then a comma after 'freedom'

2   The bloodshed, on his own testimony, set at naught all the good work of forty years. He sought, by walking in the strife-torn areas and by fasting, to allay the communal violence and hatred.

Use 'and'

3   On Friday, 30th January 1948, at about 5.10 pm, he appeared for a prayer meeting in Delhi. *He was* leaning on the shoulders of two girls. *He was* joking with them about carrot juice and punctuality.

Combine using a comma then 'leaning' alone, then another comma and 'joking' alone

4   Nathuram V Godse shot him dead at a range of two feet.

Nil

5   He murmured 'Hai Ram' (Oh God!). His feet slipped from his sandals. The Father of India was dead.

Use a comma after the second round bracket, a comma after 'sandals', then 'and'

6   Godse belonged to a particular group. *This group* considered Gandhi an impediment to Hindu control over India. *They blamed* him for giving way to Moslems.

Omit 'particular', using 'which' instead of 'this group', then change 'they blamed' to 'blaming'

7   Partition ∧ had actually occurred. *There were* streams of refugees. *They moved* in both directions. *Gandhi now wanted something. It was* non-violence and good-will in this shifting of populations. *Perhaps* people would *then* be able to stay in their traditional homes.

Use 'however', change 'there were' to 'with', 'they moved' to 'moving', then 'and what Gandhi now wanted was', then a comma after 'populations' and 'so that', omitting 'perhaps' and 'then'

8   A bomb attempt had been made on his life ten days earlier at another public meeting.

Nil

9   He had minimized the explosion. *He said*: 'Don't worry about that. Listen to me.'

Combine using a comma and 'saying' (leaving the speech alone)

10 His later comment ∧ is interesting. The assailant was caught.

Using 'when' and parenthetical commas, put the second sentence inside the first

11 In Sheean's words: 'No one should believe that he was so perfect that he was sent by God to punish the evil-doers as the accused seemed to flatter himself he was.'

Use unchanged, studying the structure

12 What did religious fanaticism claim – apart from the modern crucifixion of a great humane figure?

Nil

13   It removed from the scene ⌃ one man.   Insert 'the', then use
        He held Moslem and Hindu together.   'who'

14   It removed a symbol of unity. *This*   Use 'that', then
        symbol was accepted by both Pakistan   'and', then 'the'
        and India. Still India became a secular   instead of 'a', then
        state, without the domination of any one   'that', omitting
        religious group. Godse and his friends   'such a state'
        did not want *such a state*.

6.4 Grammar:
Various uses of the passive voice

Many verbs can be used both actively and passively; that is, the subject of the verb can actively perform the action, or the action can be passively received by the subject:

Example 1   The assassin *killed* the king.   **active**
        ▷   The king *was killed* by the assassin.   **passive**

There are various ways in which the passive form of the verb (technically known as the passive voice, as opposed to the active voice) can be used. Some are simple, the others complex. They can often have important effects upon the style and success of a piece of writing. (In a passage such as 'Assassination', variations between active and passive are particularly important, because the topic involves so much violent action: war, crime, suppression, etc.) Using the examples as your guide, work through the following exercises in various uses of the passive.

Example 2   Gavrilo Princip killed Franz Ferdinand.
        ▷   Franz Ferdinand was killed by Gavrilo Princip.

    a.   Abraham Lincoln emancipated the slaves.
    b.   Wilkes Booth shot the President.
    c.   Racial feeling motivated Booth.
    d.   A Polish student killed Czar Alexander II.
    e.   Nationalism provoked the student into killing the Czar.
    f.   Lincoln's premature death created many problems.
    g.   The writer has restricted the term 'assassination'.
    h.   The sheer weight of Northern industry, manpower and naval strength crushed the South.

Basically, a passive form is used to put something that would
normally be last into the first position in a sentence or clause. The
emphasis is reversed completely by doing this. One reason for doing
this is that the general pattern of the passage demands it – something
that might have been the object of the verb *must* be its subject. In
many such cases, the agent phrase (*by ...*) is not needed at all. The
writer and the reader are not immediately interested in who or what
did the action; it is the result, or the place, or the time that is
interesting, next to the action itself. Study the next example.

Example 3   Gavrilo Princip killed Franz Ferdinand in Sarajevo.
   ▷   Franz Ferdinand was killed in Sarajevo.

i.   The United States government emancipated the slaves in the 1860s.

j.   We classify Eichmann's crime as genocide.

k.   Wilkes Booth assassinated Lincoln in 1865.

l.   The law refers to Crippen's crime as homicide.

m.   A polish student killed Alexander II of Russia in 1881.

n.   We refer to Cromwell's involvement in the execution of
Charles I as regicide.

o.   The writer has restricted the term 'assassination' to the murder
of a major world figure.

Passive uses of the verb contain the past participle, and this element
can be used in a variety of stylistically interesting ways. It can, for
example, be used in certain kinds of compound expressions, as
follows:

Example 4   The assassins of mediaeval Persia were *addicted* to *drugs*.
   ▷   They were *drug-addicted* killers.

Complete these sentences in a similar way.

p.   The strength of the North was *based* on *industry* or on its
industries. Its strength was _____-_____ .

q.   Areas of both India and Pakistan were *torn* by *strife* in the year
of their independence. The _____-_____ areas caused
Gandhi great grief.

r.   Many of the factories were *damaged* in the *war*. Most of these
_____-_____ factories were not re-built.

s.   The space project is *financed* by the *government*. It is a
_____-_____ project.

t.   The mountains were *covered* by/with/in *snow*. He loved skiing
among the _____-_____ mountains.

u.   Both his clothes and the ground were *stained* with *blood*. They
all saw the _____-_____ clothes afterwards.

Additionally, synthesis of sentences often takes place by converting the second (passive) sentence into a phrase introduced by a past participle, as follows:

Example 5   Murder is generally a last resort. It is caused by some kind of desperation.

▷   Murder is generally a last resort, caused by some kind of desperation.

Note that the comma between the parts of the new sentence is not necessarily always used.

v.   Under the earth's crust is a layer of heavy rock. This layer is called the mantle.

w.   The army was destroyed. It was annihilated as much by climate and disease as by the country's defenders.

x.   The Emperor of Mexico died an unhappy man. He was totally rejected by the people he had come so far to rule.

y.   The attempt at assassination failed. It was betrayed by the inefficiency of the terrorist group itself.

z.   The South surrendered in 1865. It was crushed by the industrial strength and superior manpower of the North.

6.5 Grammar and vocabulary: Distinguishing particles

Words like *up*, *down*, *in*, *out*, etc, are often called 'prepositions', although they are frequently used as adverbs. For the purposes of this course, we can refer to such words generally as 'particles', which have two distinct functions: prepositional and adverbial, depending on circumstances. When such a particle follows a verb, the unit is called a phrasal verb (as practised in various earlier units of this course). We can say, therefore, that a phrasal verb consists of a verb and an adverbial particle. When such a particle precedes a noun, pronoun, etc, it is a prepositional particle and introduces a prepositional phrase. This difference can be shown as follows:

Example 1   He looked $\overrightarrow{through}$ the window.   **prepositional particle**

Example 2   He looked $\overleftarrow{out}$ sadly.   **adverbial**
(He looked out) (sadly).   **particle**

Example 3   He looked ←*out* →*through* the window.
(He looked out) (through the window).

two particles
used together,
but with
distinct
functions

It is not always easy to distinguish a particle functioning adverbially from one functioning prepositionally, especially when the same particle can behave in both ways at different times. Below you will find further examples, taken from the passage, distinguishing uses of particles. Study them, then use the same system of arrows (to the left for adverbial uses; to the right for prepositional uses) for the extracts that follow.

Example 4   ... whether we bedeck it →*in* such fancy names ... (lines *1–2*)

Example 5   ... in truth war broke ←*out* because →*of* economic rivalry ... (l. *23*)

   a. ... the term is restricted *to* meaning the killing *of* a world figure ... (ll. *10–11*)

   b. The US Civil War had come *to* an end. (l. *18*)

   c. This is amply proven *by* the subsequent failure *of* the North ... (ll. *26–27*)

   d. ... he stood resolutely *for* Negro rights ... (l. *29*)

   e. The war was *over* when Lincoln met his death. (l. *34*)

   f. The South was crushed *under* the sheer weight *of* industry ... (l. *36*)

   g. The report *of* the pistol was drowned *in* laughter. (ll. *40–41*)

   h. As a child, he had rebelled *against* his father's peaceful nature and ... (ll. *63–64*)

   i. Lincoln's death ushered *in* the suppression ... (ll. *80–81*)

   j. ... while they were riding *in* a motorcade. (ll. *88–89*)

   k. ... an ultimatum that sparked *off* the First World War. (ll. *95–96*)

   l. No doubt the war would have broken *out through* some other excuse ... (ll. *97–98*)

   m. ... famous *for* having killed and cut *up* his wife. (note 4)

   n. ... the Serbs were (and are) one *of* the ethnic groups making *up* the South Slavs ... (note 14)

6.6 Punctuation:
Organizing a passage

According to the writer of the passage, the killing of John Fitzgerald Kennedy was the fourth major assassination in modern times. The material below both describes how this came about and provides the writer's conclusions about political murder. It needs, however, to be punctuated and laid out properly.

lee harvey oswald returned to the u s from the soviet union in 1962 at the age of 23 in the words of the warren report[1] **quote** his return to the united states publicly testified to the utter failure of what had been the most important act of his life **end quote** he brought back with him a living witness to this failure his russian wife marina his adopted country russia had proved to be unsatisfactory for him and he returned to a land he had openly rejected as a child he had never known his father who had died two months before his birth but had known all too well a bitterly neurotic mother his wife accused him in front of friends of being sexually inadequate again quoting the warren report p 376 he **quote** was profoundly alienated from the world in which he lived **end quote** and as his wife admitted would not have been happy anywhere **quote** only on the moon perhaps **end quote** on friday 22nd november 1963 he shot john kennedy president of the united states the killing took place in the south in the state of texas occurring during a period of intense racial disturbance oswald was a self styled marxist and yet europeans thought immediately of a right wing plot rather than a communist one rumour had a field day meanwhile what mattered most was that a champion of the **quote** strategy of peace **end quote** had been shot from behind his skull torn away before the gaze of his wife whatever oswald resented as a loner or as one of many kennedy haters he damaged his own cause severely j f k s period at the white house had been marked by unprecedented difficulty in getting any reform measures past congress delay and obstruction attended his civil rights bill and overseas aid on the scale he proposed was resented after the killing however lyndon b johnson[2] was able to get the kennedy programme through on the strength of the nations horror regret and determination to honour a martyred hero no murder in history has created such widespread and spontaneous distress as this one in part due to modern means of communication and in part to the dynamic and attractive image of the victim like earlier assassinations oswalds act had effects quite the contrary to those intended and this is the great irony of murder as a political weapon it is clear that assassins regard themselves as fearless champions of just causes but have seldom if ever done

their causes any good notes 1 the warren report the official u s
report on president kennedys death 2 lyndon b johnson kennedys
vice president and successor

6.7 Vocabulary: Word formation

This section provides further practice with the bases of words from
everyday English as well as Latin and Greek.

Word formation: First stage

In the list immediately below you will find some bases from Latin
(and one from Greek) with their meanings beside them in everyday
English. The same material is also part of the table which follows the
list. Study both the list and the table, then use them to complete the
sentences.

hom	'man(kind); a person'
reg	'a king'
su	'oneself, himself, etc'
fratr	'brother'
gen (Greek)	'race; kind'
cid	'cut; kill'

1st base		2nd base	1st suffix	2nd suffix
hom	*i*	*cid(e)*	*al*	*ly*
reg				
su				
fratr				
infant				
gen	*o*			

a. Killing oneself is called _____ .

b. Murder is officially known as _____ .

c. The furious man looked as though he might kill someone. His
manner was _____ .

d. Killing a king is called _____ .

e. She has tried to kill herself before. She has _____ tendencies.

f.   Destroying a whole race is _____ .

g.   He drives so dangerously that he could kill himself. He drives that car _____ .

h.   Killing children is known as _____ .

i.   The North and South engaged in a _____ war, brother against brother.

j.   Destroying the language, art and culture of a people is often described as an act of cultural _____ .

Word formation:
Second stage

Study the bases in the box below. They provide a wide range of derivatives and compounds, all in some way connected with the idea of 'law'. You will find ten such words in the left-hand column that follows. Match them with their meanings in the right-hand column.

Everyday English	law
Latin base	*leg*
Greek base	*nom*

1   lawless   a.   following one's own law(s)

2   illegal   b.   the 'laws', rules or science concerned with money, living, buying, selling, etc

3   autonomous   c.   the official making of laws

4   lawyer   d.   someone who is regarded as 'beyond' or 'outside' the law

5   economics   e.   always keeping the law, behaving properly, etc

6   legislation   f.   make lawful or legal

7   legalize   g.   independence

8   outlaw   h.   not according to the law

9   law-abiding   i.   having no law or laws at all

10 autonomy   j.   one who practises law as a profession

Word formation:
Third stage

Study the bases in the box below. They are quite closely related to the previous set, and also provide a wide range of derivatives and compounds, all in some way connected with the idea of 'rules' or 'ruling'. You will find ten such words in the left-hand column that follows. Match them with their meanings in the right-hand column.

Note that, although 'rule' is an everyday English word, it is not actually of Anglo-Saxon origin. It was originally a French word, derived from the Latin form that immediately follows it in the box.

Everyday English	rule
Latin base	*regul*
Greek base	*arch*

1	ruler	a.	a person who by choice obeys no rules, and who thinks that there should be no rules to obey
2	anarchy	b.	not happening according to the proper governing rules, principles, plans, etc
3	regulator	c.	a country or institution with a king or similar person ruling alone
4	oligarchy	d.	a state or condition of having no rules, or wanting no rules
5	irregular	e.	to keep or put something right (that is, in accordance with the rules or principles that govern it)
6	monarchy	f.	official rules
7	anarchist	g.	a person or thing that makes other people or things work, operate, perform, etc, as they should (that is, in conformity with the rules)
8	regulations	h.	any person who rules
9	anarchic	i.	a small group of people who rule or control another group, a country, etc, completely
10	regulate	j.	having no rules whatever; (deliberately) chaotic or free from government

Word formation:
Fourth stage

Below is an account of the movement known as 'Anarchism'. It is not, however, completely finished. Certain words have to be formed and fitted in the various blanks. The bases for these words will be found in the right-hand margin. The first derivation is done for you as an example.

Advocates of disorder

A Frenchman founded, but a Russian gave teeth to, the (1)political movement known as Anarchism that   *polit*
sprang up in the mid-nineteenth century. The first was
the (2)_____ Pierre Joseph Proudhon, the second a   *pac*
mercurial (3)_____ called Mikhail Bakunin.   *vis*

Anarchism (4)_____ asserted that the ownership   *origin*
of property was a theft committed by grasping
(5)_____s against all mankind. It taught that if   *divid(u)*
(6)_____ would only give up ruling, then the mass   *rule*
of men, good and (7)_____ at heart, would build a   *oper*
heaven upon earth. When this (8)_____ philosophy   *idea*
met with inevitable failure even at the hands of its sister
movement, (9)_____, the Anarchists turned to   *mur*
force – or 'The Propaganda of (10)_____', as they   *act*
called it.

Whereas the Assassins of mediaeval Persia used the
knife and the Borgias in Italy used poison, the
Anarchists are now (11)_____ by the bomb.   *symbol*
Bakunin himself believed in a kind of spontaneous
combustion among the masses that would remove the
rulers, once a (12)_____ action triggered it off.   *viol*
Beginning with their (13)_____ on Kaiser Wilhelm   *tempt*
of Germany, a Spanish prime Minister, an Austrian
Empress, an American (14)_____ and the   *sid*
kings of Greece and Italy were also included in their
'kills'. As an Italian devotee, Enrico Malatesta, put it:

'It seems to me that in the (15)_____ order of   *nat*
(16)_____, violence has as much a place as the   *volut*
(17)_____ of a volcano. All great progress has been   *rupt*
paid for by streams of blood.'

This included Anarchists' blood too. The Haymarket
Tragedy in Chicago (1886), in which a (18)_____ of   *num(b)*
lives were lost due to the (19)_____ of a bomb   *plos*
thrown by an unknown hand, led to the arrest of several

(20)_____ teachers of Anarchism, four being duly
hanged and the rest receiving severe prison sentences.
There was no proof at all connecting them with the
(21)_____ , but public anger was enough to hang
and imprison them. Finally, the killing of President
McKinley in 1901 (22)_____ a law banning entry to
the USA of anyone who had any Anarchist connections
in Europe. The Anarchists (23)_____ grew to be
unloved, whether in communist or (24)_____
countries which, in view of their (25)_____
inclinations, is probably not surprising.

fess

cid

duc

gener
capit
truct

6.8 Controlled composition: 'The Hashishin'

Create a passage of several paragraphs from the basic material
printed below. It is an account (with notes) of the mediaeval Persian
sect called 'The Assassins'. A full version is provided in the answer
section to this unit. If you are not satisfied with your own version
when you compare the two, you may wish to do the work again. It
should not be forgotten, however, that your work could differ in
various ways from the version given here, without being 'wrong'.

1 schoolfellow/Omar Khayyam[1]/responsible/meteoric/rise/
   strange/mediaeval/Persian/Sect/Assassins

2 headquarters/be/valley/Alamut/remote/area/mountains/
   impregnable/fortresses/south/Caspian Sea/west/what/be/now/
   Teheran/capital/modern/state/Iran

3 from/reports/Crusaders[2]/traveller/Marco Polo[3]/we/learn/sect/
   practise/political/religious/murder/scale/that/have/perhaps/
   never/be/equal/history/except/possible/secret/society/Thugs[4]/
   India

4 they/call/-self/Nizaris/or/Ismailis/but/enemies/give/they/
   nickname/'Hashishin'/that/be/users/drug/hashish[5]

5 founder/this/order/be/Hasan-e-Sabbah

6 he/see/-self/representative/God/Earth/and/be/know/and/fear/
   throughout/Western/Asia/as/'The Old Man of the Mountain'

7 he/command/such/devotion/among/10,000/men/that/
   sentinels/will/willing/throw/-self/off/battlements/castle/into/
   abyss/below/at/one/wave/hand/in/order/intimidate/visit/
   ambassadors

8   Hasan/have/recognise/simple/political/fact/time

9   thrones/premierships/be/insecure/because/they/no/long/rest/
popular/support/or/tribal/loyalty

10   dedicated/band/men/can/be/rely/on/with/bribed/help/where/
necessary/kill/political/leader/Hasan/command/and/even/kill/
-self/same/knife/in/order/not/reveal/secrets/under/torture

11   his/men/oil/-self/make/grip/body/more/difficult/address/God/
before/plunge/knife/victim/believe/implicit/that/actions/will/
take/they/straight/Paradise

12   they/believe/this/because/they/think/they/have/already/see/
Paradise

13   it/be/say/in/Alamut/Hasan/keep/garden/which/in/all/respect/
resemble/delight/heaven/describe/Koran

14   into/this/place/young/men/drug/hashish/will/be/lead/receive/
foretaste/Paradise/to/which/future/obedient/service/entitle/
they

15   in/this/way/Hasan/create/world/first/commando unit/and/
establish/dynasty/that/rule/terror/throughout/Western/Asia/
two/century/until/it/fall/before/advance/Mongol/Hulagu
Khan[6]

16   in/this/strange/way/old/man/mountain/leave/mark/on/world/
add/new/word/its/languages/assassination

17   notes

18   1/Omar Khayyam/(1048(?)–1122)/Persian/poet/astronomer/
mathematician/author/Rubaiyat/translate/English/1859/
Edward Fitzgerald

19   2/Crusaders/members/Christian/armies/engage/in/religious/
warfare/know/as *Crusades*/or/'Wars of the Cross'/against/
Islam/for/possession/Jerusalem/Holy Land of Palestine/11th/
13th/century

20   3/Marco Polo/(c. 1254–1324)/Venetian/merchant/adventurer/
travel/Europe/across/Asia/to/China/write account/journey/
know/in/English/*The Travels of Marco Polo*

21   4/Thugs/organization/religious/assassins/who/secret/kill/
unwary/travellers/in/name/goddess/Kali/over/period/300/
year/until/they/be/break/up/between/1831/1837/by/British/
governor/general/India/William Bentinck

22   5/hashish/(literally, in Arabic, 'dried root')/name/various/
narcotic/preparations/derived/hemp plant/(*Cannabis sativa*)

23   6/Hulagu Khan/(c. 1217–1265)/grandson/Mongol/ruler/
Genghis Khan/and/destroyer/mediaeval/Persian/society/

24   fortress/Alamut/fall/Mongols/1256

UNIT 7

7.1 Comprehension and composition model: 'Chinese Food'

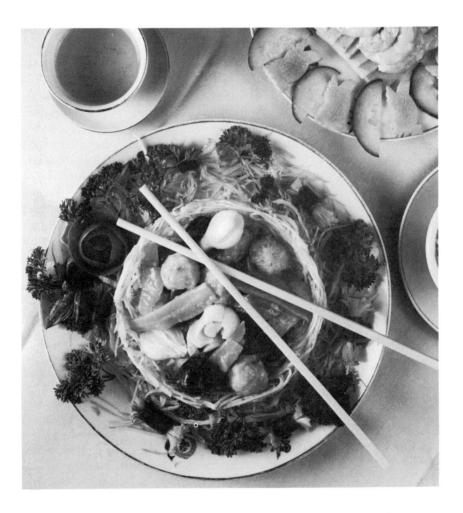

The following passage deals with the nature and international success of Chinese cooking. Read it twice, noting its grammar, style and vocabulary, the layout and the punctuation used, and the way in which its references and notes are handled (quite differently from both 'The Scale of Things' and 'Assassination'). When you have done this, proceed to the exercises and activities that follow.

'Few things in life are as positive as food, or are taken as intimately and completely by the individual. One can listen to music, but the sound may enter in one ear and go out through the other; one may listen to a lecture or conversation, and day-dream about many other things; one may attend to matters of business, and one's heart 5
or interest may be altogether elsewhere. . . . In the matter of food and eating [however] one can hardly remain completely indifferent to what one is doing for long. How can one remain entirely indifferent to something which is going to enter one's body and become part of oneself? How can one remain indifferent to 10
something which will determine one's physical strength and ultimately one's spiritual and moral fibre and well-being?'

— Kenneth Lo[1]

This is an easy question for a Chinese to ask, but a Westerner might find it difficult to answer. Many people in the West are gourmets 15
and others are gluttons, but scattered among them also is a large number of people who are apparently pretty indifferent to what goes into their stomachs, and do not regard food as having any ultimate moral effect on them. How, they might ask, could eating a hamburger or drinking Coca Cola contribute anything to 20
making you a saint or a sinner? For them, food is quite simply a fuel.

Kenneth Lo, however, expresses a point of view that is profoundly different and typically Chinese, deriving from thousands of years of tradition. The London restaurateur Fu Tong[2], for example, quotes 25
no less an authority than Confucius (the ancient sage known in Chinese as K'ung-Fu-Tzu) with regard to the primal importance of food. Food, said the sage, is the first happiness. Fu Tong adds: 'Food to my countrymen is one of the ecstasies of life, to be thought about in advance; to be smothered with loving care throughout its 30
preparation; and to have time lavished on it in the final pleasure of eating.'

Lo observes that when Westerners go to a restaurant they ask for a good table, which means a good position from which to see and be seen. They are usually there to be entertained socially – and also, 35
incidentally, to eat. When the Chinese go to a restaurant, however, they ask for a small room with plain walls where they cannot be seen except by the members of their own party, where jackets can come off and they can proceed with the serious business which brought them there. The Chinese intentions 'are both honourable 40
and whole-hearted: to eat with a capital E.'

1   from the introduction to *The Chinese Cookery Encyclopedia*, Kenneth Lo, Collins, 1974 (p. 13)
2   from Fu Tong's preface to *Chinese Cooking for Pleasure*, Helen Burke, Paul Hamlyn, 1965 (p. 6)

Despite such a marked difference in attitudes towards what one
consumes, there is no doubt that people in the West have come to
regard the cuisine of China as something special. In fact, one can
assert with some justice that Chinese food is, nowadays, the only   45
truly international food. It is ubiquitous. Restaurants bedecked
with dragons and delicate landscapes – serving such exotica as *Dim
Sin Gai* (sweet and sour chicken), *Shao Shing* soup, *Chiao-Tzu* and
Kuo-Tioh (northern style), and *Ging Ai Kwar* (steamed aubergines)
– have sprung up everywhere from Hong Kong to Honolulu to   50
Hoboken to Huddersfield.[3]

How did this come about? Certainly, a kind of Chinese food was
exported to North America when many thousands of Chinese
went there in the 19th century to work on such things as the U.S.
railways. They settled on or near the west coast, where the famous   55
– or infamous – 'chop suey joints' grew up, with their rather
inferior brand of Chinese cooking. The standard of the restaurants
improved steadily in the United States, but Lo considers that the
crucial factor in spreading this kind of food throughout the
Western world was population pressure in the British colony of   60
Hong Kong, especially after 1950, which sent families out all over
the world to seek their fortunes in the opening of restaurants. He
adds, however, that this could not have happened if the world had
not been interested in what the Hong Kong Chinese had to cook
and sell. He detects an increased interest in sensuality in the   65
Western world: 'Colour, texture, movement, food, drink, and rock
music – all these have become much more a part and parcel of the
average person's life than they have ever been. It is this increased
sensuality and the desire for greater freedom from age-bound habits
in the West, combined with the inherent sensual concept of Chinese   70
food, always quick to satisfy the taste buds, that is at the root of the
sudden and phenomenal spread of Chinese food throughout the
length and breadth of the Western World.'[4]

There is no doubt that the traditional high-quality Chinese meal
is a serious matter, fastidiously prepared and fastidiously enjoyed.   75
Indeed, the bringing together and initial cutting up and organizing
of the materials is, according to Helen Burke[5], about 90% of the
actual preparation, the cooking itself being only about 10%. This
10% is not, however, a simple matter. There are many possibilities
to choose from; Kenneth Lo, for example, lists forty methods   80
available for the heating of food, from *chu* or the art of boiling to
such others as *ts'ang*, a kind of stir-frying and braising, *t'a*, deep-
frying in batter, and *wei*, burying food in hot solids such as
charcoal, heated stones, sand, salt and lime.[6]

3 These names for Chinese dishes have been taken at random from the three
   sources acknowledged in these footnotes.

4 Lo, as cited in Note 1, p. 11

5 Burke, as cited in Note 2, p. 7

6 Lo, as cited, pp. 18–31

The preparation is detailed, and the enjoyment must therefore   85
match it. Thus, a proper Chinese meal can last four hours and
proceed almost like a religious ceremony. It is a shared experience
for the participants, not a lonely chore, with its procession of
planned and carefully contrived dishes, some elements designed to
blend, others to contrast. Meat and fish, solids and soups, sweet   90
and sour sauces, crisp and smooth textures, fresh and dried
vegetables – all these and more challenge the palate with their
appropriate charms.

In a Chinese meal that has not been altered to conform to
Western ideas of eating, everything is presented as a kind of buffet,   95
the guest eating a little of this, a little of that. Individual portions as
such are not provided. A properly planned dinner will include at
least one fowl, one fish and one meat dish, and their presentation
with appropriate vegetables is not just a matter of taste but also a
question of harmonious colours. The eye must be pleased as well as   110
the palate; if not, then a certain essentially Chinese element is
missing, an element that links this cuisine with that most typical
and yet elusive concept Tao[7]. Emily Hahn, an American who has
lived and worked in China, has a great appreciation both of
Chinese cooking and the 'way' that leads to morality and harmony.   115
She insists that 'there *is* moral excellence in good cooking', and
adds that to the Chinese, traditionally, all life, all action and all
knowledge are one.[8] They may be chopped up and given parts with
labels, such as 'Cooking', 'Health', 'Character' and the like, but
none is in reality separate from the other. The smooth harmonies   120
and piquant contrasts in Chinese food are more than just the
products of recipés and personal enterprise. They are an expression
of basic assumptions about life itself.

7   *Tao* in Chinese means 'the way' or 'the road'. It is the basic concept in the ancient
    tradition called Taoism, referring both to proper human conduct and the
    ultimate harmony of the universe.
8   from *The Cooking of China*, Emily Hahn, Time-Life Books, 1968 (p. 91)

Below are some questions about the passage. These questions can be
used for all or any of the following purposes:

1   a simple check upon your understanding of the passage
2   the basis for a group discussion of the passage
3   the basis for a brief summary of the passage, by answering each
    question in reasonable detail in the order given

a.   What is Kenneth Lo's view of food and eating?
b.   How does it contrast with the approach common among many
     Westerners?
c.   What proof is provided to show that Lo's position is typically
     Chinese?

d. What, in his view, is the difference between typical Westerners and Chinese in restaurants?

e. How has Chinese food fared in the world at large?

f. How did this come about?

g. What does Lo detect in the modern Western world?

h. What is important in the preparation of a Chinese meal?

i. What is a 'proper Chinese meal' like?

j. How is it presented to a guest?

k. What else must be pleased besides the palate?

l. Why?

7.2 Punctuation: Quotation and reference

This section deals with three aspects of punctuation which are important in more advanced styles of writing. They are:

1   the writer's own punctuation versus the punctuation used by a quoted author

2   the use of square brackets in quotations

3   the presentation of foreign expressions in a text written in English

1   The writer's own punctuation versus quoted punctuation

Compare the writer's handling of the phrase *western world* with Kenneth Lo's in the following extract from the passage on Chinese Food:

> The standard of the restaurants improved steadily in the United States, but Lo considers that the crucial factor in spreading this kind of food throughout the Western world was population pressure in the British colony of Hong Kong, which... He detects an increased interest in sensuality in the Western world: 'Colour, texture, movement, food, drink and rock music... that is at the root of the sudden and phenomenal spread of Chinese food throughout the length and breadth of the Western World.'

lines *57–73*

Clearly, the writer and Kenneth Lo are not in agreement about the use of capitals for phrases like *western world*. The writer is, however, consistent; his presentation of 'Western world' matches his presentation of 'British colony' (where Lo might have written 'British Colony'). Each writer is entitled (within reason) to his or her own punctuation system. When quoting, however, it is essential *not* to change the other person's style; give the quotation as it stands in the original work. If, for any reason, you do not want to be associated with a quoted author's usage, put the Latin word *sic*, meaning 'thus', in brackets after the offending usage.

2   The use of square brackets in adapting quotations

Consider the following extract from the passage:

> In the matter of food and eating [however] one can hardly   lines
> remain completely indifferent to what one is doing for long.   *6–8*
> How . . .

The word *however* has been placed in square brackets here because it does not appear in the original text. The writer has not quoted the whole text (as shown by the use of ellipsis), and so has needed to add this word in order to make the quotation flow properly. When one makes this kind of structural change in a quotation, one needs to mark it with square brackets.

3   The use of foreign expressions in a text written in English

Consider the following extracts from the passage:

> Restaurants bedecked with dragons and delicate landscapes   lines
> – serving such exotica as *Dim Sin Gai* (sweet and sour   *46–51*
> chicken), *Shao Shing* soup, *Chiao-Tzu* and *Kuo-Tioh*
> (northern style), and *Ging Ai Kwar* (steamed aubergines) –
> have sprung up everywhere from Hong Kong to Honolulu to
> Hoboken to Huddersfield.

> . . . Kenneth Lo, for example, lists forty methods available for   lines
> the heating of food, from *chu* or the art of boiling to such   *80–84*
> others as *ts'ang*, a kind of stir-frying and braising, *t'a*, deep-
> frying in batter, and *wei*, burying food in hot solids such as
> charcoal, heated stones, sand, salt and lime.

The simplest way of handling foreign words is to underline them (in a handwritten or typed presentation) and italicize them (in printed material). Quotation marks could be used, but this may clash with the use of these marks for English words that the author is using for a special purpose. If a writer wishes to emphasize that the foreign word or phrase is followed by a direct translation, this can be done by putting the translation in quotation marks inside brackets, thus:

> The writer discusses, for example, *Dim Sin Gai* ('sweet and
> sour chicken').

Below are five questions for you to consider. They relate to the uses of quotation marks in the passage.

a. Who is being quoted in lines 41–42?

b. Why is the phrase in quotation marks in line 56 presented in this way?

c. What is special about the way in which Lo's remarks are quoted in lines 66–73?

d. What is special about the ways in which Emily Hahn is quoted in lines 113–118?

e. What is the purpose of the quotation marks in line 119?

7.3 Punctuation and layout: Notes and bibliographies

1 Notes

In the text of Unit 5, end-notes were used for bibliographical information (that is, references to books consulted by the writer), while in Unit 6 they they were used for encyclopaedic purposes (that is, they provided additional items of information). In the text for this unit, however, footnotes occur instead, and these are both bibliographical and encyclopaedic. They could just as easily have been organized as end-notes; such matters are personal decisions relating to the style preferred by an individual, an institution, or a publisher.

In the passage on Chinese food, the footnotes have been consecutively numbered 1 to 8. This is because the text is relatively short; in a long piece of work, the footnotes would normally be numbered page by page (that is, the first footnote on a page would be '1', the second '2' and so on, then the first on the next page would be '1' again, and so on).

Notes are generally used only in academic writing. In other kinds of writing they can be more trouble than help; one should put the information directly in the text, or simply leave it out. For academic purposes, however, it is often essential to add certain kinds of information, particularly details about works consulted and quoted from. This can be done by means of notes, or a bibliography, or both.

Once information about a source has been given in a note it is not usually necessary to repeat that information when the source is mentioned a second or third time. In this unit, second and later references simply mention the writer's name, then 'as cited in Note 1' (etc), followed by the page reference in the quoted book. This is simple and clear, but some institutions prefer this to be done by means of certain Latin abbreviations, thus:

Latin abbreviation	Latin phrase	English translation
ibid.	*ibidem*	'in the same place'
loc. cit.	*loco citato*	'in the place cited'
op. cit.	*opere citato*	'in the work cited'

2   Bibliographies

A bibliography is simply an alphabetically organized list of the works consulted in the preparation of a piece of serious writing or recommended to the reader for further study. Bibliographies should be kept as simple as possible and should be consistent in their punctuation and layout. They are *not* notes, do *not* follow the sequence of the text, and each item is listed only once. There are many styles available for the proper construction of bibliographies, and it is always a good idea to check the preferred style of an institution or publisher before setting to work making a particular bibliography, especially if it contains many items. Below you will find three common bibliographical styles. Study them carefully and consider just where they differ:

Style 1:   a simple, traditional format

> Burke, Helen. *Chinese Cooking for Pleasure.* Paul Halmyn. 1965.
> Hahn, Emily. *The Cooking of China.* Time-Life. 1968.
> Lo, Kenneth. *The Chinese Cookery Encyclopedia.* Collins. 1974.

Style 2:   a common academic variation

> Burke, Helen (1965) *Chinese Cooking for Pleasure.* Paul Hamlyn.
> Hahn, Emily (1968) *The Cooking of China.* Time-Life.
> Lo, Kenneth (1974) *The Chinese Cookery Encyclopedia.* Collins.

Style 3:   A modern academic format (one among several)

> BURKE, Helen (1965)
>   *Chinese Cooking for Pleasure.* Paul Hamlyn.
> HAHN, Emily (1968)
>   *The Cooking of China.* Time-Life.
> LO, Kenneth (1974)
>   *The Chinese Cookery Encyclopedia.* Collins.

You may compare these three basic styles with those in other books and choose any particular style that suits you. Below, however, you will find some unpunctuated material. It contains the names of six works of reference for an article on styles of cooking around the world. The entries are not in alphabetical order. Punctuate and alphabetize the material in order to get a bibliography organized according to Style 1. When you have done this, re-organize the material according to Style 2 and then Style 3, so that you become accustomed to the variety of possibilities:

bon jules j the mexican cuisine I love leon amiel 1977 leonard jonathan norton latin american cooking time life 1968 brown dale american cooking time life 1968 hume rosemary and muriel downes the penguin dictionary of cookery penguin books 1966 eckley mary mccalls superb dessert cookbook random house and mccalls 1961 macrae sheila the scottish cookbook foulsham 1979

7.4 Style: Levels of formality

Academic writing is almost invariably formal in style, and easily identified as such. It is not, however, possible to divide English styles neatly into 'formal' and 'informal' compartments. The relationship is more like a continuum with two extremes, as in this diagram:

very informal 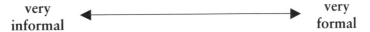 **very formal**

The general style of a text will lie somewhere on the line, and may even vary from time to time as the writer deliberately or unconsciously changes positions. Such changes in style should on the whole be deliberate; they should not be the product of carelessness, ignorance or that subtle thing called 'bad taste'. For convenience, the continuum of formality can be cut up into various compartments in order to grade various texts and styles:

very informal	quite informal	neutral	quite formal	very formal

A large number of factors (relating to grammar, vocabulary, style and punctuation) contribute towards the 'tone' of a piece of writing. Some of the more important factors are listed (and contrasted) below:

Less formal	More formal
1 Sentences are shorter. They use basic punctuation, such as commas and periods. Where necessary, they also use brackets and dashes and even exclamation marks!	Sentences tend on the whole to be longer and more complex, making use of the full range of punctuation devices, including colons and semi-colons, and tending to avoid the drama and excitement of such things as exclamation marks.
2 I am more likely to mention myself and my friends in informal material.	The use of the personal pronouns, especially 'I', is generally avoided, and personal relationships are kept in the background or ignored altogether.
3 People prefer the active voice of the verb.	The passive voice is generally preferred, especially in technical writing, along with impersonal expressions such as 'one' and the impersonal 'it', as in *It has been observed that* . . .
4 People use all sorts of short forms and ellipses, like *I'd* and *won't*, and *which* and *that* are often absent in certain kinds of clauses.	Full forms are preferred, ellipsis occurs, but not of grammatically important words, and short forms are avoided. Various special formulas of politeness, caution, etc, are often used, such as adverbs like *probably* and *apparently*, or phrases like *It would appear that. . .* and *As far as one can tell at this stage. . .*
5 Short vernacular words tend to be common, including phrasal verbs like *get up* and *put out* and vernacular compounds like *tea pot, mountain areas*, etc. We put them in all the time in the everyday use of the mother tongue.	Longer Greco-Latin material tends to be used, giving the text a more abstract quality. Verbs of Latin provenance, like *speculate* and *construe*, and polysyllabic Greek compounds like *bibliographical* and *epistemology* are common occurrences.

Less formal	More formal
6 Informal expressions are often (but not always) rather vague. Words of general meaning like *get*, *put* and *do* are common.	Formal language usually aims at precision and the avoidance of ambiguity, but sometimes it may be used simply to impress or to make a subject look more complex and important than it actually is.
7 Informal expression is often idiomatic and slangy, know what I mean?	Idioms and slang are generally avoided in formal usage, unless the writer deliberately brings them in for 'colour' or for purposes of exemplification.

Formality and informality are complex matters, but for general purposes the following scale of examples may be useful:

very informal

1 'This thing doesn't work right,' he told us.
2 He told us the thing didn't work right.
3 He told us that the machine wasn't/was not working **or** functioning properly.
4 We were informed that the machine was not functioning properly.
5 According to information received, the machine was defective.

very formal

Below are six sets containing five sentences each. The sentences are not, however, arranged in any order of formality. In front of each sentence is a set of empty boxes in which a number (from 1 to 5) can be written, indicating the proper order of formality as shown in the above example. Now organize the sets. The first one is partly done for you as a guide.

a. ☐ She told them later that she had not known about it while it was happening.
☐ Her later verbal report indicated that at the time she was completely unaware of what was transpiring.
1 'I didn't know about it while it was happening,' she told them later.
3 She informed them later verbally that she had not known about the event while it was taking place.
☐ They were informed in her subsequent verbal report that she had had no knowledge whatever of the event at the time of its occurrence.

b. ☐ He asked whether she could come and pick the stuff up at his place.

☐ He wondered if it was possible for her to come and collect the material at his house.

☐ 'Can you come and pick up the stuff at my place?' he asked her.

☐ His request was that, if possible, she should collect the material at his place of residence.

☐ She was asked if there was a possibility that she might collect the material at his house.

c. ☐ According to the astronomer, the name Capella refers to a star.

☐ 'Capella's a star,' said the astronomer.

☐ The group was informed by the astronomer that the name Capella refers to a star.

☐ The astronomer said that Capella is a star.

☐ The astronomer said Capella's a star.

d. ☐ Chinese food is tasty.

☐ The cuisine of China appeals to most people's taste buds.

☐ One's gustatory proclivities are very pleasantly stimulated by the traditional cuisine of China.

☐ Chinese food's tasty.

☐ One's taste buds are stimulated very pleasantly by Chinese food.

e. ☐ The historian said: 'Hasan-e-Sabbah trained his assassins to kill his religious and political enemies.'

☐ The assassins of mediaeval Persia were, according to the historian, trained by Hasan-e-Sabbah to kill his religious and political opponents.

☐ The historian said that the assassins were trained by Hasan-e-Sabbah to kill his religious and political foes.

☐ According to the historian, the members of the mediaeval Persian Sect of the Assassins were trained by their founder and leader, Hasan-e-Sabbah, to eliminate those who were religiously and politically opposed to him.

☐ The members of the mediaeval Assassin Sect in Persia, according to the historian, were organized so as to facilitate the liquidation of all religious and political opposition to its founder and leader, Hasan-e-Sabbah.

7.5 Composition:
Developing source material on yoga

If you set out to write a review like 'The Scale of Things', 'Assassination' or 'Chinese Food', you should follow five basic procedures:

1   Gather your raw material (through reading, interviewing people, etc.), organize your notes, then make one or more rough general plans or outlines of what you want to say.

2   Start somewhere, even if you are not sure what your first remarks should be. Work and re-work the material until it develops a satisfactory shape, leaving it from time to time so that you can come back to it a few hours or days later with a fresh mind.

3   Do not worry about it too much; many writers say that their best work almost 'writes itself'. Do not look for perfection, but do not accept carelessness from yourself either.

4   Talk about your ideas with someone sympathetic, and do not be afraid to show your work at any stage to someone who will give you an honest opinion. When you think you have finished, get an observant friend to check your work for small slips. It is surprising what we do not notice in our own work.

5   Do not be seduced or destroyed by a single opinion of a piece of work, and keep trying. All professional writers do far more work than ever appears in books or other published materials. Most of what they do is preparatory work that no one else ever sees.

As a final project for this course, some raw material on the subject of yoga is provided below. You can consult other sources if you wish. The idea is to write a systematic review of the subject, including both factual material and your personal responses. (If, for example, you want more than what is provided here, you could go to a library, a local yoga club or any other suitable source. You could even take up yoga for a time in order to get some personal 'inside' information and feelings on the subject.) Some questions to ask while organizing your review might include the following:

1   What is yoga?
2   How and where did it begin?
3   What does it do for people **or** what do certain people claim that it does?
4   How does it work?
5   What special terminology and concepts are used in yoga?

1   What is yoga?

- 'Physical or Hatha Yoga is a series of extremely well thought out postures or positions that move and improve virtually every part of the human body.'

  Lyn Marshall, *Wake Up To Yoga – The Book of the Television Series*, Ward Lock, London, 1975, p. 6

- 'Until very recently, to the vast majority of people in the West, Yoga connoted only a remote mysticism practised by Eastern holy men, involving such uncomfortable activities as lying on a bed of nails!'

  Howard Kent and Harold Orton, in their foreword to Richard Hittleman, *Yoga for Health (Based on the Independent Television series)*, Hamlyn, London, 1971

- 'We are all seeking some magic formula for good health and inner peace in a world that is charged with tension and anxiety. How do we find it? The answer is not simple, but there is a way. Through yoga.'

  Rachel Carr, *Yoga for All Ages*, Collins, London and Glasgow, 1972, p. 9

- 'Yoga is a science which teaches how to awake our latent powers and hasten the process of human evolution. This technique was discovered by the ancient teachers of Yoga through the medium of intuition.'

  Swami-Vishnoudevananda (Rishikesh, 1955, India), in his preface to Louis Frédéric, *Yoga Asanas*, translated from the French by Geoffrey A Dudley, Thorsons, London, 1959 (original French edition, 1956)

2   How and where did it begin?

- Carr: 'The tradition of yoga began in northern India over five thousand years ago among a learned aristocratic society of philosophers, scholars, and warriors who examined the ephemeral quality of life, with its inevitable sufferings and tragedies, and sought to give it deeper meaning and purpose.' (as cited above, p. 15)

- 'The word Yoga is derived from the Sanskrit root *yuj* meaning to bind, join, attach and yoke, to direct and concentrate one's attention on, to use and apply. It also means union or communion. It is the true union of our will with the will of God.'

  B K S Iyengar, *Light on Yoga – Yoga Dipika*, George Allen and Unwin, 1966 (this quotation from Mandala Books, 1976, p. 19)

- 'In its specific sense, the word *yoga* refers to that enormous body of spiritual precepts and techniques which grew up in India over several millenia and which may be regarded as the very substratum of the cultural life of Indian man. *Yoga* is thus the generic name for the various Indian paths of "unification" or the transformation of consciousness.'

  Georg Feuerstein, *Textbook of Yoga*, Rider, London, 1975, p. 3

- 'The earliest yogis sought to bind nature to their will, but to do so had first to harness their own bodies and minds. In Hindu writings the senses are often called "horses", and particularly horses that need taming ... Yoga, as we have seen, acquired its name through linking the image of yoking horses with the desire to control the body and the mind. This idea of the vehicle and the harnessed animals soon extended, however, to include the journey as well as the vehicle. Yoga came to suggest "the way to be travelled". ....'

  Tom McArthur, *Darshana: An Introduction to Yoga and Indian Philosophy*, Scotsway, Edinburgh, 1978, pp. 2–3

- yoga – an ancient Hindu system – physical and mental training under a *guru* or 'master' – years of discipline – self-control – exercises in sitting (*asanas*) – exercises in breathing (*pranayama*) – these exercises developing into a great variety of held postures, including the headstand (*sirshasana*) and the cobra posture (*bhujangasana*) – claims of supernatural powers: stopping the heart; suspended animation; survival of being buried alive; levitation; walking on hot coals, etc – meditative techniques – minority activity among holy men (*sadhus*) in India – spread in 20th century to West – particularly interested health enthusiasts, often mainly groups of women – now popular throughout the world

- **An original yoga source:** *The Bhagavad Gita*

  Of all Hindu works on religion and philosophy, the *Gita* is the most popular, both in India and abroad. It has, for example, more than fifty different published versions in English alone. It is a mystical poem, dealing with yoga, the nature of existence and how we should live our lives. Its exact age is impossible to estimate, but it is certainly more than 2,000 years old, and many of its elements go back over 3,000 years. The title is in Sanskrit, and means 'The Lord's Song'. The subject of the song is the advice that Lord Krishna gives to Arjuna, the Pandava prince, on the eve of a terrible battle between two related clans, the Pandavas and Kauravas. Arjuna is a great warrior, but suddenly he has no wish to fight his kinsmen and erstwhile friends. The god Krishna is the driver of the prince's chariot, and at this crucial moment in human history sets out to persuade Arjuna to accept life's inevitable struggles with dispassion. To do this, the prince must follow *raja yoga* – 'the path of kings' – and do his duty, constantly aware that all of life as we see it is a kind of illusion. Elements in the *Gita* allow us to compare the instructions that Krishna gives to the royal hero both with Western ideas of chivalry and, even more cogently, with the code of honour of the Japanese samurai warriors and Zen masters.

3   **What does it do for people or what do certain people claim that it does?**

- Lyn Marshall says that 'yoga can be *used* and I really do mean used in the fullest sense of the word, to improve your daily life, no matter who you are or what you do.' She adds that 'you do not necessarily have to be looking for a spiritually uplifting experience, or indeed involvement of any kind.' She then notes that yoga can be used to 'achieve' any or all of the following:

  1   lose weight – generally or in specific areas
  2   learn how to relax properly
  3   rid oneself of back problems
  4   remove mental strain and tension
  5   improve your figure
  6   strengthen and recondition your entire body
  7   stay relaxed under pressure
  8   improve one's concentration
  9   become more sensually aware of oneself and others
  10   improve circulation and breathing
  11   get relief from conditions like insomnia, headaches, migraine, sinusitis and asthma
  12   improve the condition of one's skin, eyes and hair
  13   improve one's balance and posture
  14   regain agility and youth

- Richard Hittleman says: 'For many thousands of people dreams of new life, a return to second youth, a beautiful, strong and trim body which radiates health and vitality, a wonderful peace of mind, have come true through my yoga instruction.'

  op cit, p. 3

- Rachel Carr says: '... Essentially, yoga is a search for health and well-being on two levels: physical and spiritual. It is an art of living that holds the key to youthfulness, vitality and long life. It leads to harmony and peace of mind. Its age-old teachings apply with special urgency to our needs for a calmer, healthier way of life today when tension is the number one killer in our society.'

op cit, p. 9

- 'The practice of yoga induces a primary sense of measure and proportion. Reduced to our own body, our first instrument, we learn to play it, drawing from it maximum resonance and harmony. With unflagging patience we refine and animate every cell as we return daily to the attack, unlocking and liberating capacities otherwise condemned to frustration and death.'

  Yehudi Menuhin, in his preface to B K S Iyengar, cited above.

  Note that the Latin abbreviations have been used twice so far as an example of their use, but will now be discontinued.

- 'The aim of the doctrines of Hindu philosophy and of training in yoga practice is to transcend the limits of individualized consciousness. The mythical tales [of ancient India] are meant to convey the wisdom of the philosophers and to exhibit in a popular, pictorial form the experiences or results of yoga ... Yoga is a strict spiritual discipline, practised in order to gain control over the forces of one's own being, to gain occult powers, to dominate certain specific forces of nature, or finally (and chiefly) to attain union with the Deity or with the Universal Spirit.'

  Heinrich Zimmer, *Myths and Symbols in Indian Art and Civilization*, edited by Joseph Campbell, Bollingen Series VI, Pantheon Books (a division of Random House), New York, 1946, p. 39 (from text and footnote)

- 'It is the most complete synthesis of the realities of life and living. The facets of yoga are not unique to the yoga system; it is their bringing together into a whole way of life which is so remarkable.'

  Howard Kent, editorial to the magazine *Yoga and Life* No 2, 1977

4 How does it work?

(All actual direct quotations in this section taken from Rachel Carr, pp. 16–17)

'Since nature made our bodies for constant action in walking, bending and climbing, our muscles become rigid when we do not use them. The great advantage of yoga exercises is that they bring all the muscle groups into play. This means the range of movement can be increased in the muscles, tendons and ligaments and the joints they support, with particular emphasis on stretching the spine to increase its flexibility.'

- physical poise developed through the yoga postures – series of supple, graceful movements – some appear 'deceptively relaxed, but in reality they are dynamic' – slowly stretched to full length – held in stillness – cause blood to flow evenly throughout the body

- with such movements, slow-acting and ageing glands reawakened – postures (such as the Plough, Bow, Cobra, Locust, Shoulderstand, Headstand, etc) strengthen back muscles and also act directly on endocrine glands – thus influence sexual function

- deep controlled breathing – nature's tranquillizer and rejuvenator – singers, actors and athletes benefit from this – slower respiration reduces strain on the heart – improves metabolism – transforms deposits of fat into body fuel – increases resistance of lungs to common cold and other ailments – through oxygenation, protects against fatigue and low vitality, raises levels of energy

'Most of the breathing exercises in yoga are done through the nose with the mouth closed. The reason: our nose acts as a vacuum cleaner, which sweeps in with the air fine particles of dust and bacteria. When air enters the nostrils, it passes through a labyrinth of filters that screens out dust and bacteria and warms the air before it reaches our lungs. When we exhale through the nostrils, rather than through the mouth, our lungs gain stamina, since they take a longer time to deflate.'

'Few of us are consciously aware of how our emotions influence the way we breathe. When we are excited, our heart beats faster and breathing takes on a staccato-like rhythm. When we are depressed, our body slumps and breathing becomes an effort. But when we are happy we stand to full height, the face is calm, the breathing is deeper and easier. If we breathe as nature intended, by expanding our lungs to full capacity, we can revitalize our energy, calm our nerves, induce restful sleep – and live longer.'

5   What special terminology and concepts are used in yoga?

asana	sitting; a seated position or posture; in yoga, any held position, usually accompanied by appropriate breathing
ashram	a hermitage or retreat, usually containing the home of a famous guru and the quarters of some of his disciples, a hostel for visitors, etc
guru	a respected older person, especially a father or teacher; a master of yoga; a spiritual guide, male or female, or even a book

hatha yoga	('the path of effort') the yoga of achievement through physical self-discipline
karma	action; the effects of many actions; the slow accumulation of causes and effects (over many lifetimes) that dictates every individual's future actions
karma yoga	('the path of action') the yoga of selfless action, duty, service, etc
prana	breath; the life force carried into the body by breathing; energy
pranayama	the practice of breath-control in yoga
raja yoga	('the path of kings') the path of achievement through mental self-discipline
Sanskrit	('perfected; cultivated') the classical language of India, used particularly for sacred texts, hymns and yoga treatises
sadhu	a wandering holy man; a saint; someone following a spiritual path
swami	('lord') a title for a holy man

Expressions you could use in your composition

impressive claims – evangelical fervour/enthusiasm – scientifically valid/established? – commercialize – promise the sky/earth – balanced observation(s) – justify claims by results – from remote antiquity – oriental techniques invading the West – Western proponents of yoga – secular or spiritual? – rigorous self-discipline – a personal regime of daily exercises – the 'body beautiful' or 'ultimate bliss'?

Answers

UNIT 1

1.1 a. T
b. **F**: Many people are not entirely masters of their mother tongues.
c. T
d. **F**: Many but not all of these languages have standard forms as well as regional dialects.
e. T
f. T
g. **F**: It is not a literal use of language; it is, in fact, figurative.
h. **F**: This depends on what one means by 'vast majority' and 'understand'; certainly, the passage suggests that dialect-users will have difficulty, and these must make up a large proportion of both communities.
i. **T**: The passage implies that dialect-users face problems similar to speakers of related languages.
j. **F**: The passage suggests that languages are naturally varied and makes no statement whatever about the need for control.

1.2 a. **as given**
b. (US) **as given** (Br) memorise, memorize
c. (Br) _____ (US) neighborhood
d. (Br) _____ (US) pretense
e. (US) _____ (Br) cheque
f. (Br) _____ (US) anemic
g. (Br) _____ (US) labor relations
h. (US) _____ (Br) sabre
i. (US) _____ (Br) mediaeval
j. (Br) _____ (US) kilometer
k. (US) _____ (Br) dialogue
l. (Br) _____ (US) systematize
m. (US) _____ (Br) centimetre
n. (US) _____ (Br) coloured
o. (Br) _____ (US) milliliter
p. (Br) _____ (US) encyclopedia
q. (US) _____ (Br) offence
r. (Br) _____ (US) aluminum
s. (Br) _____ (US) monolog
t. (Br) _____ (US)harbor

1.3 **Nil**

1.4 **Sentence analysis**
(The first ten sentences have been analysed.)

11 Complex sentence

A second common misconception about language <u>is</u> **that** words <u>have</u> fixed and clear meanings.

Simple sentences:
i A second common misconception about language is (this/as follows).
ii Words have fixed and clear meanings.

12 Simple sentence

This <u>is</u> – fortunately or unfortunately – far from true.

13 Simple sentence

<u>Take</u> even the apparently simple and specific English word *man*.

14 Two simple sentences joined by a semi-colon

It seems clear enough; *it* refers to an 'adult male human being'.

15 Compound sentence

Of course it <u>does</u>, **but** just <u>consider</u> for a moment the following sentences:

Simple sentences:
i Of course it does.
ii Just consider for a moment the following sentences.

16 **Apparent simple sentence/disguised complex sentence**

There <u>are</u> several men ∧ missing in that chess set.

Simple sentences:

i There are several men.
ii These men are missing.

(**Note** that the sentence is, in fact, elliptical, omitting *who are*, and so turning *missing* into an isolated present participle.)

17 **Simple sentence**

The boat <u>was manned</u> entirely by women and children.

18 **Complex and simple sentences joined by a semi-colon**

You <u>might argue</u> **that** these sentences <u>are</u> somewhat unnatural; certainly, they <u>do</u> not <u>represent</u> the everyday core meaning of the word 'man'.

Simple sentences:

i You might argue (something).
ii These sentences are somewhat unnatural.
iii Certainly, they do not represent the everyday core meaning of the word 'man'.

19 **Compound-complex sentence**

They <u>are</u>, however, legitimate extensions of that core meaning, **the second being** especially interesting **because** it <u>is</u> a verb and not a noun, **and** ∧ <u>suggests</u> **that** we <u>expect</u> adult male human beings to serve as the crews of ships, not women and certainly not children.

Simple sentences:

i They are, however, ... interesting. (**Note** that 'the second being' can be interpreted as 'and the second is', thus disguising a second clause.)
ii It is a verb and not a noun.
iii It suggests (something).
iv We expect adult ... not children. (**Note** that the construction of noun phrase and infinitive after *expect* corresponds in effect to a relative clause 'that adult male human beings should serve as ... etc.')

20 **Simple sentence**

Part of the pleasure and genius of language <u>may</u> well <u>arise</u> out of this slight 'misuse' of words.

21 **Compound-complex sentence**

After all, **if** you <u>call</u> a person a cat or a cabbage, no literal identification <u>is</u> <u>intended</u> **but** a great deal of meaning <u>is</u> nevertheless <u>conveyed</u>.

Simple sentences:

i You call a person a cat or a cabbage.
ii No literal identification is intended.
iii A great deal of meaning is nevertheless conveyed.

22 **Compound-complex sentence**

A third misconception about language <u>claims</u> **that** every language <u>is</u> – **or** ∧ <u>should be</u> – equally <u>used</u> **and** ∧ <u>understood</u> by all its practitioners everywhere.

Simple sentences:

i A third misconception about language claims (something).
ii Every language is equally used by ... everywhere.
iii Every language should be equally used by ... everywhere.
iv Every language is equally understood by ... everywhere.
v Every language should be equally understood by all its practitioners everywhere.

(**Note** the complex ellipsis.)

23 **Two simple sentences joined by a semi-colon**

Certainly, users of the standard forms of English in the United Kingdom generally <u>understand</u> their equivalents in the United States; the degree of similarity between these two major forms of English <u>is</u> great.

24 **Complex sentence**

Dialect-users, however, in these countries <u>have</u> serious problems <u>understanding</u> each other, **to the extent that** they <u>may wonder</u> **if** they <u>are</u> actually <u>using</u> the same language.

Simple sentences:

i   Dialect-users, however, in these countries have serious problems understanding each other.

ii They may wonder (something).

iii They are actually using the same language.

25 **Two simple sentences joined by a semi-colon**

Someone from Brooklyn, New York, <u>will have</u> trouble with a Cockney from London; an old-style British Army colonel <u>won't do</u> well in discussions with a Californian flower-child.

26 **Simple sentence**

Yet they all <u>belong</u> within the vast community of 20th-century World English.

(**Note** the use of a short, simple sentence to end the passage.)

1.5   **Summary continued**

(107 words as opposed to 306 in the original; only one of many possible summaries)

A second common misconception about language assumes that such everyday words as *man* have fixed, clear meanings. This is not so, however, as can be seen in the idea of 'men' in a chess set, or women 'manning' a ship. Such extensions of word meanings are legitimate, and may indeed be 'part of the pleasure and genius of language'. A third misconception claims that all the users of a language are – or should be – able to communicate with each other easily. Speakers of standard forms usually succeed in this, as for example between the U.K. and the U.S.A., but it is by no means true for dialect-users.

(**Note** the use of a direct quotation from the original, a common and recommended practice in summary-writing, as long as it is done well and not too often.)

1.6   a.   A language like English not only changes from generation to generation, but is also very diverse in geographical terms.

b.   Soccer is not only an exciting game to play, but (is) also a great spectator sport, watched ...

c.   Enthusiastic schoolboys and university students not only played various kinds of football, but also began to write out ...

d.   Nordic skiing is not only an excellent way of keeping fit, but can also be the best way ...

e.   Skiing is not only a popular winter activity with a venerable history, but (is) also nowadays a major OR is nowadays also a major factor in ...

f.   Swimming is not only a satisfying indoor and outdoor pastime, but (is) also a highly organized ...

g.   Some people not only have certain general misconceptions about language and languages, but also have a deep ...
OR
Some people have not only certain general misconceptions about language and languages, but also a deep ...

h.   Not only does a language like English change from generation to generation; it is also very diverse in geographical terms.

i.   Not only is soccer an exciting game to play; it is also a great spectator sport, watched ...

j.   Not only did enthusiastic schoolboys and university students play various kinds of football; they also began to write out ...

k.   Not only is Nordic skiing an excellent way of keeping fit; it can also be ...

l.   Not only is skiing a popular winter activity with a venerable history; it is also nowadays ...

m. Not only is swimming a satisfying indoor and outdoor pastime; it is also a highly organized ...

n. Not only do some people have certain general misconceptions about language and languages; they also have a deep ...

1.7   Compound words: First stage

a. snow trail
b. toothbrush
c. radio programme
d. school teacher
e. factory manager
f. bank clerks
g. flower pot
h. hybrid language
i. textbook
j. ski-resort, ski resort
k. snowbirds
l. steam-powered engine
m. London-based business
n. government-controlled agency
o. adding machine
p. sewing machine
q. cement-mixing machine
r. cement-mixer
s. stamp collector
t. film director
u. soap-making factory
v. snow-covered mountain
w. wedding ring
x. catfish
y. apple core
z. Sunday newspaper

Compound words: Second stage

a. 36-year-old office worker
b. 26-year-old school teacher
c. 40-year-old Chicago company manager
d. 30-year-old television [news] announcer
e. 50-year-old peace treaty
f. 11th-century Norman castle
g. ten-ton OR 10-ton snow-clearing machine
h. Spanish-language textbook
i. Saturday football match
j. World Cup soccer competition

Compound words: Third stage

a. cold-water bath
b. hot-water baths
c. slow-motion movements
d. small-scale operations OR smallscale operations
e. first-class football-player OR firstclass football-player
f. three-week holiday
g. six-month stay
h. two-year period
i. age-group swimming competitions
j. wide-angle photographic lens OR wide-angle lens

1.8   Punctuation

Many words in most languages have imprecise meanings, even ordinary words like *man*, *run* and *hot*. Such words can refer to more than one thing and have more than one use. Without a clear context we cannot always be sure just what they are meant to convey. Consider these sentences:

1) The woman shouted that the house was on fire.
2) The captain ordered his men to fire.
3) Fire!

Sentences 1 and 2 provide enough context to show what is intended by the word *fire* in each case. Sentence 3, however, presents a problem. Does it relate to the woman or the captain or to something else completely?

Notes:

1 It is also possible to indent the three sentences and the first line of the next para.

2 The brackets following the numbers 1, 2 and 3 introducing the sentences are not absolutely necessary. One could also bracket the numbers mentioned in the second paragraph to correspond with the brackets at the margin. Such things are a matter of personal choice; the main thing is that once you have chosen a style, you should continue in that style.

1.9   Nil

UNIT 2

2.1 a. **T**
b. **F**: Morris does not dispute these experts' views, but suggests that there are other factors involved.
c. **F**: Parents are not directly involved; their children are taken away from them.
d. **T**
e. **F**: Morris considers that these rites, whether we view them as barbarous or not, have a social value.
f. **T**
g. **T**
h. **T**
i. **F**: The adolescent becomes an adult, but in a subordinate position to the elders of the group.
j. **T**

2.2 1 achievement: showing success in a known course
proficiency: showing ability in something at a particular time
aptitude: showing potential ability in something
needs: showing that help of some kind is required to improve a person's performance in something

2 a. easy/tough
b. malign/benign
c. sophisticated/primitive
d. trivial/important
e. ordinary/special
f. persuaded/forced
g. gentle/severe
h. temporary/permanent
i. rejected/accepted
j. juvenile/adult

3 a. rejected/dismissed
b. behaviour/practices
c. significance/value

d. demanding/requiring
e. loyalty/allegiance
f. attachments/ties
g. obtains/gains
h. artificial/contrived
i. quite/absolutely
j. position/role

4 a. intolerable/inevitable
b. paralysis/parallel
c. exceptionally/explicitly
d. superconscious/super-tribal
e. concluded/conducted
f. assertion/assistance
g. suffuse/suffer
h. accommodates/accompanies
i. impeded/imposed
j. pre-scientific/pre-technological

5 a. regional/educational; formal; essential(ly); special; physical; psychological; genital(s)
b. population/examination; initiation; mutilation; operation(s)
c. involvement/achievement
d. efficiency/proficiency
e. latitude/aptitude
f. positive/primitive
g. urban/human
h. variety/puberty; society
i. pressure/torture
j. persistent/permanent

2.3 1 What is ... (S)
2 According to ... (S + S)
3 In the view ... (CP)
4 He argues that ... (CX)
5 In these rites ... (CP)
6 They are forced ... (CC)
7 Their bodies ... (S + S)
8 At about ... (CC)
9 These experiences ... (CC)
10 They have a ... (S)
11 Firstly, the ... (CX)
12 This provides ... (S + S)
13 The adolescent ... (CC)
14 Secondly, the ... (apparent S; disguised CX)

15 One does not ... (apparent S; disguised CX)
16 Morris in fact ... (CP, leading into quotation)
17 Thirdly, it ... (CX)
18 The intense power ... (CX)
19 The inevitable ... (CC)
20 Public examinations ... (apparent S; disguised CX)
21 No one can ... (S + S)
22 The mental anguish ... (CX)

2.4   Parachuting

Every new technology seems to produce its own sports; the military use of aircraft is no exception. Parachuting is the art of jumping successfully out of aircraft with the aid of a special canopy, and began as a dangerous wartime service for which volunteer soldiers received special training and rewards. Today, however, it is a fast-growing sport with its own unique variations: free-falling and formation sky-diving.

For many people, even the thought of jumping from a stationary balloon or a moving aircraft is horrifying, much more so than undersea swimming or Alpine skiing. It is, however, a fact that there are very few deaths and relatively few injuries in this sport. In British parachuting, for example, only ten people died between 1968 and 1974, and there is only about one injury per thousand jumps, a ratio which compares favourably with downhill skiing.

It was a woman who started sport-parachuting in England in 1948, and today, as a result, there are in that country many successful clubs and a number of full-time parachuting centres. A beginner can learn the basics of this exciting sport in one weekend training course. He or she learns how to guide a parachute, how to deal with emergencies, and how to fall in a face-to-earth position, keeping the arms and legs spread in order to prevent the body from turning in the air. When the learner actually begins, he or she jumps with a nylon line fixed to the balloon or plane, so that the line can pull the parachute open automatically in less than three seconds, but later the trainee jumps without the line, pulling his or her own 'ripcord' after a three-second delay, thus becoming a completely free agent.

2.5   Logical order: D,F,H,C,E,G,B,A

Bad weather is the enemy of traditional parachuting and has contributed towards a new activity called 'parascending'. Here, the parachutist is attached to a car by a cable and runs behind it with open chute until he leaves the ground. He is gradually lifted to about 1,000 feet, when he can release himself and do a normal descent. People who want to try this pastime can go for the same kind of weekend training as other more traditional parachutists. On Saturdays, adults and teenagers learn landing rolls and safety drills, and – for a small sum of money – are pulled off the ground on their first flights. After a series of such flights, they are allowed to release themselves and to practise steering the chute as they come down. By such means, the would-be parascender can be raised into the air and set down again remarkably gently. Parascending has its attractions as a safe and comparatively easy introduction to parachuting generally, especially for young people, and may one day become the main form of the sport.

2.6

1 a. **As given**
   b. She took the business over. She took it over.
   c. They closed the company down. They closed it down.
   d. They took the children away. They took them away.
   e. He cut the water supply off. He cut it off.
   f. They broke the old cars up. They broke them up.
   g. He chased the dogs away. He chased them away.

h. She will bring the books in tomorrow.
   She will bring them in tomorrow.
i. Hand the money over immediately.
   Hand it over immediately.
j. The workmen pulled the old building
   down. They pulled it down.

2 a. up   i. out
   b. down   j. down
   c. out   k. up
   d. out   l. out
   e. off   m. out
   f. off   n. off
   g. out   o. up/down
   h. up

2.7 Punctuation work: First stage

See Book 1 Unit 6, comprehension and composition model:
'The Marriage Market', lines 1–22

Punctuation work: Second stage

See this unit, comprehension and composition model:
'Examinations', lines 29–43

Punctuation Work: Third stage

In addition to *The Human Zoo*, Desmond Morris has written several other popular works relating to human and animal social life. These include *The Naked Ape* and *Intimate Behaviour*, both published by Cape, the first in 1967 and the second in 1971. In the latter volume, he considers the need of both animals and human beings for physical contact. He studies human social behaviour from the point of view of a zoologist, constantly comparing our actions and needs with those of our natural companions on this planet. He is not only interested in our actual capacity to touch, but also in extensions of the idea of touching that can be found in our use of language. He observes, for example:

> 'As an adult human being, you can communicate with me in a variety of ways. I can read what you write, listen to the words you speak, hear your laughter and your cries, look at the expressions on your face, watch the actions you perform, smell the scent you wear and feel your embrace. In ordinary speech we might refer to these interactions as "making contact", or "keeping in touch", and yet only the last one on the list involves bodily contact. All the others operate at a distance.'

It is clear from what Morris says that the use of words like 'touch' and 'contact' to describe activities like writing, speaking and signalling with the body is, in objective terms, rather strange. It is certainly, however, very revealing. It is as if we know, deep down inside us, that 'bodily contact is the most basic form of communication'. Morris reminds us of speakers who are said to 'hold their audiences', of 'gripping experiences' and 'touching scenes'. No physical contact is involved in any of the situations described by these idioms – and yet the metaphor is clear to us all.

Note the use of quotation within the quotation, in Morris's longer piece.

2.8 Nil

UNIT 3

3.1 a T
     b. **F:** about 20,000 years ago
     c. **T**
     d. **F:** A road passes through one of the caverns mentioned, while a small railway operates inside another, but no normal-sized railway passes through any cavern.
     e. **T**
     f. **T**
     g. **F:** They worked separately.
     h. **F:** He spent a complete period of 15 months in the cave.
     i. **F:** They did surprisingly well.
     j. **T**
     k. **T**
     l. **T**

3.2 **1 Nil**

2 1 cave wall (line 4)
   2 art treasures (ll. 8–9)
   3 Cave explorers (l. 10)
   4 limestone grottos (ll. 12–13)
   5 colour combinations (l. 15)
   6 foothills (l. 21)
   7 limestone (l. 23)
   8 electric-lit (l. 24)
   9 car park (l. 24)
  10 coal-mining (l. 28)
  11 Rouffignac Cavern (l. 30)
  12 hump-backed (l. 35)
  13 mild-faced (l. 36)
  14 Ollivier Cave (l. 43)
  15 underground living (l. 45)
  16 cave-dwelling (l. 46)
  17 Samar Cave (l. 48)
  18 self-chosen (ll. 50–51)
  19 underground conditions (l. 55)
  20 daylight (l. 63)
  21 body clock (l. 64)
  22 cave system (ll. 74–75)

3 1 took up (l. 1)
   2 twisted up (l. 5)
   3 handed down (l. 9)
   4 clamber down (l. 11)
   5 opened up (l. 12)
   6 lit up (l. 14)
   7 set off (l. 15)
   8 sealed off (l. 18)
   9 wind together (l. 23)
  10 rattles down (l. 31)
  11 came up (l. 42)
  12 carrying out (l. 44)
  13 went down (l. 48)
  14 cut . . . off (ll. 48–49)
  15 stayed on (l. 51)
  16 coming up (l. 52)
  17 taken down (l. 57)

The identification of phrasal verbs in a text is not always easy. The following list is therefore provided to show, as simply as possible, how the phrasal verbs in the passage differ from ordinary verbs that happen to be followed by prepositional phrases of various kinds. The 17 phrasal verbs are marked with an asterisk (*).

Verbs and *phrasal verbs	Prepositional phrases, etc.	Line
*took up	painting	1
crawl	through . . . passages	3
*twisted up		5
did	in the France of . . .	7
*handed down	to us	9
*clamber down	into the . . . depths	11
*opened up	the world's grottos	12–13
*lit up	by electricity	14
*set off	to best advantage	15
*sealed off		18
lies	under our feet	20
plunges	along with the river Arize into a huge cavern	22
*wind together	through tortuous limestone	23
ascends	with a guide	25
are	on display	27
is accustomed	to hearing of railways	28
used	in coal-mining	28
operates	inside the . . . Cavern	30
*rattles down	into the bowels of the earth	31

Verbs and *phrasal verbs	Prepositional phrases, etc.	Line
are covered	with a mass	33–34
drawn	over 18,000 years ago	34
set	at all angles	36
*came up	out of the Ollivier Cave	42–43
living	– separately – down in the depths	43–44
*carrying out	an experiment	44
wanted	to experience	45
*went down	into the Samar Cave	48
*cut (himself) off	from the surface	48–49
*stayed on	for another three months	51
*coming up (verb repeated)	to the light of day	52
had	with him in the cave	53
adapted	(surprisingly well) to those … conditions	54–55
suffered	(badly) from flies	55
did	(well) in the cold, *etc*	55–56
living	off the fresh fruit, *etc*	56
*taken down	with him	57
benefited	(greatly) from the processes of their decay	58–59
can live	in such conditions	60–61
confirmed	(in particular) that …	62
proceeds	(independently) at its own speed	65
was	(in fact) the case	67
removed	from caves	70
do not look	towards the stars	74
living	in tents, *etc*	76
combined	with utter darkness	78

4 Nil

3.3
a. If people travelled in outer space, they would need to …
b. If you really want to learn parachuting, you will take …
c. If one wanted to save money on skiing holidays, the best thing to do would be …
d. If X was/were equal to Y, then Y would also be equal to Z, because X equalled Z.
e. You will watch the soccer game every Saturday if you are as enthusiastic as he is.
f. If you did not feel at home in deep water, you would not want …
g. If you did not manage all the work satisfactorily the first time, you could always do it again.
h. If a person lived …, his or her body rhythms would change.

i.   If you call a person a cat or a cabbage, no literal identification is intended.
j.   If you wanted to communicate with someone, you could always find a way of doing so.
k.   Providing/Provided (that) OR Assuming (that) ...
l.   Supposing (that) ...
m. If that is the case/That being the case/If that is so/That being so ...
n.   If/When we consider ...
o.   In the event of ...
p.   If/When one considers ... OR/Taking into account/consideration ...
q.   6 If weather permits/Weather permitting OR If all goes well/All going well ...
r.   1 If ... OR
     5 Providing/Provided (that OR Assuming (that) ...
s.   **Same as m**
t.   2 If ... OR 5 Providing/Provided (that) OR Assuming (that) ...
u.   7 If there is/In the event of ...
v.   6 If all goes well/All going well ... OR If God wills/God willing ...
w.   1 ...if...OR 8 ... on condition (that) ...
x.   4 Taking into account/consideration ...
y.   3 If/When you/we consider OR one considers ... Considering ...
z.   2 If ... OR 5 Supposing ...

3.4   Compound work: First stage

a. an armchair
b. a two-hour delay
c. cathedral services
d. a London business report
e. a 15-foot brick wall
f. a New York telephone number
g. a Singapore publishing company
h. a Florida tourist centre manager
i. an 8-foot-square steel box
j. a Birmingham car factory strike

Compound work: Second stage

a. a team that engages in exploration
b. a line made of nylon
c. the cave near Mas d'Azil or at Mas d'Azil
d. the ripcord of a parachute OR the cord that serves to rip a parachute open
e. barriers relating to age
f. a pile that is 15 feet high
g. the level of the ground
h. a river that runs underground OR a river that is under the ground
i. artists who work/worked in caves/a cave
j. an explorer of caves who lives in OR comes from Nice and is 25 years old
k. a competition relating to football in a university (**Note also** football = a game played with a ball and the feet)
l. a hospital named after Queen Victoria
m. an accident on or related to a board from which swimmers dive OR a board for diving (from)
n. members of a ski patrol OR a patrol that uses skis
o. a post that is made of steel and is 25 feet high
p. the editor of a dictionary published by Oxford University Press OR someone who edits/has edited a ...
q. the director of a program related to the English language in the United States OR organized (etc) by the United States (government)
r. rites relating to (someone's) initiation at puberty
s. problems relating to the pollution of rivers and lakes
t. an operation for clearing snow

3.5   Derivational practice: First stage

(The analysis is done by separating the elements with slashes (/), and *italicizing* the bases.)

a. *Mexico*/an
b. pro/*China*/ese
c. un/*nature*/al (*nat* is the historical root)
d. *nation*/al/ist/ic (*nat* is the historical root)

e. super/*tribe*/al
f. un/control/able (*trol* is the historical root)
g. *read*/er/ship
h. *time*/less/ness
i. re/*develop*/ment (*velop* is the historical root)
j. down/*hill*
k. *inspect*/or (*spect* is the root)
l. *compete*/(it)ive/ness (*pet* is the root)
m. *milit*/ary (*milit* = soldier)
n. pre/*techn*/o/*logy*/ic/al (*techn* = art, craft)
o. tele/*vis*/ion (*vis* = seeing, sight)
p. mis/*concept*/ion (*cept* is the root)
q. *organ*/ize/(at)ion/al
r. en/*erg*/(et)ic/al/ly (*erg* = work)
s. dis/satisfy/(at)ion (*satis* is the root)
t. total/ity/ari/an/ism (*tot* is the root)

Note that it is usually possible to trace the original meaning of the root, and that it is sometimes possible to see a relationship between that root meaning and the modern use of a word. Thus, the root of *nature* and *nation* is *nat*, which in Latin signifies 'birth; being born'. Though interesting, this knowledge is not directly useful in everyday English, whereas the knowledge that *milit* means a 'soldier' will be useful when one meets, say, *militant* and *demilitarize*.

Derivational practice: Second stage

1e	3g	5i	7b	9f
2h	4c	6j	8a	10d

Derivational practice: Third stage

a. disagreed
b. re-advertising
c. pro-American; anti-British
d. overworks
e. misgovernment
f. non-scientific
g. pre-war; post-war
h. underusing
i. superstructure
j. illogical
k. unaffected
l. sub-standard

3.6   Punctuation work: First stage
Nil

Punctuation work: Second stage

The large underground caves called 'caverns' are usually found in limestock rock. Water from streams or from rainfall passes slowly through cracks in the layers of limestone. As this water, with carbon dioxide dissolved in it, trickles through the cracks, it dissolves and carries away small amounts of the limestone so that over thousands of years the cracks slowly widen into caves.

Subterranean caves may become large enough for people to go into, and some become as big as cathedrals, with side-passages and 'chapels' and even such extra marvels as underground rivers, waterfalls and lakes. Sometimes, if a cave is not far from the surface, its roof may weaken and fall in. The surface hole left by this cave-in is called a 'sink-hole' or 'sink'. Water often collects in these sink-holes, forming 'sink-hole ponds' or 'lakes'.

Limestone caverns often have slim icicle-like stalactites hanging from their ceilings, while on the ground underneath them stalagmites form as the lime-laden water drips from the ends of the 'icicles'. One can remember which of these strange terms is which by associating the 'c' of *stalactite* with the cave's 'ceiling', while the 'g' of *stalagmite* reminds us of the 'ground'. Over long periods of time, the stalactites reach down and the stalagmites reach up until they join each other in beautiful pillars.

The largest underground chamber in the world is said to be in the Carlsbad Caverns, New Mexico, in the United States of America; the most extensive cave system is probably Mammoth Cave, Kentucky, also in the U.S.A.; and the deepest caves are found in the Pyrenees, the range of mountains between France and Spain. In Britain, the largest-known caves are in South Wales, while two of the best-known caverns are Gaping Ghyll in Yorkshire, and Wookey Hole in Somerset, both in England.

3.7   Nil

3.8   'The Story of Lascaux'

Pre-eminent among the sights and tales of French caverns is Lascaux, set in a hill above the town of Montignac-sur-Vézère. The caves were discovered in 1940 by a local 18-year-old boy, who followed his dog into a hole beneath the roots of a tree that had been torn down in a storm. With two companions, this young man, Marcel Ravidat, discovered – in the light of their lanterns – vivid red, yellow and black paintings of massive animals that no longer walk the earth. Since then, many books have been written on the mysterious artists who decorated the caves, and countless visitors have entered the caverns to view these age-old masterpieces.

Disaster, however, struck in 1961.

After a particularly successful year for tourists, it was observed that a bright green OR bright-green moss was spreading over the cave walls towards the priceless paintings. By 1963, according to M. Leo Magne, the regional tourist board president, the moss had advanced more in the previous three months than in all the three preceding years, and the progress was almost visible.

The caves were closed to the public. A commission of artists, scientists and historians was sent from Paris to study the phenomenon. Wearing masks and using air-locks, like moon-explorers, the investigators studied the fast-moving moss, seeking to learn what it was, where it came from, and how to stop it. Why, after 20,000 years of tranquillity, had this strange moss only begun to wander now?

The answer was simple. The moss is the work of modern man. In all damp caves with openings to the outside world there exists a species of microscopic moss which grows larger where there is light. Under normal conditions, it resembles slime. The introduction of outside air, however, then electric light and heat, and finally the carbon dioxide breathed out by a thousand visitors a day had so encouraged this moss to grow that it (had) swept across the walls like a tide.

The closing of the caves meant economic hardship for the people of Montignac village. After their classic year of 1962, the shopkeepers had laid in large stores of photographic slides, postcards and souvenirs, while also investing in a new road to the site. The caves, however, have remained sealed off, until some adequate solution is found to the problem of protecting the ancient pictures, which have – for the time being – OR pictures which have, for the time being, returned to their equally ancient darkness.

3.9   Nil

UNIT 4

4.1 a. F: The lecturer is talking about us, not our ancestors.
  b. T
  c. T
  d. T
  e. F: They were employed to go in front of the cars, as a warning.
  f. T
  g. T
  h. F: Henry Ford did not say this.
  i. F: There is no indication that they had any effect at all on tourism.
  j. T
  k. any two of lines 3, 10–11, 13–14, 19
  l. any four of lines 2, 6–7, 8, 11, 14–17, 21, 58, 63, 69
  m. any three of lines 15–17, 25, 33, 41, 47, 58, 63
  n. any of the hyphenated words on lines 24, 27, 28, 56, 59
  o. any two of lines 41, 58, 69
  p. lines 23–24
  q. line 69
  r. lines 1–2, 5, 10, 13, 79, 81
  s. lines 1–2, 11, 67, 81

4.2 1 necessary
        necessity
        need
        needless
        needy

  2 receive   recipe
     receiver   reckless
     receptacle   reckoning
     reception   re-cycle
     receptive   reservoir

  3 syllabic   symbolism   sympathy
     syllable   symmetrical   synchronize
     syllogism   symmetry   syntax
     syllogistic sympathetic   synthesis
     symbolic   sympathize   synthetic

  4 sadden   satisfactory   Saturn
     satanic   satisfy   saturnine
     satellite   saturate   satyr
     satirical   saturation   savagery
     satirize   Saturday   say

  5 meadow   mediator   mensuration
     means   medical   mental
     measles   medicare   mentalism
     measurable   medication   mentality
     measure   medicinal   mercantile
     medal   medicine   mercurial
     meddle   meditate   mercury
     median   meditation   mermaid
     mediate   meditative   metal
     mediation   mellow   metallic

  6 automatic   mechanical   nature
     automobile   mechanism   petrify
     carbolic   mechanized   petro-chemical
     carbon   microbe   petroleum
     carburettor micro-organism polite
     colleague   microphone   political
     collective   microscope   politician
     collision   millilitre   politics
     decision   millimetre   reality
     destination million   realization
     destiny   millipede   realize
     governable   nationalist   really
     government   nationality   succeed
     governor   native   success
     machine   naturally   successful

4.3 (1) that   (11) tankful
       (2) forceful   (12) using up
       (3) When   (13) cubic
       (4) gulping down   (14) compound
       (5) as   (15) that
       (6) pouring out   (16) what
       (7) which/that   (17) although
       (8) as   (18) breathing out
       (9) poisons   (19) identical
       (10) as   (20) greatly

4.4

(1) the		(11) a	
(2) a		(12) the	
(3) ×		(13) the	
(4) ×		(14) the	
(5) the		(15) the	
(6) the/a		(16) The	
(7) the		(17) ×	
(8) the		(18) ×	
(9) a		(19) a	
(10) the		(20) the	

4.5   The logical order is: C, H, A, F, I, G, B, E, D

The punctuated passage is:

Slowly scientists became concerned about the tremendous quantities of gas, particularly carbon dioxide, released into the atmosphere through the on-going large-scale burning of fossil fuels. There was at least ten percent more carbon dioxide in the air by 1980 than there had been when the century started. Because it was being produced faster than it could be absorbed by the ocean or converted back into carbon and oxygen by plants, the carbon dioxide began to accumulate. While doing so, it produced what is called a 'greenhouse effect' in the planet's atmosphere. This allowed sunlight to come in, but effectively blocked the heat generated on Earth by the sun's rays from escaping back into space.

The inevitable result of such a blockage was an increase in temperatures all over the world. These world-wide temperature changes equally inevitably set in motion a final unthinkable change: the steady melting of the great polar ice caps. This not only raised the ocean levels more than ten feet, but also effectively solved the traffic problems of the world's great coastal cities by flooding them out completely.

In a single century, humankind had almost casually altered both air and ocean more than had happened in millions of years of geological time.

4.6   In the summer of 1940, while a group of boys were playing near the village of Montignac, in France, their dog got lost. One of them found it in a hole under a tree, a hole that was in fact the entrance to a cave. This cave is now called the Lascaux Cave. Its main hall measures 100 feet by 30 feet, and is filled with remarkable paintings of ancient animals, most of them outlined in black, but some in dotted patterns and others coloured red or brown. The animals seem almost alive; they have true-to-life shapes, and there is a very realistic scene depicting a bison wounded with a spear.

Lascaux is not, however, the only cave in Western Europe with such paintings in it. There are more than 120 caves in France, Spain and Italy with paintings in them. The painted caves of Europe are very interesting, but they are not unique, because paintings of ancient mammoths and cave bears have been found in the Kapova Cave in the Ural Mountains of Russia, and other caves in Australia contain paintings done by present-day aborigines, their style similar to the style of the ancient cave artists of Lascaux.

Note this is only one possible version of the material. Many are possible. Here, for example, is quite a different approach to the same subject:

In the summer of 1940, a group of boys were playing near the village of Montignac, in France, when their dog got lost. One of them found it in a hole under a tree, a hole that was in fact the entrance to what is now called the Lascaux Cave, whose main hall measures 100 by 30 square feet. It is filled with remarkable paintings of ancient animals, most of which are outlined in black, although some have dotted patterns and others are coloured red or brown. The animals seem almost alive, with true-to-life shapes; there is a very realistic scene depicting a bison wounded with a spear. Lascaux is not, however, the only cave in Western Europe with such paintings in it, for there are more than 120 such caves in France, Spain and Italy. The painted caves of

Europe are very interesting, but they are not unique: paintings of ancient mammoths and cave bears have been found in the Kapova Cave in the Ural Mountains of Russia, while other caves in Australia contain paintings done by present-day aborigines. The style of these paintings is similar to the style of the ancient cave artists of Lascaux.

4.7
a. Norwegian
b. Welsh
c. Iraqi
d. Peruvian
e. Dane
f. Turkish
g. Portuguese
h. Dutch
i. Hungarian
j. Swedish
k. Sudanese
l. Britons
m. Canadian
n. Egyptian
o. Finnish
p. Syrian
q. Yugoslav
r. Brazilian
s. Mexican
t. Pakistani

4.8
1 **As given**

2 pollute
polluted
pollutant
anti-pollution
etc

3 industry
industrial
industrialize
industrialization
re-industrialize
industrialist
industrious
industrially
industriously
etc

4 economy
economic
economical
economically
economist
economize
etc

5 reason
reasonable
unreasonable
reasonably
unreasonably
rational
irrational
(ir)rationally
rationalism
rationalist
rationalistic
rationalistically
reasoning
unreasoning
well-reasoned
etc

6 develop
development
developmental
re-develop
under-developed
over-developed
under-development
over-development
developing
fast-developing
etc

7 nation
national
non-national
anti-national
nationally
nationalism
nationalist
nationalistic
nationalistically
nationalize
nationalization
etc

8 resource
resourceful
resourcefully
unresourceful(ly)
resourceless
etc

9 aware
awareness
unaware(ness)
self-aware
self-awareness
etc

10 waste
wasted
unwasted
wasteful
wastefully
unwasteful(ly)
anti-waste
etc

11 material
materialism
materialist
materialistic
materialistically
non-material
immaterial
materially
materialize
materialization
etc

12 chemical
chemically
chemist
chemistry
etc

13 social
socially
anti-social(ly)
society
societal(ly)
sociable
unsociable
(un)sociably
socialism
socialist
etc

14 politics
political
politically
non-political(ly)
politic
impolitic
politician
etc

15 legal
legally
illegal(ly)
legality
illegality
legalism
legalistic(ally)
legislate
legislation
legislator
etc

4.9   a. scientists; evolution
b. distributors; commercial; transactions
c. inscription; apparently; reference
d. professor; students; re-write
e. industrialist; concessions; competitors
f. natural; assumption; completion; entirely; financial
g. Regrettably (*perhaps also* Regretfully); presidential; decision
h. intentional; concealment; information; resentment
i. declaration; beautified; tourist; attraction
j. appalling; (mis)management; faithful; employees

4.10   Nil

UNIT 5

5.1   Nil (Check the passage)

5.2   Nil (Check the passage)

5.3   1   Astronomers (line 3)
kilometres (l. 20)
astronomical (l. 35)
geocentric (l. 38)
heliocentric (l. 39)
atmosphere (l. 54)
geologists (l. 60)
biosphere (l. 98)
stratosphere (l. 105)

2   **Compounds in order:**
1   life-giver (line 3)
2   yellow dwarf (l. 4)
3   light-years (l. 8)
4   solar system (l. 15)
5   Western-style (l. 25)
6   sense impressions (l. 28)
7   20th-century (l. 45)
8   everyday (l. 47)
9   sunrises (l. 47)

10   sunsets (l. 47)
11   Flat-Earthists (l. 50)
12   home planet (l. 51)
13   earthquakes (l. 60)
14   salt water (ll. 66–7)
15   oh-so-solid (l. 67)
16   northeast (l. 68)
17   Great Lakes (l. 68)
18   North America (l. 68)
19   sea animals (l. 71)
20   time scale (l. 76)
21   onion-like (l. 77)
22   planet-spaceship (l. 89)
23   earthship (l. 94)
24   planet Earth (l. 99)
25   mankind (l. 102)
26   maximum altitude (l. 104)
27   air-borne (l. 105)
28   omnibus edition (l. 117)
29   Mother Earth (l. 119)
30   Oxford University Press (ll. 119–20)

These compounds could be classified according to how they look on the page, as follows:

hyphenated
1   life-giver
2   light-years
3   Western-style
4   20th-century
5   Flat-Earthists
6   oh-so-solid
7   onion-like
8   planet-spaceship
9   air-borne

solid
1   everyday
2   sunrises
3   sunsets
4   earthquakes
5   northeast
6   earthship
7   mankind

separate
1   yellow dwarf
2   solar system
3   sense impression
4   home planet

5 salt water
6 Great Lakes
7 North America
8 sea animals
9 time scale
10 planet Earth
11 maximum altitude
12 omnibus edition
13 Mother Earth
14 Oxford University Press

The compounds could also be classified according to the parts of speech from which they are constructed:

noun + noun
(*all making nouns*)
1 life-giver
2 light-years
3 planet-spaceship
4 northeast
5 earthship
6 mankind
7 sense impressions
8 home planet
9 salt water
10 sea animals
11 time scale
12 planet Earth
13 maximum altitude
14 omnibus edition
15 Mother Earth
16 Oxford University Press
17 sunrises ⎫
18 sunsets ⎬ also interpretable as
19 earthquakes ⎭ **noun + verb**

noun + adjective
(*making adjectives*)
1 onion-like
2 air-borne

adjective + noun
(*making adjectives*)
1 Western-style
2 20th-century
3 everyday
(*making nouns*)
4 Flat-Earthists
5 yellow dwarf
6 solar system
7 Great Lakes
8 North America

These are by no means the only ways of classifying compounds. We could also have a complex and interesting analysis of the relationships between elements (for example, *salt water* paraphrased as 'water that has salt in it', and so on). Additionally, we could look for persons such as *life-giver* and *Flat-Earthists*; specially derived forms, such as *life-giver* from the verb 'give' plus a suffix; specially coined forms in the passage alone, such as *Flat-Earthist* or the odd *oh-so-solid*, which stands very much alone; and so on.

3 **Phrasal verbs in order, with comments;**
1 point out (l. 4) – *out* suggests an extended finger, figuratively suggesting 'indicating fully or clearly'
2 make up (ll. 12 and 78) – *up* suggesting 'fully'
3 spread out (l. 30) – *out* meaning 'in all directions'
4 move upwards (ll. 79–80) – *upwards*, simple direction
5 cool down (l. 80) – *down*, meaning 'completely, so as to become (in this instance) cooler'
6 settle down (l. 81) – *down*, meaning 'completely, so as to become (in this instance) lower in position'

4 **Suffixes in order:**
i *-al*
liter*al*ly (l. 2)
anim*al*s (l. 71)
natur*al* (l. 72)
materi*al*s (ll. 79, 81)
anim*al*cules (l. 90)
terrestri*al* (l. 103)

ii *-ar*
particul*ar*ly (l. 1)
sol*ar* (l. 15)
Note that *-ar* tends to take the place of *-al* after bases with an 'l' in them: *lunar*, *polar*, *tabular*, etc

iii *-ic*
partic*ic*ularly (l. 1)
cosm*ic* (ll. 6, 24, 29, 88)
geocentr*ic* (l. 38)
heliocentr*ic* (l. 39)

scientif*ic* (ll. 46, 59)
concentr*ic* (l. 53)
dramat*ic* (l. 65)
Americ*a* (l. 68)
parasit*ic* (l. 92)

iv   *-ical*
astronom*ical* (l. 35)
pract*ical* (ll. 37, 47, 53)
scientif*ically* (l. 37)
phys*ical* (l. 62)
paradox*ical* (l. 87)
fantast*ically* (l. 103)

5   **Nil**

5.4   a.   Astronomers tell us that the star
Capella ...
b.   Most of us are not aware that the star
Antares ...
c.   Nowadays, we know that the universe is
made up ...
d.   Most people appreciate that earthquakes
and floods ...
e.   The dramatic appearance ... off Iceland
reminds us that many of today's
mountains ...
f.   Figuratively, we can say that the earth is
like ...
g.   Holes bored in its ... are proof that the
temple was ... (OR '... in the temple's
columns ... prove that it was ...')
h.   Slow changes in the earth's land masses
suggest that on its own vast time scale ...
i.   A recent geological theory proposes that
there are ...
j.   Some scientists maintain that heat deep
inside ...
k.   Astronomers tell us that the earth is like
a spaceship travelling round the sun, and
also that it does so at great speed
(**comma optional**).
l.   Some geologists maintain that there are
slow currents in the dense material under
the earth's crust and that heat deep
inside the earth ...
m.   Experimenters have confirmed that after
a few days in a cave a person ... time,
and that our body clocks ...
n.   It would appear to be true that people

can live in ... periods, and that this
experience ...
o.   Astronomers are aware that the star
Capella is ... sun, that Antares is 300
times bigger, and that the larger
'supergiants' are 3,000 times bigger.
p.   Astronomical evidence forces us to
accept that the universe ... empty space,
but also that the empty space is
predominant.

5.5   **Sentence synthesis:**

The thin outer covering of the earth on
which we live is called the crust. It does not
seem particularly thin to us, having a
thickness varying from three miles under the
sea to forty miles under the continents. This
seems reassuringly thick. Our deepest mines
go down about two miles, while our deepest
oil wells go down about five miles; therefore,
we have not yet been able to drill right
through the crust. Despite this, however, we
must accept that the crust is very thin when
compared with the thickness of the planet
itself, the distance from the surface to the
centre of the earth being very nearly 4,000
miles. Under the crust is a layer of heavy
rock called the mantle, which goes down
nearly 1,800 miles into the earth. The crust
together with the upper part of the mantle
forms what we call the lithosphere. This
rigid structure overlies the more plastic
lower mantle which is known as the
asthenosphere, on which the lithosphere
drifts. The mantle in turn surrounds the
earth's core, which is divided into inner and
outer layers. The rocks of the lower mantle
or asthenosphere are probably white-hot
where they meet the outer core. This is
apparently a molten or fluid mass of nickel
and iron which is very hot indeed, being in
the region of 2,500°C (4,600°F), while the
inner core of course is even hotter still
(removing the commas around 'of course' is
optional). This central kernel of the earth,
formed of the same substances, seems to be
squeezed solid, under such enormous
pressures that the atoms of nickel and iron
are packed together incredibly densely.

5.6 1 Logical order: E, A, C, F, D, B

2 Logical order: D, H, C, E, F, G, B, A

Soils are parts of the earth's crust in which plants can root themselves. They are made of weathered rocks and decaying animal and plant matter, and differ in depth, colour and mineral content. Whatever the soil, its uppermost layer is called 'topsoil', containing animal and plant remains in various stages of decomposition. These remains are known as 'humus'. Underneath is the 'subsoil', usually lighter in colour and reddish or brownish because of the minerals washed into it from above. It is harder for plants to grow in subsoil than topsoil, due to lack of humus. Underneath the subsoil comes the 'weathered bedrock', its colours determined by the basic rock structure of the area. Climate is also an important factor in determining what kind of soil develops in any particular part of the earth.

Note: quotation marks for technical terms not essential.

5.7 **Word formation: First stage**

1i; 2e; 3a; 4h; 5b; 6c; 7j; 8d; 9g; 10f

Word formation: Second stage

1 literally (line 2)
2 perspective (l. 12)
3 credible (l. 17)
4 appreciating (l. 18)
5 appreciation (l. 46)
6 contradict (l. 35)
7 predictable (l. 62)
8 predominates (l. 14)
9 rejected (ll. 37 and 40)
10 centuries (l. 38)
11 terrestrial (l. 103)
12 fragile (l. 111)

Word formation: Third stage

1 cosmic (l. 6, etc)
2 kilometre (ll. 19 and 20)
3 astronomers (l. 11, etc)
4 astronomical (l. 35)

5 geocentric (l. 38)
6 geologists (l. 60)
7 heliocentric (l. 39)
8 physical (l. 62)
9 biosphere (l. 98)
10 paradoxical (l. 87)

Word formation: Fourth stage

a. astr/o/nom/y – astr/o/nom/er – astr/o/nom/ic/al
b. ge/o/log/y – ge/o/centr/ic – ge/o/metr/ic/al
c. heli/o/centr/ic
d. atm/o/sphere – bi/o/sphere – lith/o/sphere – strat/o/sphere
e. agr/i/cult/ure – vin/i/cult/ure – hort/i/cult/ur/al
f. aqu/i/fer – somn/i/fer/ous – quadr/i/later/al – un/i/later/al

Word formation: Fifth stage

a. carries water
b. cultivation of gardens
c. knows everything
d. made/done by art OR craftsmanship, etc
e. many sides (to it)
f. total power
g. art/craftsmanship to make things
h. cultivating of vines; wine
i. everywhere
j. sides; three sides

Word formation: Sixth stage

a. descriptions of the earth
b. studies the heart
c. distribution of people
d. writing; light
e. heal the mind
f. study of animals/living creatures
g. writes; life
h. globe/sphere of light
i. description
j. laws; stars/study; stars

5.8 **Nil (Check the passage)**

5.9 **Nil**

UNIT 6

6.1   Nil (Check the passage)

6.2
a.   murder (line 1)
b.   fancy (l. 2)
c.   classify (l. 3)
d.   genocide (l. 4)
e.   comparable (l. 6)
f.   compulsive (l. 7)
g.   restricted (l. 10)
h.   significant (l. 13)
i.   highlight (l. 15)
j.   emancipation (l. 21)
k.   superficial (l. 22)
l.   rivalry (l. 23)
m.   resolutely (l. 29)
n.   paramount (l. 30)
o.   foredoomed (l. 39)
p.   farrago (l. 47)
q.   bestowed (l. 51)
r.   one-track (l. 54)
s.   mercenary (l. 58)
t.   excesses (l. 61)
u.   suicide (l. 63)
v.   abolition (l. 67)
w.   amendment (l. 68)
x.   even-handed (l. 78)
y.   fanning (l. 82)
z.   reactionaries (l. 91)

6.3   The assassination of Gandhi

After a lifetime devoted to human brotherhood, non-violence and national freedom, Mohandas K Gandhi was heart-broken by the Partition of British India into the new states of India and Pakistan. The bloodshed, on his own testimony, set at naught all the good work of forty years, and he sought, by walking in the strife-torn areas and by fasting, to allay the communal violence and hatred.

On Friday, 30th January 1948, at about 5.10 pm, he appeared for a prayer meeting in Delhi, leaning on the shoulders of two girls, joking with them about carrot juice and punctuality. Nathuram V Godse shot him dead at a range of two feet. He murmured 'Hai Ram' (Oh God!), his feet slipped from his sandals, and the Father of India was dead.

Godse belonged to a group which considered Gandhi an impediment to Hindu control over India, blaming him for giving way to the Moslems. Partition, however, had actually occurred, with streams of refugees moving in both directions, and what Gandhi wanted now was non-violence and good-will in this shifting of populations, so that people would be able to stay in their traditional homes.

A bomb attempt had been made on his life ten days earlier at another public meeting. He had minimized the explosion, saying: 'Don't worry about that. Listen to me.' His later comment when the assailant was caught is interesting. In Sheean's words: 'No one should believe that he was so perfect that he was sent by God to punish the evil-doers, as the accused seemed to flatter himself he was.'

What did religious fanaticism claim – apart from the modern crucifixion of a great humane figure? It removed from the scene the one man who held Moslem and Hindu together. It removed a symbol of unity that was accepted by both Pakistan and India, and still India became the secular state, without the domination of any one religious group, that Godse and his friends did not want.

6.4
a.   The slaves were emancipated by Abraham Lincoln.
b.   The President was shot by Wilkes Booth.
c.   Booth was motivated by racial feeling.
d.   Czar Alexander II was killed by a Polish student.
e.   The student was provoked by nationalism into killing the Czar. OR The student was provoked into killing the Czar by nationalism.

f. Many problems were created by Lincoln's premature death.

g. The term 'assassination' has been restricted by the writer.

h. The South was crushed by the sheer weight of Northern industry, manpower and naval strength.

i. The slaves were emancipated in the 1860s.

j. Eichmann's crime is classified as genocide.

k. Lincoln was assassinated in 1865.

l. Crippen's crime is referred to as homicide.

m. Alexander II of Russia was killed in 1881.

n. Cromwell's involvement in the execution of Charles I is referred to as regicide.

o. The term 'assassination' has been restricted to the murder of a major world figure.

p. Its strength was industry-based.

q. The strife-torn areas caused Gandhi great grief.

r. Most of these war-damaged factories were not re-built.

s. It is a government-financed project.

t. He loved skiing among the snow-covered mountains.

u. They all saw the blood-stained clothes afterwards.

v. Under the earth's crust is a layer of heavy rock called the mantle.

w. The army was destroyed, annihilated as much by climate and disease as by the country's defenders.

x. The Emperor of Mexico died an unhappy man, totally rejected by the people he had come so far to rule.

y. The attempt at assassination failed, betrayed by the inefficiency of the terrorist group itself.

z. The South surrendered in 1865, crushed by the industrial strength and superior manpower of the North.

6.5

a. to $\rightarrow$; of $\rightarrow$
b. to $\rightarrow$
c. by $\rightarrow$; of $\rightarrow$
d. for $\rightarrow$
e. over $\leftarrow$
f. under $\rightarrow$; of $\rightarrow$
g. of $\rightarrow$; in $\rightarrow$
h. against $\rightarrow$
i. in $\leftarrow$
j. in $\rightarrow$
k. off $\leftarrow$
l. out $\leftarrow$; through $\rightarrow$
m. for $\rightarrow$; up $\leftarrow$
n. of $\rightarrow$; up $\leftarrow$

6.6 Kennedy's assassin

Lee Harvey Oswald returned to the U.S. from the Soviet Union in 1962, at the age of 23. In the words of the *Warren Report*[1]: 'His return to the United States publicly testified to the utter failure of what had been the most important act of his life.' He brought back with him a living witness to this failure – his Russian wife Marina. His adopted country, Russia, had proved to be unsatisfactory for him, and he returned to a land he had openly rejected. As a child he had never known his father, who had died two months before his birth, but had known all too well a bitterly neurotic mother. His wife accused him in front of friends of being sexually inadequate. Again quoting the *Warren Report* (p. 376), he 'was profoundly alienated from the world in which he lived,' and, as his wife admitted, would not have been happy anywhere, 'only on the moon perhaps.'

On Friday, 22nd November 1963, he shot John Kennedy, President of the United States. The killing took place in the South, in the state of Texas, occurring during a period of intense racial disturbance. Oswald was a self-styled Marxist, and yet Europeans thought immediately of a right-wing plot rather than a Communist one. Rumour had a field day. Meanwhile, what mattered most was that a champion of the 'strategy of peace' had been shot from behind, his skull torn away before the gaze of his wife.

Whatever Oswald resented as a loner or as one of many Kennedy-haters, he damaged his own cause severely. J.F.K's period at the White House had been marked by unprecedented difficulty in getting any reform measures past Congress. Delay and obstruction attended his civil rights bill, and overseas aid on the scale he proposed was resented. After the killing, however, Lyndon B. Johnson[2] was able to get all the Kennedy programme through on the strength of the nation's horror, regret and determination to honour a martyred hero. No murder in history has created such widespread and spontaneous distress as this one, in part due to modern means of communication and in part to the dynamic and attractive image of the victim. Like earlier assassinations, Oswald's act had effects quite the contrary to those intended, and this is the great irony of murder as a political weapon. It is clear that assassins regard themselves as fearless champions of just causes, but have seldom – if ever – done their causes any good.

Notes

1 *the Warren Report*: the official U.S. report on President Kennedy's death

2 *Lyndon B. Johnson*: Kennedy's vice-president and successor

6.7 Word formation: First stage

a. suicide
b. homicide
c. homicidal
d. regicide
e. suicidal
f. genocide
g. suicidally
h. infanticide
i. fratricidal
j. genocide

Word formation: Second stage

1i; 2h; 3a; 4j; 5b; 6c; 7f; 8d; 9e; 10g

Word formation: Third stage

1h; 2d; 3g; 4i; 5b; 6c; 7a; 8f; 9j; 10e

Word formation: Fourth stage

1 political
2 pacifist
3 visionary
4 originally
5 individuals
6 rulers
7 co-operative
8 idealistic
9 Communism, com-
10 Action
11 symbolized
12 violent
13 attempt
14 president
15 natural
16 evolution
17 eruption
18 number
19 explosion
20 professed
21 incident
22 produced
23 generally
24 capitalist
25 destructive

6.8 'The Hashishin'

A schoolfellow of Omar Khayyam[1] was responsible for the meteoric rise of the strange mediaeval Persian Sect of the Assassins. Their headquarters was the valley of Alamut, a remote area of mountains and fortresses south of the Caspian Sea and west of what is now Teheran, (the) capital of the modern state of Iran. From the reports of the Crusaders[2] and the traveller Marco Polo[3], we learn that the sect practised political and religious murder on a scale that has perhaps never been equalled in history, except possibly by the secret society of the Thugs[4] in India.

They called themselves Nizaris or Ismailis, but their enemies gave them the nickname 'Hashishin', that is, users of the drug hashish.[5]

The founder of this order was Hasan-e-Sabbah. He saw himself as the representative of God on Earth, and was known and feared throughout Western Asia as 'The Old Man of the Mountain'. He commanded such devotion among his 10,000 men that sentinels would willingly throw themselves off the battlements of his castle into the abyss below at one wave of his hand, in order to intimidate visiting ambassadors.

Hasan had recognized a simple political fact of his time. Thrones and premierships were insecure because they no longer rested on popular support or tribal loyalty. A dedicated band of men could be relied on – with bribed help where necessary – to kill political leaders at Hasan's command, and even kill themselves with the same knives in order not to reveal his/their secrets under torture. His men oiled themselves to make gripping their bodies more difficult, addressed God before plunging their knives into their victims, and believed implicitly that their actions would take them straight to Paradise.

They believed this because they thought that they had already seen Paradise. It is said that in Alamut Hasan kept a garden which in all respects resembled the delights of heaven as described in the Koran OR of the heaven described in the Koran. Into this place young men drugged with hashish would be led to receive a foretaste of the Paradise to which future obedient service would entitle them.

In this way, Hasan created the world's first commando unit, and established a dynasty that ruled with terror throughout Western Asia for two centuries until it fell OR until its fall before the advance of the Mongol, Hulagu Khan[6].

In this strange way, the Old Man of the Mountain left his mark on the world, adding a new word to its languages – assassination.

Notes

1 *Omar Khayyam* (1048(?)–1122): Persian poet, astronomer and mathematician, author of the *Rubaiyat* (translated into English in 1859 by Edward Fitzgerald)

2 *Crusaders*: members of the Christian armies engaged in the religious warfare known as the *Crusades* (or 'Wars of the Cross') against Islam, for the possession of Jerusalem and the Holy Land of Palestine, between the 11th and 13th centuries

3 *Marco Polo* (c. 1254–1324) Venetian merchant and adventurer who travelled from Europe across Asia to China, writing an account of his journey that is known in English as *The Travels of Marco Polo*

4 *Thugs*: an organization of religious assassins who secretly killed unwary travellers in the name of the goddess Kali over a period of 300 years until they were broken up between 1831 and 1837 by the British governor-general of India, William Bentinck

5 *hashish*: (literally, in Arabic, 'dried root') the name of various narcotic preparations derived from the hemp plant (*Cannabis sativa*)

6 *Hulagu Khan* (c. 1217–1275): the grandson of the Mongol ruler Genghis Khan, and destroyer of mediaeval Persian society. The fortress of Alamut fell to the Mongols in 1256.

UNIT 7

7.1   Nil

7.2   a. Kenneth Lo
b. The writer wants to highlight an unusual name.
c. Lo is being quoted without the writer directly saying so.
d. 1 Her use of 'way' to mean the *Tao* is being highlighted.
2 The second quotation is integrated into the grammatical structure of the sentence.
e. The capitalized words are presented as if they were the titles of books or of chapters in a book.

7.3   **The punctuation of a Style 1 bibliography:**

Bond, Jules J. *The Mexican Cuisine I Love.* Leon Amiel. 1977.
Brown, Dale. *American Cooking.* Time-Life. 1968.
Eckley Mary, *McCall's Superb Dessert Cookbook.* Random House/McCall's. 1961.
Hume, Rosemary and Muriel Downes. *The Penguin Dictionary of Cooking.* Penguin Books. 1966.
Leonard, Jonathan Norton. *Latin American Cooking.* Time-Life. 1968.
Macrae, Sheila. *The Scottish Cookbook.* Foulsham. 1979.

7.4   a. 2, 4, 1, 3, 5
b. 2, 3, 1, 5, 4
c. 4, 1, 5, 3, 2
d. 2, 3, 5, 1, 4
e. 1, 3, 2, 4, 5

7.5   Nil

For further reference

The following books are recommended for both students and teachers:

Oxford Advanced Learner's Dictionary of Current English
A S Hornby and A P Cowie

Acclaimed throughout the world as the indispensable reference book for those studying or teaching EFL, this dictionary is the most comprehensive one available and gives the learner invaluable help in producing and understanding correct and appropriate English. It contains 50,000 headwords and has 1,000 illustrations, including both photographs and line drawings. Definitions have been written within a carefully controlled defining vocabulary and are reinforced and illustrated by over 90,000 contemporary example sentences and phrases. The clear layout and careful design makes the information easy to find, easy to understand and easy to use.

Hardback: 431101 5
Delux edition: 431999 9
Paperback: 431106 6

Oxford Dictionary of Current Idiomatic English
A P Cowie, R Mackin and I R McCaig

The most comprehensive and detailed survey available of this important area of English, and an ideal complement to any general English dictionary. It records and describes over 15,000 English idioms in two volumes. Volume 1 covers 8000 expressions containing verbs with prepositions and particles; Volume 2 covers 7000 general idiomatic expressions. The entries are illustrated by a wide range of examples from up-to-date sources, including newspapers and television. There is a detailed index and cross-reference system.

Volume 1: Verbs with Prepositions and Particles: 431145 7
Volume 2: Phrase, Clause and Sentence Idioms: 431150 3

Practical English Usage
M Swan

Practical English Usage is a unique reference guide which explains all those areas of grammar and usage which regularly cause difficulty to EFL students and teachers. Over 600 clear, practical entries explain specific points of vocabulary, idiom, style, pronunciation and speech. It explains typical mistakes, and gives information about the differences between British and American English. The entries are alphabetically arranged with a detailed index and cross-reference system.

Hardback: 431336 0
Paperback: 431335 2

A Practical English Grammar
A J Thomson and A V Martinet

This is the most popular intermediate-level reference grammar for students and teachers of English. All the important areas of English are covered and the use of forms is illustrated by many thousands of modern example sentences. Points which students find particularly difficult, like tense forms and auxiliary verbs, are treated with especial care and fullness.

Hardback: 431336 0
Paperback: 431335 2

Idioms in Practice
J Seidl

Idioms in Practice helps students to use, as well as understand, over 800 of the most common English idioms, including phrasal verbs, known phrases, comparisons, proverbs and cliches. Each idiom is presented in a clear, lively and often amusing context. Its meaning is explained, and it is then practised and tested in a wide variety of different exercise types. Every student or teacher who has worked through this book will use idiomatic English with greater confidence as a result. The simple arrangement, brief instructions and answer key make it ideal for private study.

432769 8

The Oxford Dictionary for Writers and Editors
Compiled by the Oxford Dictionary Department

This authoritative dictionary is an indispensable aid to writers, editors, journalists, publishers, and all those concerned with the written word. It ensures an up-to-date and consistent style in material intended for publication and gives straightforward guidance on common spelling difficulties, the use of foreign words and phrases in English, names of people and places, abbreviations, and the use of capitals and punctuation. It also provides a guide to important terms in computer typesetting.

212970 8